Evidence–Based Practice

A primer for health care professionals

Martin Dawes MD FRCGP

Professor & Chair, Family Medicine, McGill University, Canada

Philip T. Davies BA(Hons)London MA(California) MLitt(Oxon) MA(Oxon) PhD(California)

Director of Policy Evaluation, Prime Minister's Strategy Unit

Alastair M. Gray BA DPhil

Professor of Health Economics, Health Economics Research Centre, Department of Public Health, University of Oxford, UK

Jonathan Mant MA MBBS MSc FFPH

Senior Lecturer, Department of Primary Care and General Practice, University of Birmingham, UK

Kate Seers BSc(Hons) PhD RGN

Head of Research, RCN Institute, Oxford, UK

Robin Snowball BA(Hons) RMN PhD DipLibInfStud PGCE(Post-Compulsory)

User Education Manager, Cairns Library, John Radcliffe Hospital, Oxford, UK

Foreword by

Professor Alison Kitson RN BSc(Hons) DPhil FRCN

Director, Royal College of Nursing Institute, London, UK

SECOND EDITION

ELSEVIER
CHURCHILL
LIVINGSTONE

EDINBURGH LONDON NEW YORK OXFORD PHILADELPHIA ST LOUIS SYDNEY TORONTO 2005

ELSEVIER
CHURCHILL
LIVINGSTONE

First edition 1999
Second edition 2005
    Reprinted 2005

ISBN 0 443 07299 X

British Library Cataloguing in Publication Data
A catalogue record for this book is available from the British Library

Library of Congress Cataloguing in Publication Data
A catalogue record for this book is available from the Library of Congress

Notice
Knowledge and best practice in this field are constantly changing. As new research and experience broaden our knowledge, changes in practice, treatment and drug therapy may become necessary or appropriate. Readers are advised to check the most current information provided (i) on procedures featured or (ii) by the manufacturer of each product to be administered, to verify the recommended dose or formula, the method and duration of administration, and contraindications. It is the responsibility of the practitioner, relying on experience and knowledge of the patient, to make diagnoses, to determine dosages and the best treatment for each individual patient, and to take all appropriate safety precautions. To the fullest extent of the law, neither the publisher nor the authors assumes any liability for any injury and/or damage.

The Publisher

Contents

Foreword

There have been comparatively few policy initiatives in health care that have had the same impact on professional attitudes and behaviour as the evidence-based practice movement. Students of the study of the diffusion of innovations or ideas will be familiar with the ingredients that are required to make successful change happen. What is impressive about the evidence-based practice movement is that it is changing the way we think about our practice.

It starts at the beginning – how we frame our questions to our patients, how we pull together the most appropriate evidence to help us come to good decisions, how we assure ourselves and others of the effectiveness of our interventions. This means that the practitioners who choose to read this book are already a self-selecting group. Significantly, you will be individuals with a thirst for knowledge and a passion for improvement; you will also be strong enough to learn from your mistakes and knowledgeable enough to know that progress only comes through careful, continuous, dedication to improvements in practice.

The ideal, of course, is to think of ways of involving our patients in our evidence-based journeys in the future. As practitioners we have a growing duty to guarantee the evidence of our practice. But we still have the challenge of interpreting and implementing it into practice. We are beginning also to acknowledge and respect the fact that evidence does manifest itself in many guises. So the form of evidence-based practice is the discovery of knowledge but the hard part is implementation. The future no doubt will take us to more complex places but the authors have done an excellent job in plotting a course that is both accessible and scholarly. We await the next phase with expectation.

London 2004   Alison Kitson

Preface

In the last 4 years 'evidence-based' has become a term that is often heard. Frequently, the user of that term has little knowledge of how evidence about health care is gathered, the complexity of this process and the potential for harm if it is not evaluated scientifically. As health care information increases exponentially, health care professionals will need to understand the uncertainty that research might pose. At the same time, the amount of accumulated data is such that it is often difficult to ensure the successful operation of an evidence-based practice.

This edition addresses these new issues and includes all the secondary sources of appraised information. In addition, there is greater awareness of evidence-based practice today. The most up-to-date articles describing the differences between research methods have been included here.

Evidence-based practice is for all health professionals. The main focus of this book is to serve as a resource for any health professional who wants to explore and improve their practice.

Montreal, 2004   Martin Dawes

Abbreviations

ARR   absolute risk reduction
CER   control event rate
CI   confidence interval
CME   continuing medical education
EBHC evidence-based health care
EER   experimental event rate
MeSH medical subject heading
NNT   numbers needed to treat
PBL   problem-based learning
QALY   quality-adjusted life-year
RCT   randomised controlled trial
ROC   receiver-operating characteristic
RR   relative risk
RRR   relative reduction in risk
SD   standard deviation
SE   standard error
WMD   weighted mean difference
GP   general practitioner

Chapter 1

Evidence–based practice

Martin Dawes

But thou art too fine in thy evidence; therefore stand aside.
All's Well That Ends Well
Shakespeare
Real knowledge is to know the extent of one's ignorance.
Confucius

This book has been written for all primary and public health care professionals interested in evidence-based practice. Whether you are a total novice, or have some experience of searching and appraisal, it will take you through the concepts, processes and applications of evidence-based practice.

INFORMATION NEED

No matter where you work in the health service you will suffer the same snowstorm of information. My background as a general practitioner (GP) makes me especially susceptible as any information on any condition seems to get sent to me. One day I may receive a new guideline about the management of epilepsy, the next day about screening for breast cancer. Whatever the topic, the information is usually relevant and important – but rarely discusses how it should be placed in context with everything we do and never seems to be in the same format as any other information we receive.

In the last ten years we have seen the rapid expansion of information about the practice of health care. The number of papers being written, the number of journals being published and the number of postgraduate presentations have all been rising steadily.

As a result, our understanding of the nature of disease and illness has increased resulting in changes to diagnostic strategies and management of disease. A medical student qualifying in the 1950s probably knew 80% of what there was to know about medicine. Most of that knowledge would have stayed 'up to date' for 25 years. Nowadays, a medical student may leave medical school knowing 40% of medical knowledge. Half that knowledge will be out of date in ten years. The flow of information is, therefore, important in keeping health professionals aware of important changes that might affect their practice or the way they think about a problem.

This acquired data should have resulted in two changes. Our knowledge should be greater and our practice should be more effective. Unfortunately, this is not always the case.

INFORMATION AND KNOWLEDGE

Information is data that has been sorted, analysed and displayed and is communicated through spoken language, text, figures or tables. Knowledge is the meaningful link people make in their minds, between information and its application in action in a specific setting. Knowledge may be tacit or explicit. An example of tacit knowledge is the ability of a health professional to recognise when a child is ill. The child may have a temperature, be sweaty, and look pale and might be lying still. But that description might also fit a child who had a mild illness. Given this brief description of the child's illness (explicit knowledge), a health care student might not be able to recognise an ill child. Clearly there are other signs, that all added together, make severe illness highly likely in that child. However, the list is long and not all the signs are present in every child. There may be a multiplicity of signs that identify an ill child, but the basic pattern triggers the alert clinician to look for other signs. All this is done without conscious thought by experienced clinicians.

However, students may resort to using long lists of clinical signs that are checked in every patient. This approach often means the 'important' features are missed and the less 'important' features given too much attention.

For health organisations, the difference between knowledge and information and the types of knowledge are essential if health care is to be kept up to date. The context of care is critical to the type and content of the information that is delivered for it to be relevant. This is the 'needing-it-now' principle of knowledge. Two accident and emergency (A&E) doctors and three nurses are waiting in the A&E resuscitation room for a drowned patient who is *en route* by ambulance. All preliminaries have been arranged and the anaesthetist is on his/her way to the hospital. One of the doctors opens up his/her handheld computer and looks up drowning. Apart from what the doctor already knew about basic resuscitation skills, cases of drowning often have neck injuries and the spine should be stabilised with a collar (Bailes and Herman 1990). This information is applied within two minutes of receiving it. New information applied immediately is clearly of more benefit than information that waits for several months – by which time it may have been forgotten.

CLINICAL OVERLOAD

As a result of the rapid expansion of information we have been faced with a greater demand from patients as well as many politically determined structural changes in the health care system.

Our clinical responsibilities can seem saturated and we may feel that it is hard enough to stand still let alone question our practice. During our work we often feel under so much pressure that we have scarce time to consider our practice more deeply. When we do question what we do, it is difficult to find time to seek an answer to that question. This is the reason we need evidence-based practice. The aim is to use time available to its maximum potential by answering some of these questions to the best of our abilities. By doing this we are increasing knowledge but, more importantly, we are likely to change practice. This change is also likely to occur in an area of practice relevant and important to us as practitioners.

We usually see an overwhelming number of patients during the week. During each of the sessions or clinics several questions may arise concerning diagnosis, prognosis, treatment and general care. It is therefore quite possible for a practitioner to make many thousands of clinical decisions a year. When asked, general practitioners say that they generate on average two questions per three patients. Forty per cent of the questions were factual (e.g. what dose), 43% concerned with medical opinion and 17% were non-medical. One-third of these questions are answered at the time of clinical contact. On average the clinician is left with four unanswered questions per surgery or clinic (Covell and Uman 1985). We say that we get the answers to these questions mostly from printed sources (Dawes and Uchechukwu 2003) but, when observed, we get them from colleagues. Much of this information may be completely up to date and accurate, but one has no way of ensuring that this is indeed the case.

Evidence for our practice has been gathered over our professional lifetime. This will be from many sources and will depend on how long we have been in practice. The longer we have been practising, the more likely our evidence will be based on experience or information from colleagues. In addition, there will be evidence from textbooks and postgraduate lectures.

KEEPING UP TO DATE

Practitioners who, to keep up to date, regularly read their professional journals, review the passages in an occasional textbook, and attend an occasional postgraduate lecture will see only a very small fraction of the available literature. Only a few of the important studies and relevant evidence concerning common practice problems are published in such journals or textbooks.

To read everything that we need to practise efficiently we would have to read many journals. Rarely does anyone who is ill have purely one disease. As the population we look after get older, they present with additional conditions at the same time. To ensure one's knowledge is up to date for all these problems would mean reading all the key journals relating to all the various specialties. For example, to consult 30 journals a week would be an almost insurmountable achievement.

WHAT IS EVIDENCE-BASED PRACTICE?

It is against this background of information need, clinical overload and the general feeling of helplessness that evidence-based practice can offer some help. In its most basic definition it aims to provide the best possible evidence at the point of clinical (or management) contact. This book will outline how that can be achieved whilst realising the practical constraints of working in a health service. It aims at ensuring that decisions are made on evidence that has been appraised critically and presented in understandable terms rather than research jargon.

To practise evidence-based practice one needs to ask questions about the care. For example, 'Is this treatment effective?'. The next step is to break that question down into something that is answerable. The reformulated question might then contain information about the disease and the patient. The evidence answering your question would be identified and appraised and finally the evidence put into practice.

It has been suggested that evidence for more than a tiny fraction of the decisions made cannot possibly be available. Ten years ago this may have been a legitimate argument, but today it is no longer the case. There is now a wide-published database of information on many aspects of health care. This information is often published in journals with small readerships and may rarely be seen. Yet it may be extremely important. Other evidence may be published and widely disseminated, but we may be too busy too read it. More commonly, we are trying to read too much too quickly and so fail to realise the importance of certain information. Finally, even if we did see an important article, how would we remember it and apply it in our practice?

EVIDENCE

Clinical research is designed to answer specific questions. These questions fall into broad categories for which there is an appropriate research design. To determine whether smoking causes lung cancer it was inappropriate to undertake a randomised control trial. Instead a cohort of individuals (general practitioners) was reviewed over many years (Doll and Hill 1950).

The ideal, though not always possible, way to evaluate a treatment is to randomly allocate the experimental treatment or a placebo to patients (after gaining their permission). Ideally the person giving the treatment, having the treatment, and evaluating the clinical effect should not know which treatment is being used. At the end of treatment the outcome is assessed in the two groups.

The number of these randomised control trials (RCTs) is now huge (Dickersin and Scherer 1994), and those indexed on electronic databases under the umbrella of 'primary care', although still relatively small when compared with hospital medicine, have increased fivefold since 1986 (Silagy and Jewell 1994). Moreover, answers to many common primary care questions are found in research performed and published outside primary care (Silagy 1993). Thus, a computer search identified 147 randomised trials on the treatment of respiratory tract infection over the last 30 years relating to primary care or family medicine. These trials were published in 56 journals! Reading the three journals with the highest frequency of these articles (Journal of Family Practice, British Medical Journal and British Journal of the Royal College of General Practitioners) would mean you would have seen only one-fifth of those articles.

Similar increases in publication of therapeutic trials conducted by professions allied to medicine are also seen (Cullum 1997). More evidence about the cause and prognosis of diseases is also being published. There is also an increase in publications of qualitative research on the impact of disease and treatment on people as individuals.

Much high quality, relevant evidence is already there, but it remains invisible to most practitioners, even to those who have the opportunity to keep up with the mainstream journals. Having argued that the evidence is available, another barrier is that practitioners find it difficult to find the time to trace it. The move toward a more evidence-based practice does not require that every practitioner traces all the evidence on every question or appraises all the evidence.

CRITICAL APPRAISAL

Unfortunately, we cannot just accept that most articles published by reputable journals are of sufficient quality for us to believe them. Journals rely on peer review by volunteers who are often given a short time to comment on several articles. During this process there is a decision that has to be made not only about the quality of the paper but also about its potential importance. If the information is very important or topical, it may override the flaws in the research process.

For example a report in the Lancet (Kraaijenhagen et al 2000) stated in the abstract: 'We have shown that, there is no increased risk of deep vein thrombosis among travellers.' This report came out less than 2 weeks after widespread newspaper reports of a women tragically dying from a pulmonary embolus after flying to Australia. Subsequent trials have reported significant increased risk of thrombosis in patients who fly. A subsequent article in the Lancet (Scurr et al 2001) stated that: 'We conclude that symptomless DVT might occur in up to 10% of long-haul airline travellers.'These conflicting reports were published less than 6 months apart from each other. This is a typical example of the message conflicting with the facts. Critical appraisal of these articles demonstrates that there is more validity in the second than the first trial. A more recent example has been highlighted in the British Medical Journal with regard to a new form of anti-arthritic drug. This drug was shown to have fewer side-effects (Juni et al 2002). Subsequent analysis of the trial data showed that this is not exactly the result.

When teaching critical appraisal I am often asked why this occurs. The answer is not straightforward. There is a strong peer review process in all the top medical journals but, despite this, articles will appear that are severely flawed. Journals have to publish to survive and they want to publish articles that deal with topical important issues of the day. Sometimes this imperative overrides that critical review process. However, all the responsibility should not be passed onto the journals. There is also an imperative for researchers to publish: for UK-health care academics this is four articles every five years. What then should a researcher publish? I want to publish articles that will change the way readers think about a clinical problem, or change the way they practise.

However, the researcher also wants to publish material that will help other researchers in the field. These may be non-clinical in outcome but still get published in the same journals. The reason for this is that the impact factor of journals that publish these articles is also key to the furthering of my career as an academic clinician.

Thus the journals are full of articles that sometimes were initially written to help clinicians and others written to help other researchers. By the completion of the editorial stage, it is often difficult to establish a reason for publication.

Journals started out by being the notebooks of scientists that were then distributed to colleagues. For researchers, perhaps that is what we should return to, and only publish in clinical journals information likely to change the way health professionals think or act.

A piece of research may have a very meaningful outcome suggesting that one particular form of practice is better than another. However, there may be flaws in the way the research was performed. These flaws may occur anywhere along the process and not only, as some may assume, in the statistical analysis. Critical appraisal is important to examine the thoroughness of a study, and thus the amount of confidence placed in the findings.

For example, a study may not have found out what happened to every one of the patients involved (follow-up). This is often the case but in some studies the rate of follow-up may be as low as 60%. The authors may not know what happened to more than a third of patients and it may be that those patients not followed up had a different outcome to those who were described in the paper. This is one example of a methodological weakness detected by critical appraisal. Although the process is straightforward, it can take some time and if a piece of research has been through this process already, then this is very helpful.

SHORT CUTS

Some of the evidence for answering clinical questions in public health or primary care already has been tracked down, critically appraised, and packaged in easily accessible forms (See Robin Snowball's Chapter 3). The format of these publications differs in the length and style but they have one common feature. All the material has been through a rigorous, critical appraisal. The appraisal has addressed the issues of quality that are described later on.

To use journals that have filtered positively for good quality research information is a useful mechanism for general reading. The articles are often rewritten by these secondary journals in short formats. Many of these single-page abstracts and commentaries relate to public health and primary care issues. Because only about 2% of the clinical articles in the 120 journals screened for these publications pass both scientific and clinical criteria, the reading time now required to keep up with important clinical advances is a smaller, more feasible fraction of its former, unmanageable magnitude.

Another rapidly expanding resource is the Cochrane Library of Systematic Reviews. This resource, already available on computer diskette and compact disc, contains extensively and methodically searched reviews of randomised trials on the clinical and economic effects of health care, and already has become a practical resource for practitioners in all fields of patient care. However, not even all these reviews are without flaws and so need to be appraised (Olsen and Middleton 2001). Finally, for therapy there is an invaluable source called Clinical Evidence (British Medical Journal publications) that has a rigorous appraisal system and has clear well set-out evidence-based treatment recommendations for many common conditions.

LIBRARIES

Many issues in health care have not gone through this careful assembly and appraisal, and reliance on non-evidence-based reviews is risky. To address these, practitioners must spend the time required to find the evidence. The amount of time for searching will vary with each individual question, but the practitioner who can find 1 hour a week in which to search and read will start to make huge strides. Thinking about where one is likely to find the answer is critical to effective searching. Often the solution is found in searching the electronic publications described above, with the additional bonus of obviating the need to carry out the tasks of critical appraisal. But when this approach is unsuccessful, the next stage involves an electronic search of the literature, either on one's own or with the assistance of a librarian. Health libraries are very much more aware of the needs of practitioners and most can receive request for papers by telephone and fax them to the practitioner the same day. In most searches, the associated abstracts can be downloaded, and often provide sufficient information to determine the methodological approach of the research, its clinical relevance and application (McKibbon & Walker-Dilks 1994a, McKibbon & Walker-Dilks 1994b, McKibbon & Walker-Dilks 1994c).

COURSES ON SEARCHING AND APPRAISAL

Health professionals often feel that they lack the necessary skills and experience to critically appraise the evidence and determine its applicability within their locality. The experience we have gained in teaching these skills has led to this book. We feel that many of the skills can be developed by practice using various specific skills outlined here. However, appraising articles with others can be a more effective way of learning.

There is no question that being taught how to search by an experienced librarian is far more efficient than trying to practise it oneself with the minimum instruction. Therefore, to build on the knowledge gained from reading this book we also recommend attendance at one of the many courses on evidenced-based health care (EBHC). Guidelines for critical appraisal are being disseminated widely following these courses. In recognition of the importance of these skills, the examination for the UK Royal College of General Practitioners has for several years included a section requiring the critical appraisal of a clinical article.

STORING AND RETRIEVING EVIDENCE

The final hurdle facing a practitioner is that relevant evidence cannot be recalled during the consultation when the answers are required. Even if successful in solving all the foregoing, the practitioner faces the challenge of storing the results of their searches and critical appraisals in ways that can be readily accessed when they need them. Setting them aside for later filing and organisation, remains a recipe for frustration and failure. With computers on the desks of growing numbers of practitioners or hand-held electronic organisers, the potential exists for keeping these results at their fingertips, especially the evidence needed to assist their most frequent questions and decisions.

The future is here now; it just is not evenly distributed yet! Even with these solutions, there remain too many questions for an individual practitioner to answer. But collegial help is on the way. With the growing number of practitioners learning how to search and critically appraise, the opportunities for progress are rapidly increasing. For example, in the UK primary care researchers, trainers of family practitioners and postgraduate tutors cover the whole country and coordinated by University departments of General Practice are promoting a critical approach to primary care practice and research. As these and similar groups share the tasks of searching for and appraising evidence, they can collate their critical appraisals electronically in agreed formats, and make them available on the Internet to all practitioners (www.gpfaqs.com).

TIPS FOR PRACTISING EVIDENCE–BASED PRACTICE

Tip 1 Ask questions

Try asking one question per patient:
- sticky label or name –
- the problem – COPD
- the question – is spirometry an effective predictor of clinical outcome (mortality – length hospital stay)?

Put them in your pocket and look at them at the end of the week.
Select one question because there is likely to be an answer
The question has arisen:
- More than once or
- Is important.

Tip 2 Searching

Search one question every 2 weeks or every month or every quarter!
Search logically – 1st Clinical Evidence, 2nd Journal Evidence-Based Medicine, 3rd Cochrane, 4th MEDLINE
Often you will find:
- Too few articles
- They will not be in your library or they may take a long time to get
- There are too many and a systematic review is needed.

Unless you have time and the question is desperately important, move onto the next question and let someone else answer this one!
Appraise the articles that answer your question, offer the highest level of evidence and are readily available.

Tip 3 Appraisal

Look for letters about the article in subsequent issues of the journal:
- Appraise with others until confident
- Appraise using worksheets
- Or use software – CATmaker or www.gpfaqs.com

Mark (highlight) on the printed article where you found the important data.
Get someone else to check it for you.
Practise writing declarative headings – use the word 'may' a lot.

Tip 4 Share your knowledge

Try sharing uncertainty with your colleagues:
- Discuss your questions with colleagues (maybe they have answered it!)
- Find fault with the article(s) – never your colleagues
- Seek improvement in your own care
- Strive to do no harm.

References

Bailes J E, Herman J M, Quigley M R, 1990 Diving injuries of the cervical spine. Surgical Neurology 34(3):155-158

Covell D G, Uman G C, Manning P R 1985 Information needs in office practice: are they being met? Annals of Internal Medicine 103(4):596-599

Cullum N 1997 Identification and analysis of randomised control trials in nursing: preliminary study. Quality in health care 6:2-6

Dawes M, Uchechukwu S 2003 Knowledge management in clinical practice: a systematic review of information-seeking behaviour in physicians. International Journal of Medical Informatics 70(1):9-15

Dickersin K Scherer R, Lefebvre C 1994 Identifying relevant studies for systematic reviews. British Medical Journal 309(6964):1286-1291

Doll R, Hill A 1950 Smoking and carcinoma of the lung. Preliminary report. British Medical Journal ii:739-748

Juni P, Rutjes A W, Dieppe P A 2002 Are selective COX 2 inhibitors superior to traditional non-steroidal anti-inflammatory drugs? British Medical Journal 324(7349):1287-1288

Kraaijenhagen R A, Haverkamp D, Koopman M M 2000 Travel and risk of venous thrombosis. Lancet 356(9240):1492-1493

McKibbon K A, Walker-Dilks C J 1994a Beyond ACP journal club: how to harness MEDLINE for diagnostic problems [editorial]. ACP Journal Club 121(Suppl 2):A10-12

McKibbon K A, Walker-Dilks C J 1994b Beyond ACP journal club: how to harness MEDLINE for therapy problems [editorial]. ACP Journal Club 121(Suppl 1):A10-12

McKibbon K A, Walker-Dilks C J 1994c Beyond ACP journal club: how to harness MEDLINE to solve clinical problems [editorial]. ACP Journal Club 120(Suppl 2):A10-12

Olsen O, Middleton P, Ezzo J 2001 Quality of Cochrane reviews: assessment of sample from 1998. British Medical Journal 323:829-832

Scurr J H, Machin S J, Bailey-King S 2001 Frequency and prevention of symptomless deep-vein thrombosis in long-haul flights: a randomised trial. Lancet 357(9267):1485-1489

Silagy C A 1993 Developing a register of randomised controlled trials in primary care [published erratum appears in British Medical Journal Jun 19;306(6893):1660] [see comments]. British Medical Journal 306(6882):897-900

Silagy C A, Jewell D 1994 Review of 39 years of randomised controlled trials in the British Journal of General Practice. British Journal of General Practice 44(385):359-363

Walker-Dilks C J, McKibbon K A, Haynes R B 1994 Beyond ACP journal club: how to harness MEDLINE for aetiology problems [editorial]. ACP Journal Club 121:A10-11

Chapter 2

Formulating a question
Martin Dawes

Sitting at your desk one afternoon with the sun coming through the window, your mind drifts off to the holiday you have just returned from. Suddenly your patient shuffles noisily and you are brought back to the real world. This daydream may have only taken a few seconds but provides you with the energy to continue the endless stream of work.

The amount of work that we all have to complete is sometimes overwhelming and we forget what we are doing. The patient presents, you listen to the history, make an examination and, where appropriate, order some tests or start some therapy. Nothing wrong with that except: have you had time to think about alternatives? Is there a better way to listen to the history? Are the examinations appropriate and what is their clinical significance? What might be the meaning of the diagnostic tests, and which treatments are most effective for this condition? Or is it all too much and should you just carry on with occasional daydreams?

Consider a different daydream, one that would take the same length of time. Instead of drifting back to that holiday, ask yourself: what are the options here? Is this ritualistic examination of the chest of any value? Is this antibiotic going to affect outcome? Is this bandage the most effective? This questioning attitude is what makes us good professionals. Are we doing the **right** things, and if so are they being done in the **right** way and at the **right** time (Gray 1997)?

The reason we do not usually ask questions is they are so difficult to answer. This was nicely illustrated in *The Hitch Hiker's Guide to the Galaxy* when the super computer gave the answer '42' to the question: 'what does life, the universe and everything mean?' (Adams, 1994). The people asking the question were horrified and angry. The computer calmly suggested that instead of panicking they should go back and consider the question and that it would, of course, help them to do this. This is an extreme example of how a question can be so badly formed that its answer is meaningless.

It is a trap we can easily fall into in practice. I go to see a patient with asthma in the asthma clinic in our practice at the request of the district nurse. The patient is poorly controlled but stable on high doses of inhaled corticosteroids. I give a short course of oral steroids. I was in a hurry and this is the real world. I have been beset by advertisements for anti-leukotrienes and wonder if they help. I have a quick look in the British National Formulary asthma guideline and it does not mention them.

Later, while doing paperwork, I turn on my computer. The practice is connected to the Internet and I decide to use PubMed to search for articles. I type in leuokotriene and get 13 467 articles. Does this sound a familiar scenario to you? It is all very well having everything on computer, but I am still faced with the problem of finding it.

I went wrong in two places. First, my search was unstructured. This is dealt with in the next chapter. Second, what was my question? I wanted to know more about anti-leukotrienes, but why? My patient was a 38-year-old woman with poorly controlled asthma but otherwise well. She is happily married with two children. Her immediate problem was a cough and resulting sleep disturbance. It was the symptoms that troubled her and not her forced expiratory volume in 1 second (fev1).

My question should have focused on the addition of anti-leukotrienes (AL) to inhaled corticosteroids to relieve symptoms of asthma. This is the end point of my inquiry. If added to my search on anti-leukotrienes, it would now only show those papers dealing with anti-leukotrienes and symptoms of asthma and I would not be swamped quite so much with information. I am only interested now in my patient who is a young woman. My question is: 'In young women do anti-leukotrienes reduce the symptoms of asthma?'

It is becoming better but the middle part is still vague. Perhaps I should enter some of the therapeutic options I am suggesting: adding the AL to inhaled corticosteroids. My final question became: 'In a young woman with poorly controlled asthma does the addition of AL to inhaled corticosteroids reduce symptoms?' My search now reveals 181 articles which I can scan or do more refined searches as demonstrated in the next chapter.

Now I am getting somewhere. By structuring a question, the answer may be found more efficiently. It is therefore important to try to break the question down into several parts (Richardson and Wilson 1995):

1. Patient or problem
2. Intervention
3. Comparison intervention (optional)
4. Outcomes.

PATIENT OR PROBLEM

The first part is to identify the problem or the patient. Health care problems may not always seem to be about patients! For example, an administrator may want to know whether having acute medical beds in a temporary holding ward next to the accident and emergency (A&E) department is any more efficient than having conventional acute medical wards in the hospital. In this case the question is concerned with the hospital in which the administrator works. Another example is the use of nurses in out-of-hours provision of telephone advice for a medical group. In this situation, nurses may be employed in addition to receptionists to filter calls to the doctors providing out-of-hours service within primary care. In this case the 'problem or patient' may be the out-of-hours cooperative.

Make sure at this stage in the question that you are describing the problem or patients that you see. These may be patients within certain specialist settings who would respond differently from those within the community (see Chapter 16). However, if you are too specific at this stage, you may miss some important evidence and there is a balance to be struck between getting evidence about exactly your group of patients and getting *all* the evidence about *all* groups of patients.

INTERVENTION

The intervention is equally important. It may in fact be a postponement of an action such as an operation. In patients with abdominal pain lasting less than 12 hours, does an additional 24-hour delay before referral to hospital alter outcome? Most interventions are more straightforward, such as types of dressings, drug therapies or counselling. Alternatively, they can be the provision of differing environmental factors, such as the décor of waiting rooms or deal with the way in which information is given to patients (Thomas 1987).

Be as specific as possible with the intervention at this stage. You may want to backtrack later if you cannot find any evidence. What regimen of drug therapy are you interested in? If you are working in primary care, then oral methods of drug delivery will be more appropriate than intravenous. Is that therapy going to be the same as you can provide? The way in which we offer treatment to patients varies from both within and between primary and secondary care. The frequency with which we can see patients and alter doses as well as the ability to check serum levels may be different from secondary care, and all these factors may affect outcomes.

Such interventions may be quite varied and you often have to consider this quite carefully when refining the question. For example, you may have a question about the prognosis or aetiology of a condition. The intervention can be causative factors for aetiological questions. Therefore, you may want to include passive smoking as your intervention when questioning the cause of cancer. Equally, you might include certain operations for the investigation of the prognosis of a cancer.

COMPARISON INTERVENTION

Sometimes there is a comparison of the intervention. If you are already using a painkiller in normal practice you might seek papers that compare the use of that painkiller to another form as well as papers comparing the alternative painkiller to placebo. Considering whether looking for comparative studies will help when searching for that evidence.

OUTCOMES

Outcome measures are particularly important when considering the question. It is worth spending some time working out exactly what it is you want. In serious diseases it is often easy to concentrate on the mortality and miss the important aspects of morbidity. For example, the use of toxic chemotherapies for cancer may affect both aspects. Make sure you know what time period you are looking at, e.g. is the pain reduction in ear infections important in 24 hours or do you want to know the result for 5 days after the intervention?

STRUCTURING THE QUESTION

Finally, it is useful when developing the question to use a grid (Table 2.1). Initially, I start with the question jotted down on a piece of paper and stuffed in my pocket. When I examine the bits of paper later, I decide which questions I want to spend time exploring. My jottings are usually very unstructured, containing some details about the patient (usually the name so I can enter the result of the search into the patient's notes later) and the condition with something about an intervention. The next step is then to refine the question. This does take a little time and it is well worth spending a few minutes considering the various possible alternative outcomes or interventions. I write these alternatives down in the grid and then these are used to perform the searches.

Using this process I know I have developed a question that is more likely to result in a significant and useful answer. The objective is for us as clinicians to continue to ask questions. Then we will retain and increase our enthusiasm for one of the most rewarding professions.

Table 2.1 Sample grid for structuring questions

Patient or problem	Intervention	Comparison	Outcomes	Time

References

Adams D 1994 Life, the universe and everything. The hitch hiker's guide to the galaxy, 3
    Millenium (Orion) London
Gray J 1997 Evidence-based health care. Churchill Livingstone, New York
Richardson W, Wilson M 1995 The well-built clinical question: a key to evidence-based
    decisions [editorial]. ACP Journal Club 123:A12-13
Thomas K 1987 General practice consultations: is there any point in being positive?
    British Medical Journal Clinical Research Edition 294:1200-1202

Chapter 3

Finding the evidence: an information skills approach

Robin Snowball

INTRODUCTION

Information-seeking is a central and integral part of the process which we begin by formulating questions about problematic aspects of complex situations in the real world in order, ultimately, to make informed decisions or to influence change. Once we have a clear and structured question, we can work through a logical process for finding and using the best resources in our search for information which we can use as evidence to address clinical questions in health care. More than ever before, we need the key skills to search both *for* and *within* information resources of many kinds, and to identify the 'best' evidence for our particular purposes, both effectively and efficiently.

In terms of sheer quantity, we have experienced an information 'big bang'. Mulrow and Cook (1998), for example, tell us that 2 million articles are published annually in some 20 000 'biomedical' journals: a pile of paper some 500 metres high! In addition, information which could serve as good evidence may be buried even deeper, in unpublished studies, or in uncirculated publications, known as 'grey' (Europe) or 'black' (USA) literature. Our virtual new age is radically changing patterns of information recording, dissemination and access, and the resources we must use to locate research-derived information are proliferating in all disciplines and subjects, and in a bewildering variety of forms.

All the more reason, then, to take a systematic approach to finding and using the best available information resources for the various types of questions we might ask across health care practice and research. Using our own structured clinical questions, as described in Chapter 2, we will work through five key questions as a guide:

1. What type of *questions* are being asked?
2. What sort of *information* would provide the best evidence to address each type of question?
3. What type of research *study* would provide such information?
4. What types of *information resources* would give us access to (the results of) such studies?
5. How do we get the *best* out of the resources, to address each type of question?

In working through questions 2 and 3, you may want to refer to other chapters of this book. In addressing question 4, we will take a brief overview of the main types of current information resource, with examples. Addressing question 5, we will look at getting the best out of key resources, such as computer bibliographic databases and finding trustworthy World Wide Web sites. The chapter closes with a summary of the key information skills for finding evidence, and a Select List of Information Resources, items from which are indicated throughout the chapter by numbers in brackets, e.g. (35). This is a get-started list, as no such list is ever comprehensive. 'Learning the resources' is a continual task, so do enlist the expert support of those valuable human information resources: your local specialist health care librarians!

Terminology is a minefield. I use 'resources' to cover the entire range of 'sources' – both 'primary' and 'secondary' – in or from which 'information' may be discovered or constructed, in any accessible form: organisations, websites, computer databases, journals and other printed materials.

On information resources: 'information,' expressed in statements or propositions perhaps as 'facts,' is derived from 'data' (statistics, values, etc.) as its raw material; it is used to build up current, often provisional, 'knowledge.' In everyday English, we say that information can be used as 'evidence,' of varying degrees of strength, appropriate to context. So there is no essential distinction between 'evidence resources' and 'information resources'.

PUTTING TOGETHER A RESOURCES STRATEGY

Let us now work through our sequence of questions, trying out examples. It will make more sense if you run through the process after formulating your own 'clinical' or structured question as shown in Chapter 2. Searching, like research, depends on the focus of a clear, specific question, even if provisional. Of course, a preliminary search can help you to formulate or sharpen your question, before you search more thoroughly. Some simple questions – what Richardson and Wilson (1997) call 'background' questions, about the basic facts of a disease or a therapy, or a statistic – are not complex enough to have 'parts', and may best be answered from basic resources, such as textbooks or formularies. But even a 'simple' clinical question, like the leg ulcer question in Chapter 2, might have no single or simple 'answer,' or be controversial, and may be opened out by using the question structure to clarify and to ground the search for the best evidence at the outset. It is here, at the start, that so many searches go astray!

Stop now, and formulate your *own* question before you continue!

WHAT TYPE OF QUESTION IS BEING ASKED?

Richardson et al (1995), in their concise summary of clinical question formulation, checklist the main question types to help us formulate questions. We can adapt their categories, adding others if we need to, to help us 'locate' our questions, ready for the next stage:

- Intervention: Is this intervention (treatment, test, exposure, etc.) more effective (in terms of stated outcome/s) than another/others/doing nothing, etc?
- Prevention: How do we reduce the risk of this disease?
- Harm/risk: What are the side-effects, risks, etc. of this intervention? Does it do more harm than good?
- Cause/aetiology: What are the causes of this condition or state of affairs?
- Differential diagnosis: How do we distinguish condition *a* from condition *b*?
- Diagnostic testing: How accurate (sensitive/specific) is this diagnostic test (compared with another)?
- Prognosis: What is the likely outcome, course, progression, or survival time of this condition?
- Cost-effectiveness: Is intervention *x* more cost-effective than intervention *y*?
- Quality of life: What will be the quality of life for the patient(s) following (or without) this intervention, with this condition etc.?

Let's take a question about hormone replacement therapy and its effect on osteoporosis, and work through it as an example:

Q. In post-menopausal women, does hormone replacement therapy (HRT) prevent osteoporosis?

This may be, or become, a therapy question, a prevention question, a risk-benefit question or a cost-effectiveness question: we need to be clear which it is from the start. The therapy question type has served as a model in evidence-based medicine, for obvious reasons, but there is a wide range of question types across health care practice and research. A question about the 'quality of life' of those receiving treatment is a more complex 'qualitative' question type. A question about prostate cancer screening might be a cost-effectiveness question, a screening-effectiveness question or a prevention question. If we have more than one question or question type, we *must* distinguish between them. Each question may require various kinds of information for evidence, which may appear in different types of resources. We may even need a different search approach within resources, as we will see when we look at searching computer databases more effectively.

Stop now, and decide, however provisionally, the main question type of *your* **question.**

WHAT SORT OF INFORMATION WOULD PROVIDE EVIDENCE TO ANSWER THIS TYPE OF QUESTION?

We next need to be able to recognise the various types of information which may be used as evidence, from the strongest to the weakest, appropriate to our question type. The type of information we would use as the strongest evidence for a therapy question is not the same as for a question about cost-effectiveness or prognosis, or for 'qualitative' issues, such as consumer satisfaction or quality of life. So we may not find it in the same resources or in the same way. Other chapters discuss in detail the types of evidence required for these and other question types: our concern here is with using this knowledge to identify clearly the types of information resources and the search strategies appropriate to getting the best out of them.

The best evidence for a therapy question will be provided by information about defined outcomes resulting from use of the therapy in one group of patients, compared with its non-use in another. This will be stronger as systematic bias is decreased by random allocation to the groups, 'blinding' of participants, etc. (Chapter 5). The next-best evidence might be provided by information about the effects in a certain population or cohort, then about the effects in an individual, and so on down the evidence 'pyramid' – from strongest to weakest evidence – for this question type. Health economics questions (Chapters 10, 15) require a complex combination of information on effectiveness and cost. For prognosis questions, the best evidence might be provided by information about survival rates over set times, or descriptions of the course of the disease, in a specific population, with the weakest evidence (which may be all we can find, especially for a rare condition) from individual case studies.

Issues of quantitative and qualitative evidence arise here. What sort of information might serve as the best evidence for quality-of-life questions? For some types of question, including some therapy questions, qualitative factors which are difficult or impossible to quantify may be involved. Values, cultural perceptions or other types of 'soft' complexity can make generalisation between groups or populations difficult. What sort of information would provide the best evidence to address questions, such as 'What forms of terminal care interventions best meet the psychological needs of individuals with life-threatening diseases?' And what can we do about those questions where even definitions may be contested, such as 'How are crises of gender identity in adolescents most effectively resolved?'

What type of information, in general terms, would you use as the 'best' or strongest evidence (and then the next strongest, etc.) appropriate to address *your* type of question?

WHAT TYPE OF STUDY WOULD PROVIDE SUCH INFORMATION?

We must next ask what types of study or investigation will provide the information we can use as evidence, from the strongest to the weakest, for each particular type of question. We usually answer this and the previous question simultaneously, but they are logically distinct – the same information (e.g. survival rates) might be provided by different types of study, and it may help to ask the logically prior question about types of information to use as evidence first, especially in more complex areas, such as for qualitative question types. The understandable dominance of the therapy question may lead us to believe that information from randomised controlled trials (RCTs), or from systematic reviews of RCTs is the best, even the only admissible, evidence for all types of question, and that if we cannot find these, we have no evidence! A well-conducted RCT should provide the information we can use as evidence for therapy effectiveness questions, such as the use of antibiotics to treat leg ulcers. A systematic review of such trials (which may or may not include the statistical pooling of results known as meta-analysis) might provide even sounder evidence. For practical purposes, a properly 'evidence-based' clinical practice guideline (Chapter 12) might summarise for us the best evidence available for making clinical decisions. If these do not exist, we would look for non-randomised clinical trials, and so on down the pyramid of evidence studies for this type of question. If there are no trials, perhaps for a rare condition, we may find only case reports.

Toward the base of the evidence pyramid for therapy, we might have to cite the opinion of respected and experienced authorities, or we may find only 'anecdotal' evidence (but see Enkin and Jadad 1988). For a prognosis question, a cohort study might provide the best evidence; for risk or harm questions, case-control studies might provide the best evidence currently available. For our terminal care question – and for those many 'health interventions which … are not readily amenable to rigorous experimental research design' (Popay and Williams, 1998:32) – controlled trials may be all but impossible to set up, for many reasons, including ethical ones.

Qualitative research (Chapter 11) may offer the best approach where population, cultural or other contextual factors might make comparisons or generalisation difficult, or where key variables maybe impossible to quantify or control. For complex health policy decisions, Popay and Williams (1998) cite as an example Goffman's classic work (1961) on institutionalisation in mental hospitals, which greatly influenced national policy change. For terminal care questions, and other areas where trials may be difficult or impossible in certain cases, we might search (from a very wide range of information resources) for studies, for example, which narratively describe the outcomes of specific care strategies, including 'insider' phenomenological descriptions of the experience of terminal illness or its care by patients or carers, to find the best evidence available to support informed decisions, in certain cases.

But if we are clear about the information which could provide the best or strongest evidence, and the types of study which might generate it or review it, then we can search more effectively for the best information resources. And, within the resources, we can tailor specific search strategies to find them, such as *using the names of study types as search terms.*

Draft an evidence 'pyramid' of the types of research study/investigation which would best provide the type of information you would use as the strongest evidence to address *your* question type. Then, consider the next strongest, and the next – filling in any knowledge gaps from other chapters of this book.

WHAT TYPES OF RESOURCES WOULD GIVE US ACCESS TO (THE RESULTS OF) SUCH STUDIES?

First, let us recapitulate what we have established, however provisionally, by this stage. These simple strands will form our golden thread for beginning to explore the global labyrinth of resources, well beyond this chapter:

- the complete and detailed specific clinical question we want to answer
- the real 'purpose' of our question expressed as a question type
- the 'best' types of evidence to answer this type of question
- the types of study or investigation that would provide such evidence.

The sheer variety of resources in our rapidly expanding universe of information seems alarming! The types of research study we have considered briefly, and the systematic reviews which may be made of them, are accessible through a great variety of information resources. They are directly available in the so-called 'primary resources' in which original studies are published in some way, and indirectly via the 'secondary resources' which refer us (traditionally 'bibliographically' or via a reference of some kind) to the primary resources which actually hold the information on the studies. This is the distinction, for example, between the primary journal and the literature database which refers to and indexes the contents of journals, between the published book and the library catalogue, and so on – a hoary old distinction, now becoming one of function rather than of form, as many journals,for example fulfil both functions, and full-text databases increasingly deliver or link to original publications in full.

We can now begin to relate types of research study to the main types of primary resources and to the main types of secondary resources. Figure 3. 1

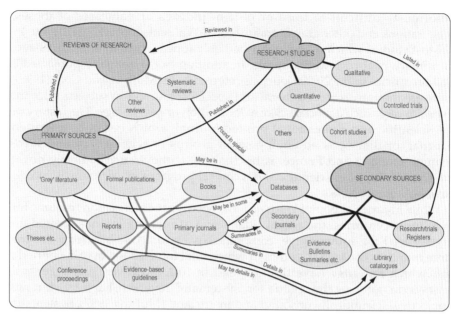

Figure 3.1 Research studies, primary and secondary resources: a concept map

attempts this in a very simplified form – it is a very complex area! – as a concept map. For those new to concept mapping, a useful learning and teaching tool (see Novak and Gowin 1984, reprinted annually since), the straight downward lines represent hierarchical relations, the lateral or bendy lines specific relations between concepts. From this, we will now take a simplified overview of the main current types of primary resources for research studies, at the same time outlining the main types of secondary resources related to them. You can find details of specific resources, under some of these (sometimes overlapping) headings in the Select List of Information Resources at the end of the chapter.

First of all, many original studies are not published (publicly issued) so that we can easily obtain them. It has been suggested (Stern and Simes 1997) that those with inconclusive or negative conclusions are more likely to be rejected by those who peer review articles for publication in journals. A 'publication bias' toward 'positive' conclusions may result, so on rare occasions we may need to know how to trace unpublished work, as systematic reviewers do, to get a more complete evidence picture. So, directories or databases of research and trials registers are an important kind of resource, increasingly available to alert us to planned, ongoing or unpublished research. They may also suggest valuable contacts, if we need them (72-74).

Second, many studies are produced, but not made widely available, such as theses and dissertations, conference proceedings, reports and other materials, often produced by health services and other key organisations. This 'grey' literature may contain the very information we need, but is notoriously difficult to trace or obtain. Indexes or databases of theses, dissertations and other grey literature can be valuable tools (13, 21, 31, etc.).

Most studies which do get published still appear, even in our virtual age, in primary peer-reviewed journals. In addition to the annually published 2 million articles in the 20 000 journals referred to by Mulrow and Cook(1998), there are thousands more general and specialist journals in subjects relevant to health care, such as social sciences, education or psychology. The history of the scientific and professional printed journal, which began as a written 'journal' or diary passed among small groups of scientists in mid-17th-century England and France, is fascinating: without such radically novel information transfer, scientific and technical progress, as we know it, would have been impossible.

While libraries of bound journals have been a key information resource for over three centuries, the recent tidal wave of information has created an urgent need for authoritative, comprehensive and accessible *reviews* of the large numbers of original studies in which vital information may be 'buried', and which few may have time to read in full. However, many general reviews do not meet the criteria for 'systematic' review (Chapter 9), but are 'subjective, scientifically unsound and inefficient' (Mulrow 1987). Systematic reviews (see Oxman 1995 for a checklist of criteria), such as Cochrane reviews – available full-text via the Cochrane Library suite of databases (12) – are now recognised to be of critical importance in gathering and synthesising evidence from original research studies. Sadly, they may not cover the topics we need them to cover. Ezzo et al (2001) also point out that the number even of Cochrane reviews, showing an intervention to have no effects or insufficient evidence, are 'suprisingly high.' The NHS Centre for Reviews and Dissemination or CRD (113) also carry out high-quality reviews, some of which appear in the DARE part of the Cochrane Library. Other reviews can be found published in primary journals, such as the British Medical Journal's Clinical reviews (free full-text on the web, like all recent British Medical Journal articles), but good reviews remain scattered and hard to find.

Journals or their contents are now increasingly accessible on the World Wide Web. Some journal websites offer searchable contents lists or references, often with article abstracts, while others offer full-text articles by subscription (which may be included in or separate from a print subscription!) or wholly or partly free of charge. (Journal websites may give more information about the contents of the recent issues of a journal than computer databases because of the time delays in database entry.) Efforts are being made to speed up the process of article publication and dissemination, widen access and perhaps reduce prices, while retaining peer review and other safeguards, with so-called 'open-access' journals, and initiatives such as BioMed Central (92) and PUBMED Central (121), (Fletcher 2002).

As the journal is still our major primary resource for research, this readily explains the crucial importance of our major secondary resource: the computer bibliographic database, the descendant of the printed bibliographic index (itself still available, and still useful). The invention of the high-capacity compact disk or CD-ROM in the 1980s enabled huge collections of bibliographical records, previously available as shelves of printed indexes, to become accessible as searchable databases on personal computers or computer networks. Now, they too are increasingly web-accessible, either free or subscription-based.

These secondary resources give us indirect access to the contents of thousands of journals and other forms of primary literature, published worldwide, and they range, as do journals, from the general to the super-specialised. Full-text databases which deliver whole articles rather than references do exist (e.g. 16, 17) – the Cochrane Library (13), for example, contains full-text systematic reviews – and more will appear in time. Web-based databases such as PUBMED (27) give links to websites where some full-text journal articles may be accessed. As they increasingly become full-text databases, and deliver the original studies directly or indirectly from the search, they will be our most important primary resource: issues of peer review, payment and copyright, rather than technology, delay this process.

On the other hand, many journals are not included in the major databases, and the true contents of original articles even of those that do appear may not be accurately or clearly described in author abstracts or by indexers. Systematic reviewers address these challenges by 'hand searching' key journals, by contacting key researchers or expert authors, and by carefully checking the reference lists at the end of articles. Any of us might miss vital information (especially if we search too few resources) when it most matters, so these are options we may need to use in certain circumstances.

Although most research in health care is still published in professional journals, these are, by today's standards, a relatively slow form of communication. The explosion of original studies published as journal articles, with a corresponding explosion of journal titles, has been mentioned. Busy health professionals do not generally have the time (or skills?) to find, appraise, sift and synthesise the primary research studies on a topic, as a reviewer would, and clearly could not do so for every clinical question that arises in practice. Health professionals badly need conveniently delivered resources which do this for them, with authority and credibility, to support clinical decision-making. McColl et al (1998) maintain, following a questionnaire survey, that promoting and improving access to evidence-based summaries would be 'the more appropriate method of encouraging evidence-based general practice' than 'teaching literature searching and critical appraisal'. Valuable information now appears in 'evidence-based' or 'effectiveness' bulletins or newsletters like the superb Bandolier (56), printed or on the Web, which may be targeted at specific groups or subjects. Such sources offer rapid and accessible communication, with critically appraised evidence summaries or digests, rather than original research studies or reviews in full. Another example is 'Hitting the Headlines' on the NeLH (110) home-page, containing quick reviews written by health researchers at NHS-CRD (113) within 48 hours of major health stories appearing in the Press. (This recently provided the quickest access to the main 'facts behind the story' about hormone replacement therapy (HRT) risks, as incompletely reported in many newspapers).

Review services such as ATTRACT, set up in Gwent, Wales following a survey which came to conclusions similar to those of (McColl et al 1998), and reviewed by Brassey et al (2001), also perform quick reviews (not claimed to be systematic reviews) on request. ATTRACT's reviews to date can be read on their website (55). Such services, offered by library systems and specialist searchers, will continue to appear, since they save the busy clinician much time and effort. Two recent major developments in this growth area are Clinical Evidence (57), a printed book series and a searchable web database, now free via NeLH (110), with critical evidence summaries to address specific health care questions and the splendid Up To Date subscription service. Watch out for more!

The 'secondary' journal (36, etc.) performs a similar function for original studies and reviews published in primary journals. Many specialist primary journals now have a similar research alerting or appraising section.

Clinical guidelines, if properly 'evidence-based' (Chapter 12), can summarise a vast amount of research, and also deal with consumer implications in a way that reviews may not be able (or be designed) to do. Sadly, many are distinctly 'grey', especially when 'local' or produced by smaller organisations, or they may be formally published, as are those from the National Institute of Clinical Excellence (NICE) (111) and the Royal Colleges. Specialist websites – NeLH is a major gateway here – organise links to these key resources (75-88). The journal Guidelines regularly summarises clinical guidelines for primary and shared care, and has a website, e-Guidelines (80). Some published guidelines can be traced in databases, such as nursing guidelines in CINAHL (11) full-text, or traced in library catalogues if published: but they are scattered, and often difficult to trace or obtain.

Reports and conference proceedings form a growing body of important literature, and may report or refer to original research. When formally published, they can be traced via specialised databases (e.g. 34, 35), key organisational websites (102) or library catalogues, but they too are scattered, and many useful reports remain distinctly 'grey'.

Finally, the published book is still a valuable tool, but because of the time it takes to publish a book (one to two years) recent or current research may not be addressed. Some databases, such as PsycInfo (28), CAB Health (8) or HMIC (20) include details of published books, which may include conference proceedings or reports. With the web come the early generations of web-based textbooks or 'e-books', such as the (free) Merck manuals of diagnosis and therapy, and geriatrics (108). As an enormously valuable and underestimated secondary resource, the web provides a host of national, organisational and university library catalogues (66-71), from which we can find details of a vast amount of both published and grey literature.

This last point confirms again the value of the Internet-based World-Wide Web, cutting across all these resources types and providing massively increased access to primary and secondary resources of all kinds: to databases, journals, research and project groups, newsletters, bulletins, health professional and consumer organisations, discussion groups, libraries and individuals. The information universe is expanding but fragmenting fast. There is no longer any central resource in which 'everything' can be found on anything at all! We have to learn to survive in, and to exploit, this new universe to our advantage.

HOW DO WE GET THE BEST OUT OF THE RESOURCES, TO ANSWER EACH TYPE OF QUESTION?

We need to be able to exploit information resources effectively, not missing the real gems, nor getting overwhelmed by dross. To do this, we must exploit the trade-off between:

1. comprehensiveness: finding everything of any relevance at all – but increasing the likelihood of retrieving irrelevant material (high sensitivity/low specificity);
2. selectivity: finding only the most highly relevant material – but increasing the likelihood of missing relevant material (low sensitivity/high specificity).

Good information skills are the key to controlling this trade-off to advantage. We will focus on two essential types of information resource: using computer bibliographic databases and, briefly, using the Internet-based World-Wide Web to find reliable starting points to access the many kinds of resources we have already begun to meet.

Computer bibliographic databases

Computer bibliographic databases are still our most important type of secondary resource. As yet, there are not enough evidence summaries or systematic reviews available for the great majority of questions in health care. Even if we do look for these *first*, we still often have to go back to the original studies and reviews published in primary resources such as journals, if we want quality evidence. The major bibliographic databases contain huge amounts of information, and we can only get at it by mastering the complex search software added by commercial vendors or others. Furthermore, since no single database covers *all* journals or other resources in any field, we may need to widen our search net and increase search sensitivity quite simply by searching several databases or other resources, rather than sticking to a standard or favourite, at least on some occasions. We should look, therefore, in some detail at searching computer bibliographic databases such as MEDLINE, EMBASE, CINAHL or the Cochrane Library. Many people find these databases difficult to search – almost always finding 'too little' or 'too much'. Others, more insidiously, do not find them as difficult as they ought to. There is evidence (McKibbon et al 1990, 1991, Shelstad and Clevenger 1994) from comparison of clinical searchers with information professionals that many searchers are not as skilled as they believe themselves to be, often entering search strategies that are far too simple to retrieve the material they need, and missing as much as half the key material retrieved by experts. They blame databases for being unnecessarily difficult to search, believe they have not found the right 'keywords' (a much misused term, but at least one that shows that most searchers know this to be the key issue), believe that search software ought, in effect, to think for them, that they lack 'computer' skills, or that they simply do not have time or need for 'fancy searching'. While the mechanics of searching have become simpler with Windows-based systems, it is good search skills and a basic understanding of databases, rather than advanced IT skills, that really make the difference.

In fact, the key to effective database searching is good search strategy skills, transferable between resources. Once again, the structured clinical question provides an elegant framework for preparing a search strategy that we can use or develop for different databases (and even for those web search engines with the advanced search features of databases). From the *search question*, we can find the best *search terms* and work out a *search strategy* which we can broaden or narrow according to need and result. Search strategy development skills should take centre stage in the search learning process, with computer operations merely the means to the end (Snowball 1997).

So let us prepare the HRT and osteoporosis question as a provisional search strategy, and test it on a key general health care database.

Q. In post-menopausal women, does HRT prevent osteoporosis?

After breaking the question into parts appropriate to an intervention question – Patient, Intervention (Comparison), Outcome – we 'brainstorm' possible search terms for each part of the question. (A quick preliminary search, scanning titles and abstracts will always produce more terms: so develop your searching as an *iterative* or cyclical process.) Less 'clinical' searches may have 'softer' terminology – less term standardisation, vagueness, ambiguity or unclear overlap between related terms – so use more variant and related terms, and never rely only on the most obvious terms. We have all missed something important in a search, perhaps the best, simply because we overlooked a good search term.

Here is the first try for our search term collection:

Table 3.1

Patient	Intervention	Outcome
postmenopausal	HRT	osteoporosis
post-menopausal	hormone replacement therapy	
post menopausal	hormone therapy	bone density
(women)	o/estrogen/s replacement / therapy	bone mineral density

We will next link these search terms into a search strategy with the universal 'Boolean operators':

- OR: to retrieve records containing **either or any** of two or more terms (union of sets)
- AND: to retrieve records containing **both or all** of two or more terms together (intersection of sets)

Here is our provisional search strategy:

postmenopaus* OR post menopaus*

AND

hormone replacement or hormone therap* OR oestrogen* OR estrogen*

AND

osteoporosis OR bone density OR bone mineral density

Note that we have also 'truncated' word-endings, with the commonly used asterix (or Dialog's dollar sign) standing for any or no characters at the end of a word: essential to catch those plural -s/-es of search terms like oestrogen/oestrogens, and other word variants: e.g. postmenopaus* for postmenopause or postmenopausal.

(Some systems also use 'wildcards,' such as the question mark to stand for one or no characters within words, such as those British/American English variants like h?emorrhage, immuni?ation, and inconsistently hyphenated terms like post?menopausal.)

These are features common to many search systems, so our seedbed of search terms linked with operators into a search strategy can be used for different databases. Specific conventions or symbols may differ according to database, or to the search interfaces added by vendors who provide access to them, so check the 'Help' facility to save time and trouble, or ask your local librarians for a practical training session!

MEDLINE (22) is an excellent, general, health care database, superb for developing search skills, and it covers all health specialties, including nursing and health management. (Brazier (1996) compares MEDLINE and CINAHL (11) for nursing searches.) We will use here the free web version of MEDLINE, PubMED (27) – from the US National Library of Medicine. In or from your libraries, you will most likely find either Silver Platter's WEBSPIRS or WINSPIRS (i.e. web or Windows) 'versions' of this and other major databases, or Dialog's, on the KA24 service for NHS users, also on the web: these are commercial vendors, who add search software and screen interfaces to the database so it can be searched.

Using the History screen, we can build up searches (as on the Cochrane Library) linking sets with the # numbers (on the left below) assigned by the system to each search line we enter. So our first try, using an amended search strategy, might be as follows:

#1 (oestrogen* OR estrogen* OR hormone*) AND (replace* OR therapy)
#2 osteoporosis OR bone density OR bone mineral density
#3 #1 AND #2

(PubMED requires AND/OR to be capitalised: so it is easier to capitalise *everything*. Truncating terms, e.g. oestrogen* – tends to over-retrieve on

PubMED, but DO use it on other systems. And there is no wildcard, so I have not used 'post?menopausal'. On many databases, too, you might replace the AND of line 1 with NEAR, to retrieve records with two or more (sets of) terms in the same sentence of title, abstract, etc. rather than anywhere in the same record, but PubMED does not allow this.)

On PubMED and on the Cochrane Library, this strategy, produces nearly four times more references than a simple two-term search, 'HORMONE REPLACEMENT THERAPY AND OSTEOPOROSIS'. On PubMED, limiting to five years and to Human, we retrieve 451 RCTs AND 16 reviews with meta-analyses, as against 126 RCTs (thus missing a series of key trials) and five reviews with meta-analyses. On the Cochrane Library, we find 148 trials and 19 systematic reviews with a simple two-term strategy, 725 trials and 44 reviews with a high-sensitivity strategy as above (although many results will not be relevant in either set: in the reviews case because we are searching their full text reviews). Think of the quality material – even one good review or meta-analysis – that we might miss with an overly simple search strategy! We are so much less likely to miss important trials and high-quality reviews and meta-analyses by starting with a larger number of retrievals. It is a very common fault to narrow database searching too much at the outset: often through lack of skill, not choice. It is not that we want them *all*, but if we want to find the *best among them*, we need to be able to construct a high-sensitivity search, especially if the literature on our topic is not large, as well as to be able to make it more specific when we need to. This is the real skill of the expert searcher – adjusting sensitivity and specificity, and being able quickly to find the *best* within the rubbish – rather than, as Lancaster and Strauss (1999) appear to accuse librarians, wanting always to find 'everything' because we have the researcher search as our only model! (Is the alternative only to find *any* sound study as the best or whole evidence? And by informed choice, or, by default, through lack of skill?) All too often, there is no magic bullet which will take you straight to the best with nothing else around it. Setting title display and eyeballing a list of titles is often the best we can do with a batch of likely references. But having 'high-specificity' search skills without 'high-sensitivity' skills would be like driving a car, but knowing only how to turn left.

The 'free-text' or 'natural language' search ('Textword' on some databases including PubMED) is the default search of most databases. And the secret is simply this: when you enter a term, e.g. 'osteoporosis', you will retrieve records *containing* that term in the various 'fields', title, abstract, etc. This is not necessarily the same as retrieving records which are significantly *about* osteoporosis! You will get 'noise' – records in which 'osteoporosis' appears in an abstract of an article which has little to do with osteoporosis (even, in an extreme case, to mention it as excluded from the study). This really is the key to understanding database searching. The system matches character-strings, nothing more. Free text sensitivity can be too high, but you need high sensitivity if few studies have been published, or if language is inconsistent or vague, as is so often the case. It is also important to realise, on the other hand, that you get only what you put in, so you may get too little: with 'osteoporosis' you do not retrieve 'bone density', or even 'osteoporotic' in a free text search. Hence the need for covering wider options with search term variants, with term truncation or with a wider search strategy.

So the next stage might be to increase search specificity. There are several ways to do this. First, you can refine your free-text search, by leaving out terms that increase sensitivity at the expense of specificity, retaining only the most relevant terms in the strategy. Second, but not on PubMED, you can replace any AND in your strategy, if it links terms you might want to relate more closely, with NEAR, to retrieve terms in the same sentence of titles or abstracts, which are thus more likely to be semantically linked (e.g. nurs* near role*). Third, you can use the Thesaurus ,Subject or MeSH search: a higher level of search on many databases, but one which remains unexplored by many searchers, who are thus missing out on a powerful and sophisticated search tool.

The Thesaurus search uses standardised terms from a 'controlled vocabulary' or 'Thesaurus' of subject headings or 'descriptors.' These are applied by trained indexers (who read the original articles) to each database record, to indicate significant subject content. So this searching by subject 'tagging' is the computer equivalent of looking up articles *under a heading*, as in printed indexes, but with valuable additional features. A useful trick is to look through the subject headings of good articles retrieved – MeSH (Medical Subject Headings) on MEDLINE, DE (Descriptor) on CINAHL, EMBASE (15) and other databases – then do a Thesaurus or Subject search for more articles with the same heading. (Lowe & Barnett 1994 explain MeSH in detail, including 'tree structures'.)

In our search, by changing Display to 'MEDLINE,' we quickly discover three useful MeSH headings in some of the best of our retrieved records. Run a MeSH search on each heading in turn, then combine them, so our History looks as follows:

#1 Estrogen-Replacement-Therapy / all subheadings
#2 Osteoporosis, Postmenopausal / all subheadings
#3 Bone-Density / all subheadings
#4 #1 AND (#2 OR #3)

Finding only records indexed with the MeSH terms generally produces a higher specificity search. In this case, the MeSH search finds 106 RCTs and 5 meta-analyses: so it may have been too specific for locating the best reviews on this topic, and our complex free text strategy is more sensitive, for *our* specific purpose of not missing key trials. Using no Limits except five years and Human, it reduces 1334 hits of the two-term strategy and 5707 hits of the complex strategy to 703. (Which is 'better?' is not the key criterion: where is the best evidence, for the job at hand?) It is difficult to compare the two approaches directly, however, since PubMED, unlike most databases, does not entirely or obviously separate the free-text and the Thesaurus search options: it is actually often running *both* of them at once in the standard search, but hidden from the searcher's view. Click on Details when you enter a search to see this 'intelligent' feature, working behind the scenes, secretly adding MeSH terms to your search (unless you use the term truncation, which switches off the MeSH search!) to make it super-sensitive. All the more reason to use the MeSH to increase specificity when necessary and safe to do so – or, better, run both types of search and compare some results, *when it really matters.*

Within the Thesaurus search, 'explosion' (usually a default option) – increases sensitivity by searching narrower headings included under broader ones. ('Exploding' Heart Diseases, for example, will search all MeSH headings for specific heart diseases, for extremely high sensitivity. In our example, the broader MeSH term Osteoprosis includes Osteoporosis, Postmenopausal, and so broadens the MeSH search.)

Finally, 'subheadings', such as 'diagnosis', 'drug therapy', etc. can be added to qualify your headings, increasing specificity (often too much) if selected singly, but increasing sensitivity if 'All Subheadings' are added. (On PubMED, by not ticking any they will all be included.) Some subheadings (therapy, diagnosis, etc.) relate directly to question types or study types, as do many MeSH headings: so here again is a strong link between question and study types and actual search strategy.

The decision about how *thorough* your search should be is always yours. Clinicians may prefer the focus and speed of the Thesaurus: researchers who want comprehensiveness will use complex free-text strategies, or (like PubMED) combine both approaches for maximum sensitivity. More often than not, it is a question of degree, not a simple either-or. Much depends on the terminology of the topic, and how consistently it is used by authors, and on the size and complexity of its literature. A higher sensitivity strategy is often needed, not to increase retrievals from 50 to 400, but from 2 to 6! There is often no useful Thesaurus term, Thesaurus terms are American–English especially for new developments and indexing quality varies. Not all databases have a Thesaurus option, so *both* types of search skills really are needed. (The Cochrane Library has both fully and partially indexed databases, so both approaches must be combined, and for each search term.) A skilled searcher is able quickly to construct and test both high-sensitivity and high-specificity searches, using free text and Thesaurus, moving skilfully between them so as not to miss that elusive gold!

On the major databases you can also use the Limit feature to separate out the RCTs, guidelines, reviews or meta-analyses by 'publication type' – our question-study-strategy link once again. (On PubMED, always Limit by Publication Year – or search MEDLINE back to 1966, by default!)

Search filters are another way of increasing search specificity. These are pre-written search strategies using research methodology terms, in free text, descriptors or Limits, designed and tested to retrieve study types appropriate to diagnosis, prognosis, therapy, or aetiology / harm / risk, some of the question types we began with – hence their other name 'methodologic filters'. Here again is a very strong link between question type and search strategy. There are usually high-sensitivity and high-specificity versions. They are downloadable from some websites (122), to be saved to disk and combined with your search. On PubMED, they are stored as Clinical Queries, along with a super-sensitive systematic review strategy. Those produced at McMaster University in Canada (McKibbon & Walker-Dilks 1993, 1994a, 1994b, McKibbon et al 1995, Walker-Dilks et al 1994) have been tested over a range of searches, and published – most recently by McKibbon, along with search filters for MEDLINE, CINAHL, PsycINFO and EMBASE (McKibbon 1999).

For those who systematically review the literature, a high sensitivity RCT filter has been developed by the Cochrane Centre (available in the Cochrane Library Handbook). (RCTs have not always been clearly identified by authors or indexers, and many have only been traced by journal hand-searches.) MEDLINE's 'publication type' of 'randomised controlled trial' only commenced use in 1991, since when many RCTs have been indexed retrospectively on MEDLINE (Dickerson et al 1995).

Using our developed HRT strategy on MEDLINE yields some excellent reviews, trials and original studies in which evidence might have remained buried. But it is *essential* to search other databases if we do not want to miss vital material. Coverage of even the larger databases is never comprehensive: MEDLINE covers nearly 4000 published journals of a potentially relevant 2000 or more! Brettle and Long (2001), for example, compare several databases for mental health rehabilitation, finding only 42% of their papers at most in any one database, and McDonald et al (1999) found that four major databases were needed to cover even 52% of 977 identified psychiatry journals. So, after MEDLINE, we must try EMBASE, a superb 'European' complement to MEDLINE, and a clear reason to use systems like KA24 which include it with MEDLINE and other databases, or CINAHL for nursing and allied health: a useful trio of databases for most health care topics, to which we might add PSYCINFO for human behaviour and psychology-related issues, AMED (3) for alternative or complementary therapies, and so on. Subject-specific databases such as POPLINE, TOXLINE, AGEINFO and discipline- or profession-specific databases, such as PEDRO for physiotherapy are increasingly available. (See Select List of Resources). For decisions about clinical interventions, we might begin with the specialised Cochrane Library databases, with their systematic reviews and trials register, and then try general or subject databases. Citation indexes such as Science Citation Index (34) trace the 'descendants' of an article by showing which other papers have cited it. 'Grey' or unpublished literature is sometimes important, so a major database, SIGLE (31), attempts to cope with the tip of this iceberg at least, and the HMIC databases (20) contain some grey health care material, as does the UK Department of Health website (102). We now have wider access to very large databases of research journals, such as Web of Knowledge (34), formerly BIDS, and the mammoth ZETOC (35). Booth (1998) gives case studies, following specific questions through various resources: a key information skill we all need to develop to cope with the new complexity.

As well as the large databases, specialised or 'value-added' databases, will continue to appear, and the boundaries will change: what, really, is a 'database'? There is an urgent need for clinical 'question-and-answer databases', containing 'frequently updated, evidence-based, peer-reviewed answers to specific common clinical questions' rather than references or even full-text journal articles. Chambliss and Conley (1996: 144) found that MEDLINE searches answered some three-quarters of their clinical questions in general practice, but that searching and appraising journal articles was 'time-consuming and expensive'. Ely et al (2002) suggest that addressing the range of 'obstacles' that medical doctors face in answering questions about patient care, which they identify and classify across the main steps in evidence-based practice (including issues about question formulation, resources access and trustworthiness, information skills and so on), would lead to better patient care by improving 'clinically oriented information resources'. Resources like MD DIGESTS (63) and INFORMED (62), in addition to the quick review and evidence summary resources already mentioned, will develop further to help clinicians keep up with key papers relevant to clinical decision-making.

National databases of *evidence-based guidelines* would also clearly be of enormous value for all clinical practitioners: NICE and NeLH have begun to make this easier in the UK. We also need to search more easily across resources, which are usually produced by different companies or organisations, and use different indexing systems and headings, so inter-database approaches, such as meta-thesauri and SignPosts are being developed (Hammond 2001). Integrated desktop information and clinical support systems, such as Doctors Desk (103) and Prodigy (120) will also further evolve, and specialised web search engines like TRIP (124) allow us to search across selected high-quality resources at a sitting, to help answer clinical questions more quickly and at point of need.

Searching the larger databases is not an arcane process, to be avoided through lack of skill,or even time! Even a quick search can produce good results, and with a moderate investment of time to learn and practise, searching becomes faster and more effective, a rewarding skill of enormous value. With practice, you as a subject expert can think through your search and find good search terms better than any current software. It can be enjoyable finding the wealth of material which is hidden from the unskilled searcher, or non-searcher. It depends far less on being 'computer-literate' than on the ability to find and test the best search terms, and to broaden or narrow a search strategy at will.

Database search skills will always be needed. As web access to databases increases, many are donning web interfaces, and looking more like web search engines, with their dangerous temptation to use single-term searching, despite the often disastrous consequences. Stern (1999) describes such 'intelligent' features as keyword access, value-added metadata, customised interfaces which make searching (appear?) easier, semantic analysis, smart-agent assistance – but reminds us that 'regardless of the technological advances, there will always be a need for critical thinking skills in order to perform an adequate database search.'

World-Wide Websites

The growth of the Internet – that staggering global interconnection of computers in over 130 countries worldwide, of which the World-Wide Web of information pages is the information heart – has fundamentally transformed the ways we disseminate and access information. Rather than a single resource that we search, like a database, it is a pervasive means of access to personal, academic, organisational, institutional and government websites, with interlinked pages of information, and with their links to further sites ad infinitum, which may contain or lead to almost every type of information resource: searchable databases, library catalogues, 'electronic' journals, evidence summaries, trials registers, guidelines, information gateways and 'virtual libraries'. Many of the good things you can find have already been described.

The basic prerequisite is a computer with a 'web-browser' (such as Internet Explorer or Netscape Navigator) which manages the operations of web-use, and web connection through a service provider. Three basic search operations are used to find, visit and move between web-pages and websites:

1. clicking on 'hypertext links' (often underlined words) on web-pages
2. typing in 'web-addresses' (technical term: Uniform Resource Locators or URLs) of specific sites
3. using 'search engines' or 'gateways' to find websites by entering search terms or clicking on headings or links.

Some search engines have Advanced Search features, using the ANDs, ORs and truncation of major databases, for higher-specificity searches. Since there is generally no equivalent to the Thesaurus search (although BIOME has MeSH indexing, and many search engines have subject lists or categories to browse), you will need creative 'free-text' search skills, trying out different search terms and term variants, to find the best. Searches on the web can be slow and time-consuming. There is no universal 'telephone directory,' so it can be difficult to get answers to specific questions. To cope a little better with the chaos, we now have sophisticated 'meta-search' engines like Metacrawler (109) AlltheWeb (89) or IxQuick (106), which use other search engines, 'intelligent' search engines like Google (104) and specialised health care search engines like BIOME (91). But no search engine searches *all* the web, so get to know more than one! Well-designed gateway sites such as OncoLink (117) offer graphical site maps and indexes. Specialised 'subject gateways' like SOSIG (123) are, in effect, virtual libraries created by experts with organised, clearly structured, hierarchical layouts, providing links to a wide variety of high-quality web resources. Directories, often confused with search engines (but the boundaries of all these things shift and blur), offer structured and browseable indexes or subject menus of links, such as Yahoo

(127). Unfortunately, very many websites are created with unhelpful design from an information-finder's perspective.

For our HRT and osteoporosis example, a quick BIOME search produces a dozen likely sites with access to tutorials, organisations, bibliographies, reviews of epidemiological studies, clinical practice guidelines, links to more sites, and journals, and this is just a start. Rather than simply using a single, favourite search engine to find miscellaneous websites of very varying quality, we can focus, to begin with, on trustworthy organisational sites, on quality subject gateways, on web databases (so many and so hard to find using search engines that the phrase 'invisible web' has been coined) and on the web journal sites, already mentioned: islands of quality and reliability in the vast sea of rubbish.

Quality of information as evidence is extremely variable: the crunch issues are authority and reliability, since anyone can set up a website, and claim almost anything. Stick to sites and sources you can trust, from academic, health service, professional or official organisations, such as the excellent NeLH (110). Use high-quality and trustworthy subject gateways (check the Pinakes (119) list), such as BIOME which vets its immediate links for quality, or TRIP, a search engine (actually a database of links) which searches across reliable 'evidence-based' resources. Do not miss Netting the Evidence, a treasure trove of evidence-based resources and links from ScHARR (122). Even so, critically evaluate websites, as you would any other information resources, carefully checking support organisations or sponsors, and their update frequency, if you intend to use or cite their information as evidence. (The BIOME site contains a comprehensive list of its own website 'evaluation questions'.)

Having said this, the range of information is truly amazing, and growing fast. For books on health care and the Internet try Kiley (1999), broader than its title suggests, and with its own website of links to a host of resources. Welsh (2001) is clear and detailed. For a health consumer viewpoint, see Kiley and Graham (2002). For a continuing update on health-related web matters, seek out the newsletter He@lth Information on the Internet (45), and for general Internet matters, try Tips & Advice Internet (54), 'your fortnightly navigator on the information highway'. They may be in your local library.

Finally, why not join a discussion list to contact experts, debate current issues, exchange information or simply 'lurk?' Check the directory of EBH-related lists at ScHARR (122).

REVIEWING THE SEARCH PROCESS

Finally, we must review and evaluate the whole search process, revisiting each stage, if necessary, and repeating those we have any doubts about. We may need to find and use further resources, or even reformulate our question, until we have the information which could be used as evidence to address it in the way we need to, or until we are reasonably certain that it does not currently exist. Evidence-based practice offers a *model* for these processes, one in which doubts or knowledge gaps can be raised and dealt with objectively and transparently. We can almost never be certain that we have not missed anything, but our certainty that there is a genuine knowledge gap only increases with the thoroughness of our search. So we need at each stage to question resource appropriateness, coverage, currency, reliability and authority – and our own skills in finding and exploiting the resources effectively.

We may return to the problematic situation, but with a clearer understanding of the evidence currently available or not available – the state of current 'knowledge'. Data which might provide information which can be used as evidence might still have to be collected or produced. (Identifying 'questions of major importance to the NHS for which good research evidence is currently lacking' is of interest to the NHS R&D Health Technology Assessment Programme [114]). But we can only feel reasonably certain of search thoroughness if we know we are truly able to find information to use as evidence from a wide range of resources, appropriate to each question type and level, and to widen or narrow our search 'net' – both for and within resources – according to need, context and result. We need to know what the key skills are, and to have practised and developed them *reflectively*, as with any other skills. We must also know our limits, and be able to seek professional, specialist search help when we need it. We need to be able to estimate how comprehensive or exhaustive we might be for a given search, and accurately evaluate the search process to assess our own success in answering the question.

Evidence-based health care practice and development are very strongly dependent indeed on the ability to find and process appropriate kinds of information to use as evidence. The key information skills are:

- formulating a clear and structured question to ground and guide the search
- identifying the type of question being asked
- recognising the type of information which could be used as evidence, from the strongest to the weakest, appropriate to each type of question
- recognising the type of study which would provide such information
- identifying primary or secondary resources which give us access to the results of such studies
- developing high-sensitivity *and* high-specificity search strategies from the question
- exploiting modern information resources by using the full capability of modern search software
- evaluating and refining the search stages until the question is answered satisfactorily, or it is reasonably certain that the data does not exist.

References

Booth A 1998 Following the evidence trail: EBHC on the Internet. He@lth Information on the Internet 1(1) (URL: http://www.wellcome.ac.uk/healthinfo/)

Brassey J, Elwyn G, Price C et al 2001 Just in time information for clinicians: a questionnaire evaluation of the ATTRACT project. British Medical Journal 322:529-530

Brazier H 1996 Selecting a database for literature searches in nursing: MEDLINE or CINAHL? Journal of Advanced Nursing 24:868-875

Brettle A, Long A 2001 Comparison of bibliographic databases for information on the rehabilitation of people with severe mental illness. Bulletin of the Medical Library Association 89:353-362

Chambliss M, Conley J 1996 Answering clinical questions. The Journal of Family Practice 43:140-144

Dickerson K, Scherer R, Lefebvre C 1995 Identifying relevant studies for systematic reviews. In: Chalmers I, Altman D G (eds) Systematic reviews. British Medical Journal Publishing, London, p 17-36

Ely J W, Osheroff J A, Ebell M H et al 2002 Obstacles to answering doctors' questions about patient care with evidence: qualitative study. British Medical Journal 324(7339):710

Enkin M, Jadad A 1998 Using anecdotal information in evidence-based health care: Heresy or necessity? Annals of Oncology 9:963-966

Ezzo J, Bausell B, Moerman D E et al 2001 Reviewing the reviews: How strong is the evidence? How clear are the conclusions? International Journal of Technology Assessment in Health Care 17:457-466

Fletcher G 2002 Averting the crisis in medical publishing: open access journals. He@lth Information on the Internet (30):6-7 – Available on BioMed Central Website: see List of Resources 92

Goffman E 1961 Asylums: essays on the social situation of mental patients and other inmates. Anchor, New York

Hammond R 2001 Negotiating the medical maze. Library Association Record 103:218-220

Kiley R 1999 Medical information on the Internet: a guide for health professionals. 2nd edn. Churchill Livingstone, Edinburgh (www.churchillmed.com/Books/MedInter/kiley.html)

Kiley R, Graham E 2002 The patient's Internet handbook. Royal Society of Medicine Press, London

Lancaster T, Straus S 1999 Practising evidence-based primary care. Radcliffe Medical Press, Abingdon

Lowe H, Barnett G 1994 Understanding and using the Medical Subject Headings (MeSH) vocabulary to perform literature searches. Journal of the American Medical Association 271:1103-1108

McColl A, Smith H, White P et al 1998 General practitioners' perceptions of the route to evidence-based medicine: a questionnaire survey. British Medical Journal 316:361-365

McDonald S, Taylor L, Adams C et al 1999 Searching the right database: a comparison of four databases for psychiatry journals. Health Libraries Review 16:151-156

McKibbon K, Haynes R B, Walker-Dilks C J et al 1990 How good are clinical MEDLINE searches? A comparative study of clinical end-user and librarian searches. Computers and Biomedical Research 23: 583-593

McKibbon K, Haynes R B, Johnston M E et al 1991 A study to enhance clinical end-user MEDLINE search skills: design and baseline findings. In: Clayton P D (ed) Fifteenth annual symposium on computer applications in medical care: a conference of the American Medical Informatics Association, Washington DC, 1991. McGraw-Hill, New York

McKibbon K, Walker-Dilks C 1993 Panning for applied clinical research gold. Online July:105-108

McKibbon K, Walker-Dilks C 1994a Beyond ACP Journal Club: How to harness

MEDLINE for diagnostic problems. [Editorial]. ACP Journal Club September/October: A10-12 (Annals of Internal Medicine 121 Suppl 2)

McKibbon K, Walker-Dilks C 1994b Beyond ACP Journal Club: How to harness MEDLINE for therapy problems. [Editorial]. ACP Journal Club July/August: A10-12 (Annals of Internal Medicine 121 Suppl 1)

McKibbon K, Walker-Dilks C, Haynes R B et al 1995 Beyond ACP Journal Club: How to harness MEDLINE for prognosis problems. [Editorial]. ACP Journal Club July/August: A12-14

McKibbon K 1999 PDQ Evidence-based principles and practice. BC Decker, Hamilton, Canada

Mulrow C 1987 The medical review article: state of the science. Annals of Internal Medicine 106:485-488

Mulrow C, Cook D 1998 Systematic reviews: synthesis of best evidence for health care decisions. American College of Physicians, Philadelphia

Novak JD, Gowin D 1984 Learning how to learn. Cambridge University Press, Cambridge

Oxman A 1995 Checklists for review articles. In: Chalmers I, Altman D (eds) Systematic reviews. British Medical Journal Publishing, London, p 75-85

Popay J, Williams G 1998 Qualitative research and evidence-based health care. Journal of the Royal Society of Medicine 91 (Suppl 35):32-37

Richardson W S, Wilson M C Nishikawa J et al 1995 The well-built clinical question: a key to evidence-based decisions. [Editorial]. ACP Journal Club 123:A12-13

Richardson W S, Wilson M 1997 On questions, background and foreground. Clinical Epidemiology and Biostatistics: 6-7

Shelstad K, Clevenger F 1994 On-line strategies of third-year medical students: perception vs fact. Journal of Surgical Research 56:338-344

Snowball R 1997 Using the clinical question to teach search strategy: fostering transferable conceptual skills in user education by active learning. Health Libraries Review 14:167-172

Stern D 1999 New search and navigation techniques in the digital library. Science & Technology Libraries 17:61-80

Stern J, Simes R 1997 Publication bias: evidence of delayed publication in a cohort study of clinical research projects. British Medical Journal 315:640-645

Walker-Dilks C, McKibbon K, Haynes R 1994 Beyond ACP Journal Club: How to harness MEDLINE for aetiology problems. [Editorial]. ACP Journal Club November/December:A10-11

Welsh S et al 2001 Finding and using health and medical information on the Internet. Aslib-IMI, London

Select list of information resources

1 Databases
2 Secondary journals
3 Evidence-based bulletins, summaries etc.
4 Library catalogues
5 Research and trials registers
6 Evidence-based guidelines
7 Web gateways and search engines – and other useful websites

1 Databases

Databases for which availability details are not given below are probably major databases, usually acquired by institutional subscriptions from a commercial or other service provider: check your **local health care library** for access to these (and others), such as the KA24 service for UK NHS staff. Bear in mind that web-accessible resources are not necessarily free; on the other hand, 'registration', when required, does not always incur a cost! (For some databases, or on some systems, 'Athens registration' is required. You can register free, if eligible, on the Athens website: http://www.athens.ac.uk/)

1 **AGEINFO CD-ROM** database produced by Centre for Policy on Ageing: www.cpa.org.uk
2 **AIDSLINE** Clinical and research aspects of AIDS, epidemiology, health policy, social issues etc. from Government reports, meeting abstracts, books and theses. Separate database until 2000, now in MEDLINE (22)
3 **ALLIED & COMPLEMENTARY MEDICINE DATABASE (AMED)** British Library database for a whole range of allied health, alternative medicine and complementary therapies from 400+ journals.
4 **ASSIA** (Applied Social Sciences Index & Abstracts) Subscription database of references from 500+ English-language journals from 16 countries on social work, sociology, social and economic aspects of health care, education, ethnic studies, mental health etc., from Cambridge Scientific Abstracts: www.csa1.co.uk

BIDS see WEB OF KNOWLEDGE (34)

5 **BIOETHICSLINE** Ethical issues, public policy, resource allocation etc. in medicine and health care, current biomedical research, from many sources. Separate database until 2000: now in MEDLINE (22)
6 **BIOLOGICAL ABSTRACTS** Enormous database of references and abstracts of articles from over 6000 journals, from 1985, on all aspects of life sciences, medical research, etc.
7 **BRITISH NURSING INDEX** Printed index and CD-ROM or web database (not free) covering some 220 English-language journals in nursing, midwifery, community health care indexed within six weeks of publication, from BNI Publications, University of Bournemouth.
8 **CAB HEALTH** Database of citations from CAB International, covering over 16 000 journals from 130 countries, plus books, research reports, dissertations and conference proceedings, on communicable diseases and disease control, tropical and parasitic diseases, nutrition and nutritional disorders, environmental and public health, etc.
9 **CENTRE FOR RESEARCH IN ETHNIC RELATIONS DATABASE** Free web database of ethnic relations (including health) issues, compiled by Warwick University Clinical Sciences Library: www.warwick.ac.uk/fac/soc/CRER_RC/search.html
10 **CHILDDATA** Subscription database from National Children's Bureau, who also produce ChildData Abstracts, a monthly listing of publications and research in child welfare topics. www.ncb.org.uk
11 **CINAHL** (Cumulative Index to Nursing & Allied Health Literature) Key database of references with abstracts and reference lists from nursing and allied health care journals, conference proceedings, standards of professional practice, guidelines (full-text), nursing dissertations, from 1982.
12 **COCHRANE LIBRARY** High-quality evidence from a 'library' of databases from the International Cochrane Collaboration (see website for information and newsletters etc.: http://cochrane.org) and the NHS CENTRE FOR REVIEWS AND DISSEMINATION (113). Cochrane Library is now free on the web from NeLH (110):
   1. Cochrane Database of Systematic Reviews (CDSR): *full-text* Cochrane systematic reviews of health care interventions: details of completed reviews, with updates; 'protocols' for ongoing reviews.
   2. Database of Abstracts of Reviews of Effectiveness (DARE): NHS Centre for Reviews and Dissemination reviews – abstracts only. (Also free on CRD (113) website.)
   3. Cochrane Central Register of Controlled Trials (CCRCT): A register of over 350 000 controlled trials, many not in other databases, many unpublished.
   4. Cochrane Review Methodology Database (CRMD): Details of articles on research synthesis, systematic reviewing etc.
   5. NHS EED (NHS Economic Evaluation Database): Economic evaluations of health care interventions. (Also free on NHS CRD (113) website.)
   6. Health Technology Assessment Database (HTA): Reviews of health care interventions: ongoing and completed assessments. (Also free on NHS CRD (113) website.)

DARE (DATABASE OF ABSTRACTS & REVIEWS OF EFFECTIVENESS) see COCHRANE

LIBRARY (12) and **NHS CENTRE FOR REVIEWS AND DISSEMINATION** (113).
DoH-DATA see **HMIC** (20)

13　**DISSERTATION ABSTRACTS** Database of 1.6 million citations with abstracts to doctoral and masters' theses and dissertations from international educational institutions, in all disciplines, with full-text access to 100 000 dissertations – from ProQuest Digital Dissertations at: wwwlib.umi.com – subscription database and services, with some free searching.

14　**ECONLIT** Database from American Economic Association, containing citations from 400+ economics and related journals, books, book reviews, conference proceedings and working papers, from 1969 www.econlit.org

15　**EMBASE** Key database covering all aspects of medicine and health care (strong on drug information and pharmacology) with citations and abstracts from 4000 journals (up to two-thirds not on MEDLINE) from 70 countries, 1980 onwards, with strong European journal coverage. Produced by Elsevier Science: www.elsevier.com

16　**EXTRAMED CD-ROM** database of full-text articles from over 300 biomedical journals from 61 Third World countries, updated monthly. Started in 1993 as a WHO initiative, now produced by its founder's company Informania Ltd. Covers tropical diseases, traditional medicine, biodiversity, communicable diseases, health development studies, etc.

17　**HEALTH-CD** Full-text subscription database from UK Stationery Office (TSO The Information Management Company: www.tso.co.uk/site.asp?), with WinSPIRS search software. Unique source of legislation, guidance notes, newsletters, UK health management reports and other 'grey' literature.

18　**HEALTH PROMIS** The free web-based national public health database for England: evidence-based public health, health promotion and health inequalities, with references and document links to books and journal articles: http://healthpromis.hda-online.org.uk

19　**HEALTHSTAR** Health care policy, planning, administration, delivery and economics, health services research, clinical practice guidelines, health care technology assessment, etc. from journals, books, official reports, conference papers and newspaper articles. Separate database until 2000: now in **MEDLINE** (22).

20　**HMIC (HEALTH MANAGEMENT INFORMATION CONSORTIUM)** Set of three databases: DoH Data (Dept. of Health), HELMIS (Nuffield Institute of Health), until recently, and King's Fund Library database. Health service policy, management, organisation, finance, quality of care etc., worldwide from 1983, from journals, books, reports, official publications and 'grey' (unpublished) literature.

HTA (HEALTH TECHNOLOGY ASSESSMENTS) DATABASE see **COCHRANE LIBRARY** (12) and **NHS CENTRE FOR REVIEWS AND DISSEMINATION** (113).

INDEX TO SCIENTIFIC & TECHNICAL PROCEEDINGS see **WEB OF KNOWLEDGE** (34)

21　**INDEX TO THESES** Comprehensive listing of theses with abstracts accepted for higher degrees by universities in the UK and Ireland – printed index, with web access via personal or institutional subscription: www.theses.com

22　**MEDLINE** Database version of printed indexes Index Medicus and International Nursing Index, produced by US National Library of Medicine. Key general health care database, covering medicine, allied health, health management, nursing and midwifery. References (80% with abstracts) from 4500 journals worldwide, from 1966. Includes material from 2001 previously on **AIDSLINE, BIOETHICSLINE,** and **HEALTHSTAR** databases. Free web access as **PUBMED** (27).

23　**NATIONAL LIBRARY OF MEDICINE (NLM) GATEWAY** Access to several databases and US National Library of Medicine resources, including **TOXNET** (33), **ClinicalTrials.gov** (72), **NLM** Library catalogue etc. www.gateway.nlm.nih.gov

24　**NHS NEED (NHS ECONOMIC EVALUATION DATABASE)** see **COCHRANE LIBRARY** (12) and **NHS CENTRE FOR REVIEWS AND DISSEMINATION** (113).

25　**PEDRO (PHYSIOTHERAPY EVIDENCE DATABASE)** Abstracts of systematic reviews and randomised controlled trials in physiotherapy, free on the web at: ptwww.cchs.usyd.edu.au/pedro

26　**POPLINE** Billed as 'the world's largest reproductive health database' with 'citations with abstracts of the worldwide literature in the field of population, family planning and related health issues'. Covers books, reports, journal articles, theses and more: http://db.jhuccp.org/popinform/index.stm

27 **PUBMED** Free web version of **MEDLINE** (22) at http://www.pubmed.gov

28 **PSYCINFO** Database from the American Psychological Association with references and abstracts of articles from 1300 journals from 50 countries – and from published books, reports and dissertations – on psychology, psychiatry, mental health, human behaviour and many related disciplines.

29 **ReFeR (RESEARCH FINDINGS ELECTRONIC REGISTER)** Free web database for quality assured information on research findings that emerge from completed projects funded by the **DEPARTMENT OF HEALTH** (102), including the NHS Executive: www.info.doh.gov.uk/doh/refr_web.nsf/Home?OpenForm

30 **REGARD** Web-accessible free database from University of Bristol, funded by Economic and Social Research Council (ESRC), for details of ESRC-funded research awards and projects in wide range of social sciences and related research, including health-related, with details of publications: www.regard.ac.uk

SCIENCE CITATION INDEX see **WEB OF KNOWLEDGE** (34)

31 **SIGLE** (System for Information on Grey Literature in Europe) British Library database produced by EAGLE (European Association for Grey Literature Exploitation), a consortium of major European libraries, of reports, dissertations and other 'grey' literature not formally published, and difficult to identify and obtain. All subjects, with availability details, including British Library shelfmarks.

SOCIAL SCIENCE CITATION INDEX see **WEB OF KNOWLEDGE** (34)

32 **SOCIOLOGICAL ABSTRACTS (SOCIOFILE)** Subscription database of research in sociology, social and behavioural sciences, social policy, social aspects of health etc. from over 2600 journals, plus conference proceedings, books and dissertations, from Cambridge Scientific Abstracts: www.csa1.co.uk

33 **TOXNET: (TOXicology Data NETwork)** Free web database covering toxic and other effects of drugs, chemicals, and physical agents; adverse drug reactions, carcinogenesis, environmental pollution, food contamination, water treatment, pesticides, herbicides, risk assessment etc., from **NATIONAL LIBRARY OF MEDICINE (NLM) GATEWAY** (23): www.gateway.nlm.nih.gov

34 **WEB OF KNOWLEDGE** (WoK) (Formerly BIDS Databases) Web-based suite of very useful databases at http://wok.mimas.ac.uk – (Athens registration required) –
   1. Citation Databases for general searching of large numbers of journals or tracing journal article citations: Arts & Humanities Citation Index, Science Citation Index, Social Sciences Citation Index;
   2. Other WoS Databases: Index to Scientific and Technical Proceedings (ISTP): Science and technology conferences, seminars, workshops, and conventions. (Covers only publications in which the proceedings are published for the first time – and only those containing complete papers, not just abstracts); Journal Citation Reports database (JCR): Journal citation data, impact factors and title changes in science, technology, social sciences.

35 **ZETOC** (Electronic Table of Contents) In partnership with MIMAS and JISC, a huge British Library database of citations to some 20 000 research journals, 2.5 million conference papers, etc., in all subjects, very strong in health care. Free web access via NeLH (110) – but if accessed outside NHSNet, Athens registration is required (see Note above).

2 Secondary journals

Primary journals with a strong research/review, methodology or effectiveness emphasis, or an Internet interest.

36 **ACP JOURNAL CLUB** Secondary bi-monthly journal from American College of Physicians, containing summaries of significant articles 'that warrant immediate attention by physicians attempting to keep pace with important advances in treatment, prevention, diagnosis, cause, prognosis and economics of the disorders managed by internists' from 80 major medical and other health care journals, with expert commentary on practice perspectives and editorials on evidence-based practice issues. www.acpjc.org

37 **CLINICAL EFFECTIVENESS IN NURSING** Quarterly journal published by Elsevier Science. Peer-reviewed articles with peer commentaries on clinical interventions and outcomes in all nursing, midwifery, health visiting and allied health specialties, with emphasis on the 'impact on patients and clients. www.harcourt-international.com/journals/cein

38 **CONTROLLED CLINICAL TRIALS** Official monthly journal of the Society for Clinical Trials, published by Elsevier Science six times annually, with articles on design, methods, operational aspects of controlled clinical trials and follow-up studies, and associated operational, methodological, legal and ethical problems and solutions. www.elsevier.com/locate/issn/01972456

39 **DISEASE MANAGEMENT AND HEALTH OUTCOMES** Monthly journal published by Adis International to provide practical information on the latest developments in disease management and health outcomes assessment based on best evidence. Focus on 'total disease management', disease management programmes and tools, and clinical and economic outcomes measurement. www.adis.co.uk

40 **EVIDENCE-BASED CARDIOVASCULAR MEDICINE** Quarterly secondary journal published by Harcourt International, with summaries of and commentaries on key, high-quality articles from 'over 70 of the most authoritative and respected journals in the field', and with educational articles on evidence-based practice. www.harcourt-international.com/journals/ebcm

41 **EVIDENCE-BASED HEALTH CARE** (formerly EVIDENCE-BASED HEALTH POLICY AND MANAGEMENT) Quarterly secondary journal published by Harcourt International, with summaries of high-quality research articles on organisation and management of health care, and evidence-based practice, to provide managers with the best available evidence. www.harcourt-international.com/journals/ebhc

42 **EVIDENCE-BASED MEDICINE** Bi-monthly secondary journal published by BMJ Publishing Group and American College of Physicians, to 'alert clinicians to important advances' in a wide range of medical and health care disciplines, with summaries of key original and review articles from the literature, and commentaries by clinical experts. Website of EBM Online, with full-text: http://ebm.bmjjournals.com/current.shtml

43 **EVIDENCE-BASED MENTAL HEALTH** Quarterly secondary journal in mental health issues from BMJ Publishing Group, for clinicians, therapists, managers and policy makers.

44 **EVIDENCE-BASED NURSING** Quarterly secondary journal, published by RCN Publishing Company and BMJ Publishing Group, with the help of the Health Information Research Unit (**HIRU** see (105) below) at McMaster University, Canada. Each issue identifies and appraises 24 high-quality, clinical research articles or reviews published in primary journals, with critical abstracts, and commentaries by nurses to place the research in context. http://ebn.bmjjournals.com

EVIDENCE-BASED PURCHASING See (60) below.

45 **HEALTH INFORMATION ON THE INTERNET** Published six times per year by the Royal Society of Medicine Press. Original articles, news, hints and tips, new sites, reviews. www.hioti.org

46 **INTERNET RESOURCES NEWSLETTER** Free monthly newsletter from Heriot-Watt University Library of Web resources for academic users. www.hw.ac.uk/libWWW/irn

47 **JOURNAL OF CLINICAL EPIDEMIOLOGY** Monthly journal from Elsevier Science, concerned with research in chronic illness, encompassing clinical epidemiology, clinical medicine and biostatistics, including Pharmacoepidemiology Reports for rapid publication of clinical epidemiologic investigations of pharmaceutical agents. Articles also on methodological issues, such as design and analysis of trials: and observational studies, evaluation and measurement, statistical techniques and computer applications. www.elsevier.com/inca/publications/store/5/2/5/4/7/2/index.htt

48 **JOURNAL OF CLINICAL GOVERNANCE** (formerly Journal of Clinical Effectiveness) Quarterly multidisciplinary journal from Radcliffe Medical Press, Abingdon, Oxon. (www.radcliffe-oxford.com), aims to inform 'people involved in clinical governance about effective methods and innovations', with a strong primary care focus.

49 **JOURNAL OF EVALUATION IN CLINICAL PRACTICE** Quarterly journal from Blackwell Science Ltd, promoting critical enquiry into, and evaluation of, clinical practice in medicine,

nursing and other health professions; clinical audit, outcome measurement and guidelines are also considered.www.blacksci.co.uk

50   **JOURNAL OF FAMILY PRACTICE** Monthly journal from Dowden Health Media which publishes original research, clinical updates, brief reports and 'applied evidence' articles – and POEMs (Patient-Oriented Evidence that Matters), for which the editorial team reviews some 90 journals each month, 'and identifies articles you need to know about to stay up to date.' Website JFP Online provides e-mail discussion of issues raised by articles, EBP Newsletter, primary care links etc. www.jfponline.com

51   **JOURNAL OF QUALITY IN CLINICAL PRACTICE** Quarterly journal published by Blackwell Publishing as the official journal of the Australian Council on Health care Standards and the Australian Medical Association, with original articles 'addressed primarily to the factual reporting of peer review activity within hospitals and health care institutions', health policy and clinical review. www.blackwellpublishing.com/journals/jqc

52   **NT RESEARCH** Sister journal to Nursing Times, published bi-monthly by Emap Health care, with original clinical research papers on a wide range of nursing and related areas 'to encourage evidence-based practice and improve the quality of patient care', with review articles and critical commentary by academic peers. (Link from Nursing Times website: www.nursingtimes.com)

53   **QUALITY AND SAFETY IN HEALTH CARE** (Formerly QUALITY IN HEALTH CARE) A quarterly interdisciplinary journal from BMJ Publishing and Institute for Health care Improvement, with original articles, quality improvement reports, case studies, and reviews on all aspects of improving quality and safety of health care, medication safety, patients' perspectives and consumer views, organisational learning and management, and relevant research from other fields: http://qhc.bmjjournals.com/misc/about.shtml

54   **TIPS & ADVICE INTERNET** 'Your fortnightly navigator on the information highway' in printed newsletter form or on the Web, by subscription: www.indicator.com/BIT

3 Evidence–based bulletins, summaries, etc

55   **ATTRACT** Check out the quick reviews done to date, and find out about the project at www.attract.wales.nhs.uk

56   **BANDOLIER** Monthly Internet journal from Pain Research at Oxford 'about health care, using evidence-based medicine techniques to provide advice about particular treatments or diseases for health care professionals and consumers. The content is 'tertiary' publishing, distilling the information from (secondary) reviews of (primary) trials and making it comprehensible'. Contains summaries (title refers to 'bullet points') on drug and treatment interventions and on many matters of interest in EBP. Read it free at: www.jr2.ox.ac.uk/bandolier

57   **CLINICAL EVIDENCE** A printed book series, published six-monthly, from BMJ Publishing and American College of Physicians, a 'compendium of evidence on the effects of common clinical interventions' with summaries of the 'current state of knowledge, ignorance and uncertainty about the prevention and treatment of a wide range of clinical conditions, based on thorough searches of the literature'. Now available as a free web database from **NeLH** (110).

58   **EFFECTIVE HEALTH CARE BULLETIN** Bi-monthly bulletins for decision-makers which examine the clinical effectiveness, cost-effectiveness and acceptability of specific health care interventions, based on systematic review and synthesis of research. Available free and full-text (including 10 years of back-issues) from their new publishers: **NHS CENTRE FOR REVIEWS AND DISSEMINATION** (113).

59   **EFFECTIVENESS MATTERS** Occasional peer-reviewed free printed bulletins, to complement **EFFECTIVE HEALTH CARE BULLETIN** by **NHS CENTRE FOR REVIEWS AND DISSEMINATION** (113), providing updates on the effectiveness of important health interventions for practitioners and decision-makers, 'in a shorter and more journalistic style,' and summarising the results of high-quality systematic reviews. Can be read on **NHS CRD** website (113) – future of bulletins currently under review.

60   **EVIDENCE-BASED PURCHASING** Bi-monthly digest of evidence about effective care, reviews of materials, resources, journal articles and databases, published by the UK NHS: www.doh.hov.uk/research/swro/rd/publicat/ebpurch/index.htm

61   **HEALTH EVIDENCE BULLETINS WALES** 'Signposts to the best current evidence across a

broad range of evidence types and subject areas'. Search completed bulletins at: http://hebw.uwcm.ac.uk

62 **INFORMED** Quarterly newsletter from Institute of Clinical Evaluative Sciences (ICES), Toronto, Canada. Aims to 'put health services information and clinical research together in a clear and concise format to give practising physicians' and other health professionals ... 'material that is directly relevant to their practice'. Printed newsletter by subscription. Read it free at www.ices.on.ca

63 **MD DIGESTS** A service from HealthStream 'designed to keep the busy practitioner up to date on the most recent advances in clinical medicine.' Each week the MD Digests editor selects two relevant journal articles from the top five general medical publications (Annals of Internal Medicine, BMJ, JAMA, Lancet, New England Journal of Medicine) and summarises the articles, focusing on the practical aspects of the research and patient care issues, with links to related resources on the web, plus librarian-prepared MEDLINE searches for further research. Free e-mail alerting service. www.healthstream.com/mddigests

64 **UPTODATE** A subscription-based clinical information resource for physicians on an individual, group or institutional basis. Designed 'to get physicians the concise, practical answers they need at the point of care' using topic reviews written exclusively for UpToDate by physicians for physicians, with a peer review process. www.uptodate.com

65 **US NATIONAL INSTITUTE FOR HEALTH CONSENSUS STATEMENTS** The NIH Consensus Development Program is 'the focal point for evidence-based assessments of medical practice and state-of-the-science on behalf of the medical community and the public'. Major conferences produce 'consensus statements and state-of-the-science statements on controversial issues in medicine important to health care providers, patients and the general public'. http://odp.od.nih.gov/consensus

4 Library catalogues

66 **BRITISH LIBRARY** http://blpc.bl.uk

67 **BRITISH MEDICAL ASSOCIATION** www.bma.org.uk

68 **COPAC** Free access to the merged online catalogues of 22 of the largest university research libraries in the UK and Ireland, plus the British Library. www.copac.ac.uk

DEPARTMENT OF HEALTH see (102) and HMIC (20)

69 **NATIONAL LIBRARY OF MEDICINE** Search the catalogue and use many other resources from the vast US National Library Medicine at http://locatorplus.gov/ – or see **NATIONAL LIBRARY OF MEDICINE (NLM) GATEWAY** (23) to add even more resources.

70 **ROYAL COLLEGE OF NURSING** http://rcn-library.rcn.org.uk/

71 **ROYAL SOCIETY OF MEDICINE** http://www.rsm.ac.uk/

WORLD HEALTH ORGANIZATION see (126)

5 Research and trials registers

72 **CLINICALTRIALS.GOV** Register of clinical trials from **NATIONAL LIBRARY OF MEDICINE (NLM) GATEWAY** (23) or direct at: http://clinicaltrials.gov

COCHRANE CENTRAL REGISTER OF CONTROLLED TRIALS see **COCHRANE LIBRARY** (13)

73 **CURRENT CONTROLLED TRIALS** Website from Current Controlled Trials Ltd. dedicated to promoting the exchange of information about controlled trials in all areas of medicine and health care. Includes searchable metaRegister of Controlled Trials (mRCT), Controlled Trials Links Register, Publications (trial protocols and reports; trial-related journals and databases), and Services for trials groups. Free registration at www.controlled-trials.com/

74 **NATIONAL RESEARCH REGISTER** Free web access to a set of databases of details of ongoing and recently completed research projects funded by, or of interest to, the UK NHS. Includes the National Research Register Projects Database, MRC Clinical Trials Directory, Register of Reviews from the **NHS CENTRE FOR REVIEWS AND DISSEMINATION** (113) and Abstracts of Reviews from the **COCHRANE LIBRARY** (13). www.update-software.com/National

6 Evidence-based guidelines

See also guideline sites list from **ScHARR** (122)
www.shef.ac.uk/~scharr/ir/guidelin.html and from Medic8 at
www.medic8.com/ClinicalGuidelines.htm – and check Royal Colleges websites.

75 **AGENCY FOR HEALTH CARE POLICY & RESEARCH (AHCPR)** Free web database containing practice guidelines in full form, clinicians' Quick Reference Guides and consumer versions. www.ahcpr.gov

76 **BMJ GUIDELINES** Full-text guidelines free from BMJ journal.
http://bmj.com/cgi/collection/guidelines

77 **CANADIAN MEDICAL ASSOCIATION CLINICAL PRACTICE GUIDELINES DATABASE AND CANADIAN TASK FORCE ON PREVENTIVE HEALTH CARE** www.cma.ca/cpgs

78 **CANCERBACUP** Treatment guidelines for cancer from the UK's leading cancer information service. www.bacup.org.uk

79 **CENTRES FOR DISEASE CONTROL AND PREVENTION (CDC) GUIDELINES DATABASE** Free web database of up to date and archived guidelines and recommendations approved by the CDC (USA) for the prevention and control of disease, injuries, and disabilities. www.phppo.cdc.gov/cdcRecommends/AdvSearchV.asp

80 **eGUIDELINES** Website for printed handbook Guidelines (published three times annually, by subscription) summarising clinical guidelines for primary and shared care, and for online Guidelines in Practice, dealing with developing guidelines. Free registration for health professionals to search these resources on the website: www.eGuidelines.co.uk

81 **eMJA** Clinical guidelines published by the Medical Journal of Australia.
www.mja.com.au/public/guides/guides.html

82 **NATIONAL electronic LIBRARY FOR HEALTH** (NeLH) For NeLH Guidelines Finder, a database of some 450 clinical guidelines – see (110)

83 **NATIONAL GUIDELINES CLEARING HOUSE** Free public web resource for evidence-based clinical practice guidelines sponsored by the US Agency for Health care Research and Quality in partnership with the American Medical Association and the American Association of Health Plans. www.guidelines.gov

84 **NATIONAL INSTITUTE FOR CLINICAL EXCELLENCE (NICE)** – NICE Guidelines and Technology Appraisals, and background information – see NICE (111)

85 **NEW ZEALAND GUIDELINES GROUP** www.nzgg.org.nz/index.cfm

86 **PRIMARY CARE CLINICAL PRACTICE GUIDELINES** From University of California: http://medicine.ucsf.edu/resources/guidelines/index.html

87 **SIGN (SCOTTISH INTERCOLLEGIATE GUIDELINES NETWORK)** Scotland's national guidelines database. www.sign.ac.uk/guidelines/index.html

88 **US HEALTH SERVICES TECHNOLOGY ASSESSMENT TEXT** Free web database of full-text clinical practice guidelines, technology assessments and health information. http://text.nlm.nih.gov

7 Web gateways and search engines – and other useful websites

89 **ALLTHEWEB** A very powerful meta-search engine, which uses other search engines to search the web (and which, like any other search engine, does *not* search the entire web!): www.alltheweb.com

90 **ALTA-VISTA** General search engine, with Advanced Search feature: http://altavista.com

91 **BIOME** For 'quality Internet resources in the health and life sciences' from the University of Nottingham – a free, searchable catalogue of Internet sites and resources which have been checked against strict evaluation criteria (which can be viewed on the site). You can also select OMNI (116), to restrict to health and medicine resources, excluding wider life sciences. http://biome.ac.uk

92 **BIOMED CENTRAL** An 'independent publishing house committed to providing immediate free access to peer-reviewed biomedical research'. Free journals on the web: http://www.biomedcentral.com

93 **CAIRNS LIBRARY**, Oxford. Links to sites in this list and others, a table of search engines,

database search guides and more: www.medicine.ox.ac.uk/cairns

94 **CASP** Critical Appraisal Skills for Purchasers: premier site, now based at the NHS Public Health Resource Unit, for critical appraisal skills issues, resources, workshops, links: www.phru.org.uk/~casp/index.htm

95 **CENTRE FOR EVIDENCE-BASED CHILD HEALTH**, Institute of Child Health, Great Ormond Street Hospital for Children, London. www.ich.ucl.ac.uk/ebm/ebm.htm

96 **CENTRE FOR EVIDENCE-BASED DENTISTRY** An independent body, linked to the Institute of Health Sciences, Oxford, whose aim is 'to promote evidence-based dentistry worldwide'. www.ihs.ox.ac.uk/cebd

97 **CENTRE FOR EVIDENCE-BASED MEDICINE**, Oxford. Aims 'to promote evidence-based health care and provides support and resources' related to learning, using and teaching EBM, EBM toolbox, links to other EBHC sites, news, conferences, and more. http://cebm.jr2.ox.ac.uk

98 **CENTRE FOR EVIDENCE-BASED MENTAL HEALTH**, Department of Psychiatry, University of Oxford. Aims to promote and support the teaching and practice of evidence-based health care for psychiatry and mental health. http://cebmh.warne.ox.ac.uk/cebmh

99 **CENTRE FOR EVIDENCE-BASED NURSING** Based at University of York. 'Concerned with furthering EBN through education,research and development.' Links, details of research, staff contact. www2.york.ac.uk/healthsciences/centres/evidence/cebn.htm

100 **CENTRE FOR PSYCHOTHERAPEUTIC STUDIES** Based at the Mental Health Section of ScHARR (122), a large resource of links, mental health research and publications, hosted and affiliated projects, e-mail discussion groups and more. www.shef.ac.uk/~psyc

101 **CLINIWEB INTERNATIONAL** Provides identification and topical indexing of nearly 10 000 clinically oriented web pages using a portion of the National Library of Medicine's (NLM) Unified Medical Language System (UMLS) and the disease and anatomy portions of the Medical Subject Headings (MeSH) classification. Direct links to PUBMED (27). Enter search terms in any of five European languages: www.ohsu.edu/cliniweb

102 **DEPARTMENT OF HEALTH (UK)** 'The latest on the work of the Department, as well as health and social care guidance, publications and policy.' Go to Publications for COIN (Circulars Library), POINT (Publications Library), Research Publications, Statistical Publications, Bulletins etc. (See also ReFeR (29) above). www.doh.gov.uk

103 **DOCTORS DESK** A free web portal from St. George's Hospital Medical School, London, with links to useful sources of evidence-based medicine relevant to general practitioners – includes an 'EBM meta-evidence search engine that searches across multiple publications of secondary review': http://drsdesk.sghms.ac.uk

104 **GOOGLE** A new generation of Internet search engines, claiming links to 3 billion websites, with 'intelligent' search features. (Check out the Advanced Search tips.) www.google.com

105 **HIRU (HEALTH INFORMATION RESEARCH UNIT)** Based at McMaster University, Canada, 'conducts research in the field of health information science', health and clinical information problems and development of new information resources, to support evidence-based health care. http://hiru.mcmaster.ca

106 **IXQUICK** Claims to be 'the world's most powerful,' and 'the fastest growing since 1999', meta-search engine! www.ixquick.com

107 **MEDBIOWORLD** Claims, with 25 000 links, to be 'the largest medical reference site', with links to 6000 medical and biological science journals and the home-pages of 4000 medical associations, plus medical glossaries, disease databases, clinical trials and guidelines, and many other resources. http://medbioworld.com

108 **MERCK MANUAL OF DIAGNOSIS AND THERAPY** From Merck, a not-for-profit web-accessible textbook; Merck Manual of Geriatrics and others also available at www.merck.com

109 **METACRAWLER** A powerful meta-search engine: www.metacrawler.com

110 **NATIONAL electronic LIBRARY FOR HEALTH (NeLH)** A wonderful free access, web-based virtual library being developed by the UK NHS Information Authority 'to provide health care professionals and the public with knowledge and know-how to support health care-related decisions'. Free access to databases such as **COCHRANE LIBRARY** (12), **ZETOC** (35) and to a wide range of information resources such as **CLINICAL EVIDENCE** (57), to 'portals' for specific health professions, to virtual branch libraries in mental health, child health, cancer, health

screening etc., to evidence-based summaries on current health care issues in its 'Hitting the Headlines' section, and to much more. www.nelh.nhs.uk

111 **NATIONAL INSTITUTE FOR CLINICAL EXCELLENCE (NICE)** Set up as a Special Health Authority for England and Wales by the UK NHS 'to provide patients, health professionals and the public with authoritative, robust and reliable guidance on current 'best practice''. NICE Clinical Guidelines and Technology Appraisals, links, news, events, and more, in English and Welsh, at www.nice.org.uk

NATIONAL LIBRARY OF MEDICINE (NLM) GATEWAY See (23) above, for NLM library catalogues, databases and more.

NETTING THE EVIDENCE See ScHARR (122)

112 **NEW JOUR** From University of California, San Diego Libraries, the Internet list for new journals and newsletters available on the Internet: http://gort.ucsd.edu/newjour

113 **NHS CENTRE FOR REVIEWS AND DISSEMINATION (CRD)** Based at University of York, produces and disseminates reviews on effectiveness and cost-effectiveness of health care interventions: search CRD Databases – now also on **COCHRANE LIBRARY** (12) – **DARE, NHS EED** and **HTA**; also publications, bibliography, links: www.york.ac.uk/inst/crd/welcome.htm

114 **NHS R&D HEALTH TECHNOLOGY ASSESSMENT PROGRAMME** The HTA programme is 'a national programme of research established and funded by the Department of Health's Research and Development Programme to ensure that high-quality research information on the costs, effectiveness and broader impact of health technologies is produced in the most effective way for those who use, manage and provide care in the NHS'. (For HTA Database see (13) and (113) above.) Details of programmes, Suggestion Page, Calls for Proposals, Publications Page, Correspondence Page and more on HTA website at: www.hta.nhsweb.nhs.uk

115 **NMAP** 'Your guide to quality Internet resources in Nursing, Midwifery and the Allied Health Professions' from the **BIOME** (91) stable: http://nmap.ac.uk

116 **OMNI** The health and medicine part of the BIOME subject gateway for health and life sciences: see entry above at (91). http://omni.ac.uk

117 **ONCOLINK** A well-designed site for oncology-related searching, with Cancer News, Cancer Trials, Treatment Options, Ask the Experts, a wealth of links, health consumer information and a search engine: www.oncolink.com

118 **OXFORD PAIN INTERNET SITE** From the excellent **BANDOLIER** (56) Library, for 'anyone with a professional or personal interest in pain and analgesia … firmly based on the principles of evidence-based medicine' with lots of systematic reviews with pain as an outcome. www.jr2.ox.ac.uk/bandolier/booth/painpag/index.html

119 **PINAKES** A gateway to high-quality subject gateways. www.hw.ac.uk/libWWW/irn/pinakes/pinakes.html

120 **PRODIGY** A developing, complex support system from SCHIN (Sowerby Centre for Health Informatics at Newcastle), University of Newcastle, with funding from the Department of Health Primary Care Computing Branch and **NICE** (111). Provides direct clinical guidance and authoritative management advice to general practitioners in the consultation on prescribing and other treatment options and referral, based on up to date evidence and guidelines on some 120 medical conditions; patient leaflets, background and training materials, e-mail lists and user groups are also available: http://prodigy.nhs.uk

121 **PUBMED CENTRAL** The 'US National Library of Medicine's digital archive of life sciences journal literature… free and unrestricted': www.pubmedcentral.nih.gov

122 **ScHARR (SHEFFIELD CENTRE FOR HEALTH & RELATED RESEARCH)** A health services research department within the University of Sheffield, involved in finding, appraising and producing the evidence. Their NETTING THE EVIDENCE – a goldmine of EBHC resources – gives access to a listing of information resources, organisations, learning resources, and an evidence-based virtual library with links to articles on all aspects of research and evidence-based practice (including the famous User Guides to the Medical Literature from Journal of the American Medical Association or JAMA). Check EBHC mailing lists at www.shef.ac.uk/~scharr/ir/email.html. Netting the evidence website (check Index to find sites to download search filters): www.shef.ac.uk/~scharr/ir/netting

123 **SOSIG** (Social Science Information Gateway) Free web-based online catalogue of, and links to,

thousands of selected high-quality Internet resources, including statistics sources, over a wide range of social science and related areas: http://sosig.ac.uk

124   **TRIP** (Turning Resource into Practice) A superb search engine which searches over 75 sites of high-quality medical and health care information to give direct access to 'evidence-based' material on the web from key evidence-based practice sources such as BANDOLIER (56) and selected primary journals. A limited company from 2001, now at www.tripdatabase.com

125   **UK HEALTH CENTRE** Claims to be 'the web's most comprehensive and up to date index of UK health and medical internet resources' with the resources indexed for use for the general public, health care professionals, health and service providers. www.healthcentre.org.uk

126   **WORLD HEALTH ORGANISATION** Search the Library Database (WHOLIS) or the Guide to Statistical Information (WHOSIS), as well as checking Publications, Research Tools, News, Bulletins and more: www.who.int/en

(See also WHO Regional Office for Europe at: http://www.who.dk)

127   **YAHOO** General search engine, browseable subject links: www.yahoo.com

(No mention of any product or website in these lists constitutes an uncritical endorsement or advertisement.)

Chapter 4

Introduction to critical appraisal

Martin Dawes

Many clinicians feel that research is something only clever people do. This is not true. The people who undertake clinical research do so because it interests them just as clinical practice and areas of clinical speciality are of interest to various specific groups of individuals. A nurse working in a coronary care unit has more knowledge of critical care of patients with heart disease than a doctor working in a dermatology unit. This does not mean that one is cleverer or more intelligent than the other. It is the interest in the subject that leads to acquisition of knowledge.

Doctors and nurses doing research are no more or less intelligent than their colleagues on the wards. This book is an exploratory introduction to research and it explains the short cuts that can be taken when evaluating research projects. When buying a second hand car one needs only a little knowledge to avoid the bad deals. That knowledge does not make you skilful enough to make a living buying and selling second-hand cars but it gives you the edge over those who have not learnt the five key areas to consider when looking at a used car and also will often prevent you from buying a dangerous vehicle.

The aim of critical appraisal is to identify the quality of an article. There are three key issues to think about when appraising any paper:

- are the results of the study valid?
- what are the results?
- are the results relevant?

It can be hard to get any research published. Before the paper gets sent to a journal it will often have gone through eight or nine drafts with each author changing the contents and the appearance. The paper then arrives at the journal and is sent for a brief scrutiny to assess originality, serious scientific flaws, and the presence of an important message relevant to the journal's readers. This will decide whether it then enters the process of peer review and as many as half the papers fail at this stage.

If it passes this first scrutiny, it will be sent to several people who work in the same field for their opinion. This opinion is usually classified into several areas, such as originality, statistical quality and methodological quality. The journal then decides whether to accept the paper. The reviewers will certainly have made some comments and the journal will ask the authors to rewrite the paper incorporating those comments. These may range from very minor changes to major analysis and rewrites. Finally, the paper is accepted and is published.

Given this process why do we need appraisal? Surely this rigorous approach would ensure that all research published is of good quality. To begin with, there may be journals that are less rigorous in their approach to peer review. This is not the case for the majority of journals and certainly not the most prestigious ones. So why not accept research published in a major journal? The chief reason is that the reviewers may not check the methodology in a systematic way. Unlike the system described in the next few chapters, there is often no standard reviewer's checklist to ensure simple research processes have been performed adequately, though individual journals may circulate their own guidance.

Is all published research flawed? The answer is categorically no. The process of designing a study and ensuring that it will answer the posed question is very time-consuming and costly. Funding bodies will scrutinise research protocols before money is awarded just as rigorously as journals assess papers relating to it. However, not all research is externally funded and so may not go through this process.

In one's enthusiasm to develop an idea or share a discovery, certain factors affecting the research can be overlooked. Finally, hindsight is a wonderful tool. We should not forget that the researchers are working without the benefit of this!

So how do you start? First, it may be easier to try to do it with someone else. Second, it is very hard to appraise a paper if you have not read it. That may sound obvious. When we run workshops we ask people to read a paper before the session. Very few of the tutors, let alone the students, have managed to find time to do this. So for any session appraising a paper always allow 10 or 15 minutes at the beginning for reading the paper. Third, start with easy questions. For example, have the authors answered the question the research was designed to study? A simple question, but often you see studies that outline a finding that was discovered by accident during the process of data collection. Fourth, do not stop appraising once you find flaws in the work. There may still be useful information in the study.

Fifth, review your appraisal. You will be amazed how easy it is to 'rubbish' a paper. You are using hindsight and tools/checklists that may have been designed after the research was published. The art of appraisal is to assess not whether the paper is 'rubbish', but whether there is so much potential bias that the results are no longer valid. That is a slightly odd sentence but does contain the essence of appraisal. When you start appraising there are many difficulties. Being unfamiliar with research papers is the first.

All this sounds like it will take far too long and be far too difficult. To start with, it will feel uncomfortable. If you think about everyday life, you are judging the information you receive all the time for its completeness and trustworthiness, in newspaper articles, for example, or information received from people you meet. Undertaking a critical appraisal is really using your everyday skills, and applying them in a more structured and systematic way. After you have read the following chapters and you have increased your understanding, you will feel more confident and be able to start developing your skills. Once you read one or two articles a week your confidence (and speed) will pick up. Not only that, but your knowledge and practice may even change as well!

Chapter 5

Randomised controlled trials
Martin Dawes

One of the best sources of information that I consult regularly is the British National Formulary (BNF). It contains most of the drugs that I use in everyday practice and I can find my way around it very easily. I use it several times each day to check dosages, side-effects, drug interactions and also to review prescribing guidelines for various chronic conditions such as epilepsy. Its advantages are that the layout for each drug is similar, the book comes with a certain authority, and most UK health professionals use it. In comparison, the identification of information from a research article is much harder. The layout is frequently different, depending on the journal you are reading. You are often relying on the editorial board of the journal as well as the people who reviewed the article to have ensured the quality of the article. There may be confusing statistics that make interpretation of the data seem difficult. These problems seem to be very daunting when you are trying to identify information that may affect the care of a patient.

One problem is the time it may take to read through and identify all the major features of an article. The aim of the next section is to speed up the process whilst ensuring quality. If you can assess the quality of a paper very quickly, then you can decide whether or not to continue the process of appraisal.

CONTENTS OF ARTICLES ON THERAPY

Treatment articles do not always use a consistent format when describing their results. It has taken many years for articles in scientific journals to reach a reasonably similar format of presentation. An article usually contains the following sections: abstract, introduction, methods, results, discussion and references. Even so the layout of the articles differs from journal to journal. So what information can you gather from the abstract? After all, this is the part of the article you are most likely to read (usually going directly to the last line in the conclusions section!).

A general practitioner (GP) is seeing a woman for a routine post-natal check-up. She mentions that she is having a little bit of urinary incontinence. He asks whether she has been doing the pelvic floor exercises and she replies she has not had time. He notes that she had a large baby and states confidently that the exercises will help. After she leaves, he has doubts and finds this article in response to his structured question. He tried looking for systematic reviews first but none were specifically about women after delivery. He finds this article by Chiarelli and Cockburn (2002) from the British Medical Journal and he reads the abstract.

Abstract

Objectives:

To test the effectiveness of a physiotherapist-delivered intervention designed to prevent urinary incontinence among women 3 months after giving birth.

Here the authors clearly define that they are looking at safety as well as effectiveness of treatment. This is particularly important when comparing experimental treatment with placebo.

Design:

Prospective randomised controlled trial with women randomised to receive the intervention (which entailed training in pelvic floor exercises and incorporated strategies to improve adherence) or usual post-partum care.

This describes what was done and how. However, we will need more information about the randomisation and the intervention.

Setting:

Post-partum wards of three tertiary teaching hospitals in the Hunter region, New South Wales, Australia.

This describes where the study took place. It helps us decide whether the study is relevant to our practice, which may be in a different setting (see Chapter 16).

Participants:

Women who had forceps or ventouse deliveries or whose babies had a high birth weight (4000 g), or both; 676 (348 in the intervention group and 328 in the usual care group) provided end point data at 3 months.

From Chapter 2 we know we should have a three-part question comprising (1) the patient, (2) the intervention and (3) the outcome. We can see here whether the patients in this study match those of the GP's hypothetical question.

Main outcome measures:

Urinary incontinence at three months measured as a dichotomous variable.[1] The severity of incontinence was also measured. Self-report of the frequency of performance of pelvic floor exercises was recorded.

How was all this done? Was self-reporting accurate?

Results:

At 3 months after delivery, the prevalence of incontinence in the intervention group was 31.0% (108 women) and in the usual care group 38.4% (125 women); difference 7.4% (95% confidence interval 0.2%-14.6%, $P = 0.044$). At follow-up significantly fewer women with incontinence were classified as severe in the intervention group (10.1% vs 17.0%), difference 7.0%, 1.6%-11.8%). The proportions of women reporting doing pelvic floor exercises at adequate levels was 84% (80%-88%) for the intervention group and 58% (52%-63%) for the usual care group ($P = 0.001$).

This is the stage at which many of us get confused. The first line usually contains the meat of the paper. Here the author states clearly the difference in incontinence rates but also tells us the rate on placebo. What is startling is the high number of women with incontinence. Certainly it appears that symptoms improved when they did their exercises. The interpretation of results will be dealt with in Chapter 14.

Conclusions:

The intervention promoting urinary continence reduced the prevalence of urinary incontinence after giving birth, particularly its severity, and promoted the performance of pelvic floor exercises at adequate levels; both continence and adherence to the programme were measured at 3 months after delivery in women who had forceps or ventouse deliveries or babies weighing 4000 g or more.

Finally, the authors write a conclusion that describes their opinion of the results. Having read this synopsis, would the GP now continue to recommend this treatment to women? What questions form in the GP's mind

---

1 A variable with one of only two possibilities – i.e. present or absent.

while reading the article? There is a lot of information carried in the abstract but not enough to completely check the validity of the article. Secondary questions occur as to the types of delivery and the likelihood of incontinence. This is normal whenever doing any reading. More questions arise and it is important to remain focused on the question you originally decided on. However, some of these secondary questions may in themselves be important and it is worth jotting a few of them down.

In this study the methods section is remarkably thorough (long). There is a sample size calculation (see later), the development of the intervention, collection of baseline data in hospital, a description of the intervention and the usual care as well as a description of follow-up. They also tell exactly what incontinence means in great detail, for example, 'leaked even small amounts on your way to the toilet'. We need this level of description to understand what a trial is about. It is not useful just to say the end point is pain – how do the authors define pain?

The results section should describe clearly the demographic features of the patients in terms of age, sex and other relevant characteristics. It should then outline the specific characteristics of the problem that the research addresses, for instance the severity of the disability in whatever measure has been used. Finally, it should present in tabular form the main results of the intervention. Included in this table should be not only evidence of clinical effectiveness, but also statistical significance. The latter should enable you, as a reader, to determine whether this finding may have happened by chance, and whether the same finding is likely to occur if the research was performed again in other populations.

So where does this leave the GP? Does he believe the results? Is the

---

Box 5.1 Guidelines for appraising a therapeutic article

1. Did the authors answer the question?
2. What were the characteristics of the patients?
3. Were the groups similar at the start of the trial?
4. Aside from the experimental treatment, were the groups treated equally?
5. What was the treatment?
6. What was the comparison (placebo)?
7. Were all patients who entered the trial accounted for at its conclusion? Were they analysed in the groups to which they were randomised? (Intention to treat) (See Chapter 14)
8a. Was the assignment of patients to treatments randomised?
8b. Was the randomised list concealed?
9. Were patients and clinicians kept 'blind' to which treatment was being received?
10. Was the length of study appropriate?
11. Is the context of the study similar to your own? (See Chapter 16)
12. Did the treatment work? (See Chapter 14)

research of sufficiently good quality for him to believe? It may be helpful at this stage to introduce a list of useful questions to ask of any therapeutic article (Box 5.1). These questions are derived from several sources including what are known as the Journal of the American Medical Association (JAMA) guidelines (Guyatt et al 1993).

The advantage of the BNF is that familiar layout and relevant information can be found quickly. Only by practising appraisal skills can we gain that familiarity with research papers. Chapter 3 on Finding the Evidence dealt with the types of papers that would be likely to contain information relevant to therapy.

These are the questions that are important when considering a paper on therapy.

DID THE AUTHORS ANSWER THE QUESTION?

Each article written has an introduction in which the authors put forward the context of the problem and justify their research by demonstrating the lack of evidence within the literature. At the end of this section you will often find described the exact question that the research has been designed to answer. Sometimes authors put this into the abstract while others leave it to the discussion. Finally, some authors leave you guessing as to what the original question might have been.

WHAT ARE THE CHARACTERISTICS OF THE PATIENTS?

These include a description (usually found in the methods) of the patients and how they were recruited. In this case it was women with babies greater than 4000 g, or a ventouse or forceps delivery.

ARE THE COMPARISON GROUPS SIMILAR AT THE START OF THE TRIAL?

To determine whether bias has occurred in the selection procedure certain potentially relevant characteristics of the two populations should be displayed in tabular form. Usually these include age, sex, duration of illness and other demographic and functional characteristics. If the treatment is studying the effect of a drug on mortality, for example, then the age and gender of the subjects in either arm of the study will have an effect on the overall rate of mortality. A paper describing two options of therapy will usually have a table describing the characteristics of each group and may evaluate whether any differences between the groups are statistically significant.

For example, Table 5.1 outlines the characteristics of the two groups (Chiarelli & Cockburn). A brief view of this table will then enable you to ensure that the groups are similar. In this table there are no statistics. As the purpose of this table is for the reader to assess whether there is a clinically significant difference (as apposed to statistically significant) this is entirely appropriate. I would have liked to have seen the average weight of the women in each group as that would have an effect on incontinence. However, the absence of this data is not critical – but something to bear in mind when looking at the results.

WERE THEY TREATED EQUALLY APART FROM THE INTERVENTION?

In this section you want to make sure that, apart from the advice and physiotherapy, they did not have any other treatments or types of care. For example, a new drug might require more blood tests and so the patient may be called back to the clinic more frequently than the patients in the control group. Just this frequency of seeing the nurse may improve symptoms. In this study there were no additional processes of care.

Table 5.1 Patient characteristics

Charcteristics of women randomised to receive an intervention designed to prevent urinary incontinence after giving birth and controls. Values are numbers (percentages)		
	Intervention (n=348)	Usual care (n=328)
Age group		
15–19	15 (4)	27 (8)
20–24	69 (19)	62 (18)
25–29	128 (35)	125 (36)
30–34	118 (32)	92 (26)
35–39	34 (9)	41 (12)
40–44	6 (2)	3 (1)
No of pregnancies		
One	198 (54)	187 (53)
Two	98 (27)	85 (27)
Three	60 (16)	44 (13)
Four or more	14 (4)	24 (7)
Marital status		
Married or cohabiting	397 (91)	306 (87)
Single	31 (8)	40 (11)
Widowed, divorced or separated	2 (1)	2 (1)
Other	0 (0)	2 (1)
Education		
Not completed high school	141 (38)	145 (42)
Completed high school	86 (23)	64 (18)
Tertiary	143 (39)	141 (40)

WHAT WAS THE TREATMENT? WHAT WAS THE COMPARISON (PLACEBO)?

It is important that all the processes of the intervention are described. Who is providing the care, what sort of dressing, when the treatment is given and for how long. Placebos are inactive versions of the treatment. Even though they are pharmacologically inert they still have an effect on the disease (see Chapter 14). Studies investigating a therapy should be designed so that the patients are unaware (single-blind) of whether their treatment is experimental or control. If the trial is of a medication that can be given in tablet form, the pharmaceutical company involved will usually provide both placebo and experimental treatments to the researcher already packaged and sealed so that the researcher cannot know which they are giving. If there is a trial of medication that may have large cost implications, companies do not analyse the data themselves but give the analysis over to a third party such as a university department of statistics. In this way, bias is excluded all the way from the clinician down to the presentation of the results.

To determine the impact of an intervention on patient health you need to define clearly the outcome that needs to be measured. This sounds straightforward enough but can take up a larger amount of the preparation time of the research. What is meant by outcome measure? An outcome measure is any feature that is recorded to determine the progression of the disease or problem being studied. A large number of studies are undertaken to evaluate the impact of therapies on arthritis. The outcome measure that is presented in the paper may not be the most relevant to the patients. Restriction in mobility may be of more importance than the presence or severity of pain although both are clearly related. Thus, a paper only describing pain relief may not necessarily have answered the question about mobility. Researchers often assume the most important clinical features of a disease which may not be the same as those most relevant to the day-to-day lives of our patients. It is one of the reasons that qualitative research is so important in determining what is relevant to the patient.

When the outcome measure used in the research appears appropriate, examine the thresholds of that measure used to determine severity. In terms of ability to walk, we may ask patients how far they can walk or we may give them options, such as 50 yards, 100 yards or 150 yards. The researcher may then make an arbitrary decision that the ability to walk 1 mile is the aim of the therapy. The researcher will then present results in terms of how many patients reached that threshold. Another question might be about the assessment of the distance walked. Was it the patient or clinician judging it, or was there an objective measurement? What is not so desirable is the researcher who finds that the therapy is effective in enabling patients to walk $1/2$ a mile, but not 1 mile and so uses $1/2$ mile retrospectively as the threshold for improvement. It is difficult, if not impossible, to detect whether this has taken place. Critical appraisers will determine what threshold they would have used for walking distance and see whether the one used in the paper approximates to their own choice.

Other authors will describe the mean walking distance before and after treatment. They can then describe statistical significant improvements in walking distance. What this description does not tell you is the number of patients who have improved. The use of means or averages hides important information about the characteristics of patients who have improved and perhaps, more importantly, those who have got worse. The presentation of data is therefore critical to the use of a paper. When examining a paper in detail, check back to the introduction and title to determine whether the author really has addressed the problem properly in the results.

In this study the description of the intervention by the physiotherapist are very clear and well described. The comparison was with normal care.

WERE ALL PATIENTS IN THE TRIAL ACCOUNTED FOR AT ITS CONCLUSION? WERE THEY ANALYSED IN THE GROUPS TO WHICH THEY WERE RANDOMISED?

The undertaking of a clinical trial is usually time-consuming and difficult to complete properly. A good clinical trial requires the complete follow-up of patients in both the placebo and experimental treatment groups. If less than 80% of patients are adequately followed up, then the results may be invalid. To assess the thoroughness of the article check that follow-up was discussed. The American College of Physicians has decided to use 80% as its threshold for inclusion of papers into the ACP Journal and Evidence-Based Medicine (ACP Journal Club 1994). If the 20% not followed up had the opposite outcome, then the overall results would be unlikely to vary substantially. (Intention to treat, see Chapter 14.)

During any study it is extremely difficult to follow up all the individuals in the study. In the UK, the turnover of the patient list of an average family practitioner is 7% per year; that is 7% of all registered patients each year will have moved out of the area, transferred to another practitioner or died. This indicates the difficulty in tracing patients entered into a study that lasts for anything longer than a few weeks.

The other major feature affecting the follow-up is patient compliance. A large proportion of patients may never complete the treatment. I am sure that very few patients will complete a 5-day course of an antibiotic. Not because of side-effects or the treatment did not work, but because life is too hectic. It is often not convenient to attend the clinic or the hospital to have a repeat assessment of the illness and further investigations, particularly if you are feeling better.

The compliance with the quite rigorous follow-up requirements of drug trials is a major problem. Patients are not paid to be included in a study and therefore have to have some other incentive for attending. They may have a difficult illness that has not responded to therapy. This means that those not attending may not have responded to the treatment as well as those who have responded, or vice versa.

This is the reason that researchers strive to get the maximum response rate in order to avoid bias. When evaluating results of their study researchers will often include non-attendees in the analysis by giving them the worst possible outcome studied (Schulz et al 1996). This reflects more accurately what will happen in the real world when you give a treatment, rather than in some super-compliant population. For a study into the role of a treatment to reduce pain from arthritis, researchers would include in the analysis the patients who had not returned for their evaluation as having the maximum pain after treatment.

The follow-up was 97% in this study and a very clear flow diagram showed the number of patients at all stages of the trial.

WERE THE GROUPS RANDOMISED AND WAS RANDOMISATION CONCEALED?

The major reason for randomisation is to prevent bias. Alternative methods of allocation are to use the day of the week, birth date or patient identification number. These non-random methods may result in biased results. The day of the week that patients can attend the doctor varies with work and home circumstances. Thus, selecting alternate days may introduce a bias. Some diseases are related to season of birth, and high-registration numbers are likely to be given to people who have recently moved into the area. Although we could stratify patients for important factors that we know about, we cannot stratify for the factors we do not know about, e.g. genetic susceptibility.

Randomisation is usually done by using columns of random numbers. One method is to start at any point on the table. If that number is even the patient gets the experiment. If it is odd they get the control. The same is done with the next consecutive number in the table and so on.

True random allocation can result in some differences occurring between the two groups through chance. This can lead to difficulty when analysing the results if, for instance, there was an important difference in severity of disease between the two groups. This can be addressed at the early stages of a study by using 'stratified randomisation'. The researcher identifies the most important factors relevant to that research question and stratifies by these factors.

The largest potential cause of bias in research about effectiveness of an intervention is: if the patients allocated to the treatment group are different from those participating in the control group in a deliberate way (that might influence outcome). To reduce this bias as much as possible, the decision as to which treatment a patient receives should be determined by random allocation, the result of which is concealed from the recruiting clinician.

Why is this important? Consider a practitioner allocating hypertensive patients to experimental or placebo treatment. The practitioner has the patients' best outcome in mind. When patients with very high ranges of blood pressure come in he may be wary of using placebo and if he knows, by looking at the random list of allocation, that the next patient is getting placebo, he will not mention the trial to the patient. This introduces a large deliberate bias. This is not blinding as that occurs after randomisation. This effect occurs during the recruitment phase of the trial.

For this reason, it is preferable that the randomisation list is concealed from the clinicians. This can be done by using sealed sequentially numbered opaque envelopes or a central computerised randomisation process. In the latter, once the patient has agreed to enter the study and if they meet the entry requirements, the investigator rings the central organisation which, after taking the details, tells them whether that patient is in the experimental or control group.

In this study a computer-generated randomisation list contained the identification numbers for women in the trial. The allocation to intervention or control group was placed by a research assistant in a sealed opaque envelope marked with the corresponding study identification number. This was the optimal process of randomisation.

PATIENTS AND CLINICIANS BLINDED

If the outcome relies on the judgement of the clinician and she/he knows that the patient has had the experimental treatment, the clinician's interpretation of clinical findings may be exposed to bias. As researchers, we put forward a hypothesis and aim to prove or disprove that hypothesis using research. Inevitably, we have staked some intellectual investment in the outcome of the study and wish for a positive result. It is therefore extremely hard to be totally unbiased in the clinical evaluation of the outcome, when aware of the intervention that the patient has undergone. This also extends to the evaluation of clinical findings recorded by others in the notes. Researchers identifying positive outcomes may search harder through the notes for an indication of that outcome if they are aware of the treatment. Consequently, it is preferable for both clinicians and their patients to be blind (double-blind).

In this study the patient was not blind, but the results were obtained by telephone interview by someone who was blind. In some circumstances, patients often say something that might 'give it away' so there is a small possibility of some lack of blinding.

LENGTH OF STUDY

The length of the study is critical in determining the clinical significance of the results. For a disease of short duration, for example, an acute infectious disease, the period of the study need only be long enough to cover the course of that infection. Where the disease is more progressive and lengthy, the duration of the study needs to reflect that. The question that the research is trying to answer will also be helpful in deciding the appropriate length of the study. In the example of a patient with acute painful arthritis the question might be about pain relief from that acute attack in which case the research need only be quite short. Another question might be the impact that a drug might have on the mobility of the patient following a prolonged period of treatment. This study would need to be of sufficient length to address that aspect.

Table 5.2 Appraisal answers

Did the authors answer the question?	Yes
Characteristics of the patients?	Women with babies greater than 4000 g, or a ventouse or forceps delivery
Were the groups similar at the start of the trial?	Yes – but unsure about weight
Aside from the experimental treatment, were the groups treated equally?	Yes
What was the treatment?	Physiotherapy and advice on exercise
What was the comparison?	Normal Care
Were all patients who entered the trial accounted for at its conclusion?	Yes – 93% follow-up
Was the assignment of patients to treatments randomised?	Yes
Was the randomisation list concealed?	Yes
Were patients and clinicians kept 'blind' to which treatment was being received?	Patients not blind but evaluator was
Was the length of study appropriate?	Yes

A study is set up to look at the effect of antibiotics on children with ear infections. The study aims to determine whether the use of antibiotics shortens the duration of symptoms, including pain and fever. The study is performed and clearly demonstrates that at three days antibiotics have reduced both of these characteristics. From this evidence it is clear that antibiotics have a role in the treatment of ear infections in children. However, what has not been demonstrated is that at seven days there is no difference between the two groups in pain or fever. This further information may affect your protocol for treatment of this condition.

In order to determine the appropriate length for a study one must understand the natural progress of the disease.

In this case follow-up was three months which seems very appropriate.

SUMMARY

Are these factors important? In a review of studies investigating the importance of blinding, randomisation, concealment of randomisation, Juni et al (2001) found that lack of concealment of randomisation may produce a 30% increase in effect size, and lack of blinding a 20% increase. As many interventions have an effect size that is less than 20%, this is very important. If the randomisation is not concealed and shows an effect size of 15% reduction in events, this may be as a result of the lack of concealment and the intervention may be harmful rather than beneficial.

Although this work may seem very complicated, it can be broken down into manageable chunks. To start appraising for the first time, try working with two or three other people. Look at each of the questions described above relating to a paper you have chosen and write down your comments (see Table 5.2).

At the beginning of appraisal many people new to it are surprised at the number of flaws in papers, even from established journals. It is therefore quite easy to 'rubbish' a paper. This will give you confidence to begin with. The skill of appraisal is not only to answer these quality questions, but later to evaluate how these flaws might influence the results. Would 78% follow-up significantly alter the results in this paper? By examining critically you seek to assess the inference of bias produced during the research, on the eventual results. It is possible to value and use results that contain bias. That is the real skill of appraisal.

References

ACP Journal Club 1994 120(3): A9-10

Chiarelli P, Cockburn J 2002 Promoting urinary continence in women after delivery: randomised controlled trial. British Medical Journal 234:1241-1247

Guyatt G, Sackett D, Cook D 1993 Users' guides to the medical literature. II. How to use an article about therapy or prevention. A. Are the results of the study valid? Evidence-Based Medicine Working Group. Journal of the American Medical Association 270:2598-2601

Juni P, Altman D, Egger M 2001 Systematic reviews in health care: Assessing the quality of controlled clinical trials. British Medical Journal 323(7303):42-46

Schulz K, Grimes D, Altman D, Hayes R 1996 Blinding and exclusions after allocation in randomised controlled trials: Survey of published parallel group trials in obstetrics and gynaecology. British Medical Journal 312:742-744

Chapter 6

Studies assessing diagnostic tests

Jonathan Mant

Diagnoses are usually made through interpreting and combining information from a combination of the clinical history, examination findings and the results of investigations, such as blood tests and X-rays. An important component of evidence-based health care is working out how useful these different pieces of information are in making a diagnosis. For example, if you test a patient's urine and find protein in it, how likely is it that this represents kidney disease? Or if you find sugar in it, how likely is it that the patient has diabetes? A test result needs to be interpreted in the light of how accurate you think the test is, and what you already know about the patient. We will look at how to combine your knowledge about the test and the patient in Chapter 13. In this chapter, we consider the types of studies that are carried out to assess how good a test is, and how to critically appraise them.

What is meant by test accuracy? Usually, this is expressed in terms of the sensitivity and specificity of the test. Sensitivity reflects the ability of a test to identify people who have disease and specificity reflects the ability of the test to identify 'normality', or people who do not have disease. These terms are discussed in greater detail in Chapter 13, together with other terms that are also used to summarise test accuracy, such as predictive value and likelihood ratio. Here, we are concerned with how a study might be done to assess the accuracy of a test, and how a reader can judge whether or not the study has been done well. To illustrate the principles, we will use a specific example, namely a study performed to assess how good is clinical assessment at making a diagnosis of deep-vein thrombosis (DVT) (Wells et al 1995).

EXAMPLE: STUDY TO ASSESS ACCURACY OF CLINICAL ASSESSMENT OF DEEP-VEIN THROMBOSIS

In this study, Wells et al wanted to find out how useful clinical history and examination are in making the diagnosis of DVT. The patients in the study were those who had been referred to out-patient clinics in three hospitals (two in Canada and one in Italy) for the evaluation of suspected DVT. Out of 887 consecutive patients who were referred for this reason to these hospitals, 529 were included in the study. In the out-patient clinics, patients were seen by physicians who regularly assess people for this problem. The clinicians summarised their clinical assessment by categorising the patients into three groups: high, moderate and low probability of DVT. This was done by looking for explicit features in the history and examination (Table 6.1), and considering whether or not there was an alternative diagnosis. Patients were assessed as having a high probability of DVT if they had no alternative diagnosis and either at least three major points or two major and two minor points suggestive of DVT (Table 6.1). Other possible combinations of major and minor points and presence or absence of alternative diagnoses were assessed as being of moderate or low probability of DVT according to an explicit scoring system (Wells et al 1995). Venograms were then performed on all the patients. Venography is generally recognised to be the most accurate way to make the diagnosis. The results were interpreted by a panel of at least three observers who were unaware of the patient's clinical history and of the results of any other diagnostic test (in this study, most of the patients also had ultrasound).

The results are analysed by comparing those obtained by the diagnostic test(s) being evaluated (in this case, clinical assessment) with a 'reference standard' test (in this case, venography). An ideal reference standard test (see below) is one which always gives the correct answer. In other words, it always tells the truth. The result of the comparison of clinical assessment with venography is shown in Table 6.2. This shows, if we accept that the venogram is always right, that 26% of the patients referred with suspected DVT actually turned out to have one. It also shows that clinical assessment was by no means perfect. Some patients (n = 16) who were thought to have a low probability of DVT turned out to have DVT, and some patients who were thought to have a high probability of DVT (n = 13) did not have one. Nevertheless, the clinical assessment did reasonably well, in that someone assessed as having a high probability of DVT actually turned out to have an 85% chance of having DVT. Likewise, someone assessed as having a low probability of DVT did indeed have a low probability of having a positive venogram (5%). Formally, the accuracy of clinical assessment of DVT can be summarised using a number of different terms, as shown in Table 6.3. The significance and meaning of these terms is described in Chapter 13.

Table 6.1   Features of history and examination used in clinical assessment of DVT

	History	Examination
Major points	Active cancer Paresis or immobilisation of legs Recently bedridden (>3 days) or major surgery within 4 weeks Strong family history of DVT	Local tenderness along deep venous system distribution Swelling of thigh and calf
Minor points	Recent injury of symptomatic leg Hospitalisation within 6 months	Pitting oedema only on symptomatic leg Dilated superficial veins only on symptomatic leg Erythema

Adapted from Wells et al (1995)

Table 6.2   Comparison of clinical assessment of DVT with venography in 529 patients with suspected DVT

	Venography result		
	Positive (%)	Negative	Totals
Clinical assessment			
High probability of DVT	72 (85)	13	85
Moderate probability of DVT	47 (33)	96	143
Low probability of DVT	16 (5)	285	301
Totals	135 (26)	394	529

Adapted from Wells et al (1995)

However, it is important not to just take the results of a study at face value, but to decide for yourself whether or not you think the study was sufficiently well performed that you can trust its results. A guideline for how studies of diagnostic tests should be reported has been developed by the Standards for Reporting of Diagnostic Accuracy (STARD) steering group (Bossuyt et al 2003). This comprises a checklist of 25 criteria which aims to 'help readers judge the potential for bias and to appraise the applicability of the findings'. The criteria are summarised in Table 6.4. This important reference guide, if adhered to by authors, should lead to an improvement in both the standards and usability of diagnostic test studies. However, in order to consider the basic principles of appraising such studies, it is useful to have a simpler framework, such as that shown in Box 6.1 (Jaeschke et al 1994). We will now consider what these criteria mean, why they are important, and discuss them in terms of the DVT study.

Table 6.3   Summary measures of accuracy of clinical assessment of DVT as compared to venography

Sensitivity	72/135	53%
Specificty	381/394	97%
Positive predictive value	72/85	85%
Negative predictive value	381/444	86%
Likelihood ratio (+ve)	0.533/(1 - 0.967)	16.1
Likelihood ratio (-ve)	(1 - 0.53)/0.97	0.5

Calculations are done for clinical assessment of 'high probability' of DVT
Calculated from data provided by Wells et al (1995)
See example at end of Chapter 13 for further details of calculation

---

Box 6.1 Questions about the validity of studies evaluating diagnostic tests

1. Was the reference standard appropriate?
2. Were the reference standard and the diagnostic test interpreted independently of each other?
3. Was the reference standard applied to all patients?
4. Was the test evaluated on the right sort of patients?
5. Is it clear how the test was carried out?
6. Is the test result reproducible?

Adapted from Jaeschke et al (1994)

WAS THE REFERENCE STANDARD APPROPRIATE?

To start with, we need to find out how the study found out what the 'truth' really was about patients. That is to say, how did the investigators know whether or not someone really had a disease? To do this, they will have needed some reference standard test (or series of tests) which they know 'always' tells the truth.

Examples of reference standards that have been used to assess some diagnostic tests are shown in Table 6.5. Sometimes, there may not be a single test that is suitable as a reference standard. In such situations, a battery of tests may need to be performed, and an 'expert' panel may need to decide whether disease is present or absent. For example, in the study by Mushlin et al (1993) of the accuracy of magnetic resonance imaging (MRI) for the diagnosis of multiple sclerosis, a single reference standard could not be used since there is no perfect test for multiple sclerosis. Instead, Mushlin et al asked a panel of experts to review all the clinical data about the patients, with the exception, of course, of the MRI result! (If the MRI scan result had been included, this would most likely have resulted in overestimation of test

Table 6.4   The STARD checklist for reporting diagnostic accuracy studies

Topic		Description
Title	1	Identify as study of diagnostic accuracy
Introduction	2	What is/are the research question(s)?
Participants (methods)	3	What is the study population?
	4	How were the participants recruited?
	5	How were participants sampled?
	6	How were data collected?
Diagnostic test (methods)	7	What is the reference standard?
	8	How are index test and reference standard test performed?
	9	How are the results of the index test and reference standard test defined?
	10	Who perfromed the index test and reference standard tests?
	11	Were the readers of the index test and refrence standard 'blind' to the results of the other test?
Statistical methods	12	How were the results analysed?
	13	Was test reproducibly assessed?
Participants (results)	14	When was the study done?
	15	What were the characteristics of people who took part?
	16	How many eligible patients did not undergo index test or reference standard?
Diagnostic test (results)	17	How long between index test and refrence standard? Any treatment received in between?
	18	What was the distribution of severity of disease being tested for, and what other diagnoses were present in people without this disease?
	19	How well did the index test perform against the reference standard?
	20	Did any adverse events occur in performing index test or reference standard?
Estimates	21	How much statistical uncertainty is there for the estimates of diagnostic accuracy of index test?
	22	How were indeterminate results of tests handled?
	23	Did diagnostic accuracy vary between readers, centres or groups of patient?
	24	What were the results of test reproducibility?
Discussion	25	Are the study findings applicable?

Adapted from the STARD checklist for reporting diagnostic accuracy studies, Boussuyt et al (2003)
Index test: test being evaluated by the study
Reference standard: 'gold' standard against which index test is being compared

Table 6.5   Examples of diagnostic tests and possible reference standards

Diagnostic test	Reference standard	Reference
Mammography for breast cancer	Biopsy for test positives; clinical follow-up for test negatives	UK Trial of Early Detection of Breast Cancer Group (1992)
Doppler ultrasonography for carotid artery stenosis	Carotid arteriogram	Carpenter et al (1995)
Urinalysis using test strip for urinary tract infections	Culture of urine in the laboratory	Winkens et al (1995)
Electrocardiograph for diagnosing heart failure	Echocardiography	Davie et al (1996)
Magnetic resonance imaging for multiple sclerosis (MS)	Review by panel of two neurologists specialising in MS and a neuroradiologist of: –clinical history, examination findings, and follow-up –all laboratory and neurophysiological tests	Mushlin et al (1993)
Ventilation/perfusion (V/Q) scan for pulmonary embolus	Pulmonary angiogram or clinical follow-up for 1 year	PIOPED Investigators (1990)

accuracy: a phenomenon referred to as incorporation bias.) Included in this data was follow-up information concerning any clinical developments after the patients had their MRI scan.

Sometimes, it is not possible to carry out the same reference standard test for all the patients in the study. For example, the Prospective Investigation of Pulmonary Embolism Disease (PIOPED) Investigators (1990) used two reference standards in their assessment of ventilation/perfusion (V/Q) scanning as a test for pulmonary embolism. They used pulmonary angiography or they used clinical follow-up for 12 months. Pulmonary angiography is highly accurate and is the recognised reference standard for this diagnosis. However, it is an invasive investigation with a risk of complications. It is difficult to justify on ethical grounds carrying out this investigation on people who you do not think have had a pulmonary embolus, such as those in the study with a normal V/Q scan. Therefore, the PIOPED investigators used a different reference standard for those patients in whom pulmonary angiography could not be performed. They followed them up for 12 months without treatment for pulmonary embolus, and observed whether any of them developed any clinical evidence of pulmonary embolus.

Similarly, it would have been neither ethical nor practical for the UK Breast Cancer Group (1992) in their assessment of the accuracy of mammography as a screening test for breast cancer to carry out their reference standard investigation (breast biopsy) on women who had a normal mammogram. Instead, they classified 'interval cancers', i.e. cancers occurring within 12 months after the screening, in patients who had a normal mammogram as evidence of a false negative result. There is a potential problem with using a different reference standard for people who had a negative test (referred to as verification bias), which is discussed below in the section 'was the reference standard applied to all patients'?

When considering the validity of a study looking at a diagnostic test, you need to consider whether the reference standard used is sufficiently accurate, i.e. that it gives a good approximation to the truth. If it does not reflect the truth, then the results of the study will be difficult to interpret. In the DVT study, the reference standard was venography. This is the generally accepted reference standard. It is accurate, but has problems of expense, invasiveness and risk of complications, and it is not technically possible to carry out on every patient (Anand et al 1998). Nevertheless, in this context, 'appropriateness' is essentially about accuracy, so the venogram can be taken to be an appropriate reference standard.

WERE THE REFERENCE STANDARD AND THE DIAGNOSTIC TEST INTERPRETED INDEPENDENTLY OF EACH OTHER?

If the study investigators know what the result of the reference standard is, this might influence their interpretation of the diagnostic test and vice versa. Suppose we wanted to evaluate how good auscultation (listening with a stethoscope) of the chest is to diagnose pneumonia. A simple reference standard we could use might be a chest X-ray. It is much easier to hear crackles in the chest if we have seen changes on the X-ray. We might be more likely to consider a chest X-ray abnormal if we knew that there were abnormalities on auscultation. Therefore, to ensure that the results of one test are not influenced by the results of the other test, it is important that each is carried out independently of the other. The person interpreting one test should be blind to (i.e. does not know) the results of the other test.

In the study of the accuracy of clinical assessment of DVT, the clinical assessments were carried out before the venograms, and the venograms were interpreted without knowledge of the clinical assessment (Wells et al 1995). Therefore, in this example, the reference standard and the diagnostic test were indeed interpreted independently of each other.

WAS THE REFERENCE STANDARD APPLIED TO ALL PATIENTS?

Ideally, both the test being evaluated and the reference standard should be carried out on all patients in the study. However, this may not be possible for both practical and ethical reasons, as was discussed above. In many cases, the reference standard test may be invasive and may expose the patient to some risk and/or discomfort. It would usually be ethical to use such a test in a patient in whom you had grounds to suspect that it might be positive, but it would not be ethical if you thought that the test would be negative (i.e. if the diagnostic test being evaluated had been negative). Therefore, when reading the paper you need to find out whether the reference standard was applied to all patients, and if it was not, look at what steps the investigators took to find out what the 'truth' was in patients who did not have the reference test. Examples have been given above – pulmonary angiography as a reference standard for pulmonary embolus, and biopsy for breast cancer – where it is not possible to carry out the preferred reference standard on all patients. In each of these cases, the studies cited followed up their patients for a period of time to see if any signs of the disease developed as an alternative.

If the reference standard is not applied to all patients, there is the danger of verification bias if the decision to perform the reference test is based on the result of the diagnostic test being studied. There are two types of verification bias. Differential verification bias occurs when a different reference standard is used to verify a positive diagnostic test as compared with a negative test, as in the examples given above for pulmonary embolus and breast cancer. In general, the effect of differential verification bias is to artificially inflate both the sensitivity and the specificity of the diagnostic test. The reason for this can be understood by considering the pulmonary embolus example, where people who had negative ventilation/perfusion scans were followed up clinically in an attempt to differentiate the 'true' negatives (i.e. people who genuinely had not suffered a pulmonary embolus) from the 'false' negatives (i.e. those people who definitely had a pulmonary embolus). There is likely to have been some residual mis-classification of 'false' negatives as 'true' negatives, in that some people with small emboli may have recovered with no further symptoms, and therefore, were classified incorrectly as a 'true' negative. This will lead to an artificially low number of people in the study that had pulmonary emboli that were not detected (and therefore increase the apparent sensitivity of the test), and an artificially high number of people without pulmonary emboli that were 'correctly' labelled (thereby raising test specificity).

Partial verification bias is where most of the positive results and a smaller proportion of the negative test results are verified through the reference standard, and the rest are omitted from the study. In general, the effect of this is to raise the apparent sensitivity and lower the apparent specificity. Punglia et al (2003) illustrate this with an example of diagnosis of coronary heart disease by exercise testing with confirmatory testing by coronary angiography. All the people who had positive exercise tests went on to receive angiography, but less than half of the people with normal exercise tests. Whereas Punglia et al estimate that the true sensitivity is 44% and the true specificity 87%, the apparent test performance uncorrected for verification bias gives a sensitivity of 67% and a specificity of 73%. The reason for this is that by ignoring many people who test negative, the number of both false negatives and true negatives in the study is reduced. The former raises sensitivity while the latter reduces specificity. (The mathematical definitions of sensitivity and specificity are covered in Chapter 13, so you may find it useful to revisit the effects of verification bias when you are familiar with these terms.)

In the study by Wells et al (1995) 635 patients were in fact eligible for the study, but only 529 patients had the reference standard applied. This was either because patients did not give consent to take part in the study, or because a venogram could not be performed. Rather than use an alternative reference standard, the investigators excluded patients who did not have venograms from the study. Since their exclusion was not on the basis of the clinical assessment of probability of DVT, this is not a serious problem and significant partial verification bias is unlikely to have occurred.

WAS THE TEST EVALUATED ON THE RIGHT SORT OF PATIENTS?

The STARD checklist includes several questions about the study participants (Table 6.4) (Bossuyt et al 2003). Ideally, the study should be performed in people in whom the diagnostic test would be carried out in real life, i.e. people in whom the relevant disease is suspected, but not already proven. The study sample should be a consecutive series of patients or a random sample of such patients.

An important complication is that a test may perform differently depending on the sort of patients on whom it is carried out. For example, the more severe a disease is, the easier it tends to be to detect. Thus, you might find that testing for protein in the urine might be better at detecting kidney disease when evaluated in patients who attend a renal clinic, than in those attending a general practice surgery. This is because people with kidney disease who attend a renal clinic, in general, will be more symptomatic and lose more protein in the urine, making it easier to detect. This problem is referred to as spectrum bias (see Chapter 13). A test is going to perform better in terms of detecting people with disease (i.e. higher sensitivity) if it is used to identify it in people in whom the disease is more severe, or advanced. Similarly, the test will produce more false positive results (i.e. have lower specificity) if it is carried out on patients with other diseases that might mimic the disease that is being tested for.

The issue to consider when appraising a paper is whether the test was evaluated on the typical sort of patients in whom the test would be carried out in real life. For example, it would not make a lot of sense to evaluate a diagnostic test on someone you already know has the disease, since this would not be done in clinical practice – if you know they have the disease, then there is no point in carrying out further tests! Furthermore, such patients are likely to have more advanced disease than people who have not yet had the diagnosis made, so the study would overestimate sensitivity because of spectrum bias (see chapter 13). This is a particular problem if the study is designed as a case-control study (see Chapter 8). In a case-control study, rather than evaluate test performance on a single population, the study is carried out in two populations: people with the disease being investigated ('cases'), and people without the disease ('controls'). Such a design will tend to overestimate specificity as well as sensitivity, as the healthy controls are likely to have a lower prevalence of diseases that might lead to false positive results.

The participants in the study by Wells et al (1995) were the right sort of patients in that they did not include people with already proven DVT, everyone in the study had been referred for assessment because of suspected DVT, and consecutive patients were considered. An issue to consider here is the selection of patients for the study. Only 72% (635/887) of patients referred with suspected DVT were considered eligible for the study, and only 60% (529/887) were actually included in the study. It is important to scrutinise the reasons for their exclusion to see if they might have resulted in spectrum bias. The principal reasons for exclusion were previous history of DVT or pulmonary embolism, and clinical findings not compatible with DVT; the reasons for non-participation of eligible patients were lack of consent and inability to carry out venography. These explanations are not directly related to severity of disease or risk of false positives, so spectrum bias is unlikely to have been introduced.

IS IT CLEAR HOW THE TEST WAS CARRIED OUT?

To be able to apply the results of the study to your own clinical practice, you need to be confident that the test is performed in the same way in your setting as it was in the study. In the study by Wells et al (1995) 'clinical assessment' was not left as an implicit judgement, but clearly defined criteria were written down as to what constituted high, moderate and low probability of DVT. Therefore, it should be feasible to use the same clinical model in your own practice and achieve similar results.

IS THE TEST RESULT REPRODUCIBLE?

This is essentially asking whether you get the same result if different people carry out the test, or if the test is carried out at different times on the same person. Many studies will assess this by having different observers perform the test, and measuring the agreement between them by means of a kappa statistic. The kappa statistic takes into account the amount of agreement that you would expect by chance. For example, if two observers make a diagnosis simply by tossing a coin, you would expect them to agree for 50% of patients. A kappa score of 0 indicates no more agreement than you would expect by chance, a negative score less agreement; a positive score, more agreement than you would expect by chance. Perfect agreement would give a score of 1. Generally, a kappa score greater than 0.60 indicates good agreement (Altman 1991).

If agreement between observers is poor, then this will undermine the utility of the test. The extent to which the test result is reproducible or not may to some extent depend on how explicit the guidance is for how the test should be carried out (see 5 above). It may also depend on the experience and expertise of the observer. If the test is found to have poor reproducibility, then it is likely that this will be reflected in poor test accuracy in terms of sensitivity and specificity.

Wells et al (1995) repeated the clinical assessment of 34 of their patients by a different clinician on the same day as the original assessment. They reported that the level of agreement was 'excellent' (kappa = 0.85).

CONCLUSION

When considering a study assessing a diagnostic test, it is important to decide whether or not you think the results of the study will be valid. In this chapter, we have explored a series of questions (summarised in Box 6.1). The most important question is the first one: was the reference standard appropriate? If the answer to this is 'no', then the study will be very difficult to interpret. If you can answer 'yes' to all the other questions, then you can think about what the results mean, and how they might be applied to your patients (see Chapter 13). However, no study is perfect, and if the answer to one or more of the questions is 'no' (apart from the first one), this does not mean that you should automatically throw the study away. Rather, the results need to be interpreted in the light of the bias(es) that might have been introduced. In general, weaknesses in study design tend to lead to overestimates of test accuracy. Lijmer et al (1999) found that the two design weaknesses that were associated with the greatest inflation of estimates of test accuracy were when case-control designs were used, and when differential verification bias was present (different reference standards used for positive and negative test results).

References

Altman D G 1991 Practical statistics for medical research. Chapman & Hall, London, p 403-409

Anand S, Wells P S, Hunt D et al 1998 Does this patient have deep vein thrombosis? Journal of the American Medical Association 279:1094-1099

Bossuyt P, Reitsma J, Bruns D et al (STARD steering group) 2003 Towards complete and accurate reporting of studies of diagnostic accuracy: the STARD initiative. British Medical Journal 326:41-44

Carpenter J, Lexa F, Davis J 1995 Determination of 60% or greater carotid artery stenosis by duplex doppler ultrasonography. Journal of Vascular Surgery 22:697-705

Davie A, Francies C, Love M et al 1996 Value of the electrocardiogram in identifying heart failure due to left ventricular systolic dysfunction. British Medical Journal 312:222

Jaeschke R, Guyatt G, Sackett D L 1994 For the evidence-based medicine working group 1994 Users' guides to the medical literature III. How to use an article about a diagnostic test: A. Are the results of the study valid? Journal of the American Medical Association 271:389-391

Lijmer J, Mol B, Heisterkamp S et al 1999 Empirical evidence of design-related bias in studies of diagnostic tests. Journal of the American Medical Association 282:1061-1066

Mushlin A, Detsky A, Phelps C et al 1993 The accuracy of magnetic resonance imaging in patients with suspected multiple sclerosis. Journal of the American Medical Association 269:3146-3151

PIOPED Investigators 1990 Value of ventilation/perfusion scan in acute pulmonary embolism: results of the Prospective Investigation of Pulmonary Embolism Diagnosis (PIOPED). Journal of the American Medical Association 263:2753-2759

Punglia R, D'Amico A, Catalona W et al 2003 Effect of verification bias on screening for prostate cancer by measurement of prostate specific antigen. New England Journal of

Medicine 349:335-342

United Kingdom Trial of Early Detection of Breast Cancer Group 1992 Specificity of screening in United Kingdom trial of early detection of breast cancer. British Medical Journal 304:346-349

Wells P, Hirsh J, Anderson D et al 1995 Accuracy of clinical assessment of deep-vein thrombosis. Lancet 345:1326-1330

Winkens R, Leffers P, Trienekens T, Stobberingh E 1995 The validity of urine examination or urinary-tract infections in general practice. Family Practice 11:290-293

Chapter 7

Case series and reports

Martin Dawes

Not all evidence comes from neatly packaged meta-analyses or randomised controlled trials. The initial discovery may have been one or two cases where an observant health professional started questioning. These questions may have been published as observations. These papers are 'case reports'. If several cases have been observed to show the same features, then they may be published as a case series.

How then does one assess the validity of a case or case series report? An example of a case report is shown below (Grimson T 1977 Reactions to cimetidine [letter]. Lancet: (8016):858 © by The Lancet Ltd).

Reactions to cimetidine

Sir, I wish to report the two cases of a possible reaction to cimetidine. A 50-year-old man was admitted with acute exacerbation of pain due to reflux oesophagitis. Two days after admission cimetidine was started at 200 mg three times daily and 400 mg at bedtime. He was discharged 9 days later and inadvertently given two bottles, one labelled cimetidine and the other labelled Tagamet (trade name of cimetidine). The instructions on each bottle were to take three tablets per day with meals and two at bedtime, so he took double doses of cimetidine for 48 hours. He felt light-headed and dizzy and noticed some pain down the right side of his neck. He started sweating profusely together with flushing and was mentally confused. The symptoms disappeared 24 hours after he reverted to a normal dose.

A 54-year-old man was admitted with an acute exacerbation of pain due to reflux oesophagitis of some 3 years duration. Two days after admission, cimetidine 200 mg was given three times per day with meals and two other tablets at bedtime. After he had been on treatment for 4 days he was told that a patient had accidentally taken double the dose resulting in symptoms, but he was not told the nature of the reaction. He was asked whether he would take a double dose to see what happened and this he did. Twenty-four hours later he became dizzy, drowsy, and confused with flushing and sweating. The double dose was reduced to the original dose and his symptoms gradually disappeared, and 24 hours after reduction of the dose he was normal. He had no memory for the event.

Cimetidine is said to be well tolerated, but some patients may get diarrhoea, muscular pain, rash and dizziness. No other drugs of significance were taken by either patient. Dr Y of Company Z tells me that double doses had been taken during some clinical trials without these side-effects.

This letter was written on the basis of only one case of confusion and other symptoms arising from an excessive dose of this drug. The doctor had then confirmed the finding in a second patient and reported the finding. What are the important features of this letter that help the reader decide whether these cases are important (see Box 7.1)?

Not only has this doctor described all these factors but he has also gone on to repeat the increased dosage. The details he has given allow the reader to make an informed opinion of the case. There is no degree of analysis of the pharmacological cause of the mental disturbance nor any suggestion of bias. The plain facts are displayed. So how does this differ from a case series?

Two years later a case series was published in the Lancet (Schentag et al 1979). It first described 15 cases of confusion associated with cimetidine. It then described the mental state of 36 elderly ill patients on cimetidine with their levels of cimetidine in the bloodstream. The article describes six of the 36 patients as having severe mental reactions. It demonstrated that all six patients had concentrations of cimetidine that were greater then 1.25 µg/ml, whereas only two of the non-confused patients had levels above this threshold.

So what characteristics were important in determining the quality of this research? Some of the questions (see Box 7.2) are similar to those in appraising other sorts of trials.

In this study, the authors have raised the awareness of this drug's potential for causing confusion while admitting that their patients had multiple health problems and were elderly. The next step was a review of the literature that

---

Box 7.1 Main features of a case report

- Age
- Diagnosis
- Symptoms
- Treatment
- Dosage
- Duration
- Onset of event
- Duration of event
- Outcome of event
- Action taken during course of event
- Author origin

> **Box 7.2 Guidelines for appraising a treatment trial**
>
> - Were all patients accounted for at the end of the study?
> - Were the characteristics of the patients described fully?
> - Was the treatment of all patients consistent?
> - Were evaluations of symptoms or clinical findings blinded?
> - Were the methods used for measurement of symptoms or clinical findings valid?
> - Were the results consistent (in this case was there a dose response, i.e. the higher the level in the bloodstream, the more likely that there was confusion)?
> - Was there potential for bias (recruitment of more severely ill or confused patients)?

took place in 1991 (Cantu & Korek 1991). The limitations of case series and case reports are many. It is very difficult to be at all certain that what you are observing is not associated with a totally different action than the one that has been suspected. Most clinicians will start to suspect abnormality when several cases occur.

In the case of AIDS this occurred after the admission of a few, young, previously fit men to hospital in California with life-threatening, immune-related disorders. These were reported in two small articles describing three cases and then another four cases in 1981. The next event was the publication of three case series together in the New England Journal of Medicine in December 1981 (Gottlieb et al 1981, Masur et al 1981, Siegal et al 1981). An epidemic was declared after 26 cases were described. This shows the rapid publication of information about potentially serious conditions. Although we may be frustrated about the time that it takes for certain information to reach the light of day, in this case at least the delay was minimal.

A more recent example is that of new variant Creutzfeldt-Jakob disease (CJD) reported first by Will et al in 1996. They described 10 cases, yet the cause of this case series and those that followed are still being debated (Venters 2001). It is clear that major parts of the medical profession are still not certain from the evidence presented in these series what exactly is happening in these patients.

The data contained in case reports must always be evaluated on the basis of the scientific evidence that they are presenting. Does the observation match the data presented? The examples I have cited are well known and often used as illustrations describing the history of discovery. However, many case reports and case series have not led to eventual discoveries. Case series and case reports have to be examined very critically even when all the above criteria have been met.

References

Cantu T, Korek J 1991 Central nervous system reactions to histamine-2 receptor blockers. Annals of Internal Medicine 114(12):1027-1034

Gottlieb M, Schroff R, Schanker H et al 1981 Pneumocystis carinii pneumonia and mucosal candidiasis in previously healthy homosexual men: evidence of a new acquired cellular immunodeficiency. New England Journal of Medicine 305(24):1425-1431

Grimson T 1977 Reactions to cimetidine [letter]. Lancet i(8016):858

Masur H, Michelis M, Greene J et al 1981 An outbreak of community-acquired Pneumocystis carinii pneumonia: initiamanifestation of cellular immune dysfunction. New England Journal of Medicine 305(24):1431-1438

Schentag J, Cerra F, Calleri G, DeGlopper E, Rose J, Bernhard H 1979 Pharmacokinetic and clinical studies in patients with cimetidine-associated mental confusion. Lancet i(8109):177-181

Siegal F, Lopez C, Hammer Get al 1981 Severe acquired immunodeficiency in male homosexuals, manifested by chronic perianal ulcerative herpes simplex lesions. New England Journal of Medicine 305(24):1439-1444

Venters G 2001 New variant Creutzfeldt-Jakob disease: the epidemic never was. British Medical Journal 323:858-861

Will R, Ironside J, Zeidler M et al 1996 A new variant of Creutzfeldt-Jakob disease in the UK. Lancet 347(9006):921-925

Chapter 8

Case–control and cohort studies

Jonathan Mant

In contrast to experimental studies, such as randomised controlled trials where treatments are assigned by researchers, the other major group of clinical research studies are observational studies, where the treatment or exposure occurs without any intervention on the part of the researchers (Grimes & Schulz 2002). Grimes and Schulz sub-divide observational studies into uncontrolled descriptive studies, such as case series (see Chapter 7) and analytical studies that are characterised by the use of a comparison group. There are two major types of analytical observational study that are used in epidemiology: case-control studies and cohort studies. In this chapter, we shall explore the principles of design and critical appraisal of these studies by looking at how the different research designs would approach the same research question, and the potential pitfalls of each design. We will also take a brief look at cross-sectional studies which, while predominately a type of descriptive study, can be used to serve an analytical function.

As discussed in Chapter 2, clinical questions can be characterised as having three or four elements: a patient; an outcome; an intervention and possibly a comparison intervention. In Chapter 3, these questions were characterised into different types, such as those concerning effectiveness, prognosis and harm. Case-control and cohort studies have been used to answer questions of effectiveness, for example, in the field of cancer screening (Connor et al 1991); however, their role in addressing questions of this type is dwarfed by the randomised controlled trial (Chapter 5). This is because randomisation is the best technique to eliminate bias that arises from confounding (see below). Nevertheless, observational studies have a role in the assessment of the effectiveness of medical treatments, since there are several circumstances where it is either unethical or impractical to perform randomised controlled trials. Also, there may be concerns about the applicability of the results of randomised trials to the general population owing to the selective nature of recruitment to trials (see Chapter 5). It is a lot easier to recruit representative populations to observational studies. For example, Nichol et al (2003) carried out a cohort study involving nearly three hundred thousand people to explore whether vaccination against influenza might reduce risk of hospitalisation for heart disease and stroke. The cost of a randomised trial of this magnitude would have been prohibitive, and many people would probably not have given their consent to take part. Furthermore, given that it is already known that influenza vaccination protects against influenza, it would be difficult ethically to justify actively withholding the treatment from half of the participants.

Case-control and cohort studies really come into their own when the question involves harm. For example, does air pollution cause or worsen asthma in children? Does eating meat increase the risk of cancer? It is usually not feasible or ethical to conduct a randomised controlled trial to answer this sort of question, so alternative designs must be used. Cohort studies are also of particular value in addressing questions of prognosis and natural history. For example, what is the chance that someone who is HIV-positive will develop AIDS in a given period of time?

DIFFERENT STUDY DESIGNS

In a cohort study that is concerned with addressing questions of harm, people are classified on the basis of their exposure to the agent under investigation and followed up over time to see if they have developed the disease or diseases of interest. For example, in a cohort study investigating whether hormone replacement therapy (HRT) is associated with breast cancer, participants were defined in terms of whether or not they took HRT, and then followed up over time to see if they developed breast cancer (Million Women Study Collaborators 2003). The analysis compared the rate of breast cancer in users of HRT with the rate in non-users of HRT.

In a case-control study, two groups of people are identified: people who have the disease of interest ('cases'), and people who do not ('controls'). For both groups of people, exposure to the relevant risk factor is measured, and the extent to which one group is exposed is compared with the other group. For example, in a case-control study looking at whether mobile phone use was associated with brain tumours, cases were people admitted to hospital with a brain tumour and controls were people who were admitted to hospital for a reason unrelated to cancer (Inskip et al 2001). Use of mobile phones was ascertained by interview and compared in cases and controls.

In a cross-sectional study, the outcome of interest and exposure is measured at the same point in time. For example, Titan et al (2001) were interested in exploring the association between number of meals and snacks per day and blood cholesterol level. Participants had a blood sample taken, and completed a questionnaire. Participants were classified on the basis of the number of meals/snacks per day they ate, and analysis compared the serum cholesterol levels in these different groups. It was found that people who had the most meals had the lower serum cholesterol levels. Cross-sectional studies in general are a weak design for analytical epidemiology. They have the same potential biases as case-control and cohort studies (see below), but have two further important potential limitations. First, by definition, they deal with prevalent cases of disease rather than incident cases of disease. In other words, they identify already existing cases rather than new cases. The problem is that with potentially lethal conditions (such as myocardial infarction), a prevalence survey will miss the fatal cases, and simply pick up the survivors. Thus, the cases found are not representative of the spectrum of disease in the population. This is not a problem in Titan et al's study since the outcome under study is not a rapidly fatal disease, but a chronic risk factor for disease. Second, because the information on exposure and outcome is elicited at the same time, it can be difficult to distinguish the time sequence. For an exposure to cause a disease, it has to precede it. It is unusual to be able to elicit this in a cross-sectional survey. Thus, in Titan et al's study, do extra meals lead to lower cholesterol levels, or do lower cholesterol levels lead to extra meals?

EXAMPLE: HORMONE REPLACEMENT THERAPY AND VENOUS THROMBOEMBOLISM

The key differences between these designs are illustrated in Figure 8.1 using this example which we will explore in greater depth: does 'exposure' to hormone replacement therapy (HRT) increase the risk of thromboembolism? In a cohort study, you identify people before they have a disease, characterise them in terms of whether or not they are exposed (in this case to HRT), and then follow them forward in time to see whether or not they develop the disease. In a case-control study, you identify a group of people with the disease, and a group of people without the disease, and then you look back in time to try to identify what was different in the history of people who developed the disease as compared with those who did not. In a cross-sectional study, you measure both disease status (thromboembolism) and exposure status (past use of HRT) at the same time, and observe whether or not one is associated with the other.

In order to illustrate the principles of cohort and case-control studies, we will now explore these two designs in more detail, using the example of HRT and thromboembolism. It is now generally accepted that one of the complications of hormone replacement therapy (HRT) for peri- and post-menopausal women is that it increases the risk of deep vein thrombosis (DVT) and pulmonary embolus (venous thromboembolism). However, as recently as 1995, this was not thought to be the case. Textbooks reported that there was little risk of venous thromboembolism from HRT (Vandenbroucke

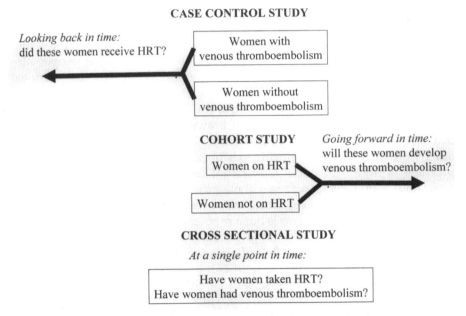

CASE CONTROL STUDY

Looking back in time:
did these women receive HRT?

Women with
venous thromboembolism

Women without
venous thromboembolism

COHORT STUDY   *Going forward in time:*
will these women develop
venous thromboembolism?

Women on HRT

Women not on HRT

CROSS SECTIONAL STUDY

At a single point in time:

Have women taken HRT?
Have women had venous thromboembolism?

Figure 8.1 Summary of design of cohort, case control and cross-sectional studies

and Helmerhost 1996), and the British National Formulary (1995) advised that 'evidence of an increased thrombotic risk associated with HRT is questionable'. What changed the clinical consensus was the publication of three case-control studies and a cohort study in the Lancet in 1996 (Mant and Vessey 2002).

Cohort study

A cohort study that looked at the association between HRT use in post-menopausal women and pulmonary embolus was the Nurses' Health Study (Grodstein et al 1996). Over 120 000 female registered nurses in the USA were recruited to this study in 1976. A baseline questionnaire was sent at that time which included questions on HRT use, past medical history and menopausal status. Follow-up questionnaires, including further questions on HRT-use were sent at 2-yearly intervals thereafter until 1992. On this basis, it was possible to categorise the women into three categories in relation to HRT-use: never users; current users and past users. New cases of pulmonary embolus were identified from the post-1976 questionnaires, or, in the case of deaths, from the National Death Index. If a woman reported a pulmonary embolus or the National Death Index revealed a suspected cardiovascular death, then the medical records were reviewed. If there was confirmatory evidence of a pulmonary embolus (from a ventilation perfusion scan, pulmonary arteriogram or post mortem), then the diagnosis of pulmonary embolus was accepted. Primary pulmonary emboli (no strong predisposing factors) were distinguished from secondary pulmonary emboli (predisposing factors for pulmonary emboli were cancer, trauma, surgery and immobilisation).

The analysis was restricted to post-menopausal women who had no history of cardiovascular disease, and focused on the occurrence of primary pulmonary emboli. The incidence of primary pulmonary embolus in current users of HRT was compared with the incidence in past users and never users. An incidence is a rate, and as such comprises a numerator (the top line of a fraction) and a denominator (the bottom line of the fraction). In this case, the numerator is the number of primary pulmonary emboli, and the denominator is the number of person years. This is the typical denominator for a cohort study. It has two important advantages over the other possible denominator (number of people). First, in a long-term follow-up study like this, some people will have been lost to follow-up. For example, a woman may have responded to the questionnaires in 1976, 1978 and 1980, but not thereafter. In this case, the women would have contributed 4 years to the denominator, whereas other women followed up through the whole study would have contributed 16 years. Second, women may have changed exposure category during the study. For example, if a women took HRT from 1976 to 1982, but not thereafter, for 6 years she will have been a 'current user', and for 10 years a 'past user'. If the denominator is person years, then this change of exposure over time can be taken into account, rather than assuming that the exposure category stays the same throughout the study. The incidence rates are compared by dividing one by the other – this comparison of incidence rates is termed relative risk. The derivation of relative risk in the Nurses' Health Study is shown in Box 8.1. In this case, the incidence in current users and in ex-users is compared with the incidence in never users. The relative risk in current users is 1.7 and in ex-users 1.4. Taken at face value, this implies that HRT-users have a 70% higher risk of a pulmonary embolus than women who have never taken HRT.

Box 8.1 Derivation of relative risk for a cohort study

Exposure category (HRT use)	Number of Pulmonary Emboli	Person years	Incidence (per 10,000 person years)	Relative risk (compared to never users)
Never user	27	320,339	27 ÷ 320,339 =0.84	1.0
Current user	22	155,669	22 ÷ 155,669 =1.41	1.41 ÷ 0.84 = 1.7
Past user	19	157,809	19 ÷ 157,809 =1.20	1.20 ÷ 0.84 = 1.4

Data from Grodstein et al (1996)

Case–control study

One of the case-control studies looking at the association of HRT with venous thromboembolism was the study by Daly et al (1996). Women in this study, aged 45-64, admitted to hospital over a two-year period with supected thromboembolic disease, were identified through screening the relevant hospital wards. Women were excluded if they had a past history of thromboembolic disease, stroke, myocardial infarction, or a history of a recent event predisposing to thromboembolic disease, such as surgery, trauma or illness necessitating bed rest for over 1 week. The medical notes of each possible case were reviewed and classified into four categories according to

---

Box 8.2 Derivation of an odds ratio

The results of a case control study can be summarised by means of a two by two table:

	Cases	Controls
Exposed	a	b
Not exposed	c	d
Totals	a+c	b+d

The odds of disease (i.e. being a case) in people exposed is given by a/b.
The odds of disease in people not exposed is given by c/d.
Therefore, the odds ratio is given by a/b ÷ c/d (which is the same as ad/bc).

Using the example in the text, cases would have been patients with venous thromboembolism (VTE) and 'exposed' would have meant that they had received hormone replacement therapy (HRT). Thus, the results of the Daly et al study might have looked like this:

	VTE	Controls
Current HRT user	44	44
Non–HRT user	59	134
Totals	140	280

The odds of VTE in people given HRT is 44/44, and the odds of VTE in people not on HRT is 59/134. Therefore, the odds ratio is (44/44) ÷ (59/134), or (44 x 134)/(59 x 44), which comes to 2.3.

You will notice that in the text, the odds ratio is given as 3.5. In the published study, the data were analysed to take account of the matched design and were adjusted for other confounding variables, and a crude odds ratio as calculated above was not reported.

Box 8.3 Critical appraisal of an observational study addressing questions of harm

Are the results valid?	1	Have potential confounding factors been identified and dealt with appropriately?
	2	Is it likely that there is selection bias?
	3	Is it likely that there is information bias?
What are the results?	4	What is the size of the odds ratio or relative risk?
	5	How large are the confidence intervals around the odds ratio or relative risk?
Are the results relevant?	6	Is it likely, if an association is observed, that the relationship between exposure and disease is causal?
	7	How big is the risk?
	8	Is exposure of patients in the study similar to the exposure of your own patients?

explicit criteria: definite, probable and possible thromboembolic disease and other disease (that were then excluded). Up to two controls were selected for each case. These comprised women with the same exclusion criteria as the cases who were admitted to hospital with a diagnosis judged to be unrelated to HRT-use. The controls were matched (see below) to cases for age, date of admission and district of admission. Next, cases and controls were interviewed while still in hospital to obtain information about past and present HRT-use and other factors that might confound (see below) any association between HRT-use and thromboembolism.

The principal analysis involved the calculation of an odds ratio, which compares the odds that cases received HRT with the odds that controls received HRT. In this study, the odds ratio was 3.5. In other words, the odds that a case was on HRT was three and a half times higher than the odds that a control was on HRT. An odds ratio is a different statistic from relative risk, but can be interpreted in the same way: an odds ratio of 1 or a relative risk of 1 would mean that there is no association between HRT and thromboembolism; an odds ratio or relative risk greater than 1 would mean that there is an association (the higher the odds ratio/relative risk, the stronger the association); and an odds ratio or relative risk of less than 1 would suggest that HRT was protective against thromboembolism. The derivation of an odds ratio is shown in Box 8.2.

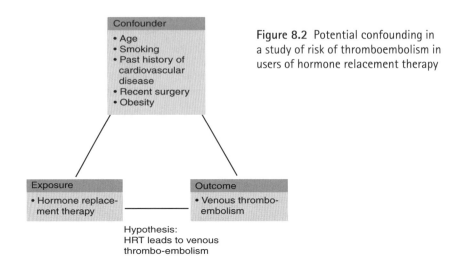

Figure 8.2 Potential confounding in a study of risk of thromboembolism in users of hormone relacement therapy

Both the cohort and case-control study concluded that there was an association between HRT and thromboembolic disease. In deciding how much weight to attach to this conclusion, it is important to consider how well you think the studies have been performed. There are three key issues to think about when appraising any paper: Are the results of the study valid? What are the results? And are they relevant? For observational studies addressing questions of harm, these key questions can be sub-divided into eight more detailed questions, as shown in Box 8.3.

1. Have potential confounding factors been identified and dealt with appropriately?

A confounding factor is something that is associated with exposure to the risk factor under study and that independently affects the risk of developing disease (Hennekens & Buring 1987). Possible confounders of the relationship between HRT and venous thromboembolism are illustrated in Figure 8.2. Each of these factors is likely to be associated with both use of HRT, and risk of venous thromboembolism. For example, women are most likely to take HRT around the menopause and in the few years immediately following the menopause, and the risk of thromboembolism increases with age. Thus, age is a potential confounder, since it is associated both with HRT-use and with the outcome of interest. Similarly, smoking is known to be associated with increased risk of thromboembolic disease. If smoking were more (or less) likely in HRT-users than in non-users, then this too would confound the relationship between HRT and thromboembolism. If you do not take account of these factors in some way, you cannot be sure that any association you observe between HRT and venous thromboembolism is a result of the influence of the confounder, rather than an effect of HRT. Thus, if you find that thromboembolism is more common in HRT-users than in non-users, it

Table 8.1 Strategies to deal with confounding in an observational study

Design	Analysis
Restriction	Stratification
Matching	Multivariate analysis

may simply reflect that HRT-users smoke more, rather than any harmful effect of HRT. In this example, smoking would be exaggerating any positive association that might exist between exposure and disease. However, a confounder can also disguise a true association between exposure and disease.[1] In the cohort study outlined above, the study population was post-menopausal women. Older women in this category are less likely to take HRT, but more likely to have a thromboembolism. In this situation, HRT-users might be found to be less likely than non-users to suffer a thromboembolic event. This would not reflect that HRT-users were protected against such events, but simply that they were younger than non-users. In other words, confounding can work in two ways: it can cause an apparent relationship between a risk factor and a disease when there is not one, or it can conceal a real association.

Confounding can be taken into account either in the design or in the analysis of an observational study, as shown in Table 8.1. In the case-control study by Daly et al (1996), a matched design was used. What this means is that for each case, the controls (up to two per case in this study) are specially selected to 'match' the case for the confounding factor. In this study, matching was for age, district of admission and date of admission. Thus, for a 50-year-old woman, two controls would be selected who were the same age (within a 5-year age group) and admitted to hospital in the same area and during a similar time period (from 2 weeks before to 4 weeks after) as the case. Matching is unusual in a cohort study, and indeed was not employed by Grodstein et al. However, both studies used a restricted design, in that they excluded women with a prior history of cardiovascular disease (including thromboembolism) or cancer. By excluding such people, the possible confounding effects of these factors is nullified.

Alternatively, one can deal with confounding in the analysis of an observational study, either by stratification or multivariate analysis. It is beyond the scope of this book to give details of these techniques. In essence, their purpose is to derive an odds ratio or relative risk that has been adjusted to take account of confounding factors. Thus, in Daly et al's case-control study, the odds ratio was adjusted for body mass index, history of varicose veins and socioeconomic group. They reported an unadjusted odds ratio of

---

1 To distinguish between these opposite effects of confounding, sometimes the terms 'positive' and 'negative' confounding are used. Unfortunately, there is no consistency in the literature as to which is which!

Table 8.2 Summary of how possible confounders were dealt with in a case control and cohort study

Case control study – Daly et al (1996)

Confounding factor	Strategy to address confounder			Not taken into account	
	Matched design	Restricted design	Analysis	Measured	Not measured
Age	✓				
Socio-economic status			✓		
Time period	✓				
Area	✓				
Prior CV disease (inc VTE)		✓			
Cancer		✓			
Immobility/surgery/trauma		✓			
History of varicose veins			✓		
Parity					✓
Body mass index			✓		
Smoking status				✓	
Alcohol use				✓	
High blood pressure					✓
High serum cholesterol					✓

Cohort study – Grodstein et al (1996)

Confounding factor	Strategy to address confounder			Not taken into account	
	Matched design	Restricted design	Analysis	Measured	Not measured
Age			✓		
Socio-economic status					✓
Time period			✓		
Area				✓	
Prior CV disease (inc VTE)		✓			
Cancer		✓			
Diabetes			✓		
Immobility/surgery/trauma		(✓)			
History of varicose veins		(✓)			
Parity			✓		
Body mass index			✓		
Smoking status			✓		
Alcohol use					✓
High blood pressure			✓		
High serum cholesterol			✓		

VTE = Venous thromboembolism; CV = Cardiovascular

2.9 and an adjusted odds ratio of 3.6. In other words, the effect of the confounders had been to disguise the association between HRT and thromboembolism. Thus, it may be that people in a higher socioeconomic group are more likely to take HRT and less likely to have a thromboembolic event. In the Nurses' Health Study, the relative risk was adjusted for age, smoking, body mass index, diabetes, high blood pressure, high serum cholesterol, parity, and time period, to give an adjusted relative risk of 2.1 (as compared with a crude unadjusted relative risk of 1.7 – see Box 8.1).

Table 8.2 summarises how the two studies dealt with the various confounding factors. There is considerable overlap between which factors were taken into account in the two studies, but also, some factors were taken into account by one study, but not by the other. Thus, the cohort study did not take account of socioeconomic status, and the case-control study did not take account of level of blood pressure. The reader needs to form a view as to how important it is that such factors were not taken into account. With regard to critical appraisal, the key questions to consider are: first, have important confounders been identified and measured? The reader must have some knowledge of the disease to be able to answer this question. Some confounding factors are not immediately obvious and this part of the appraisal does require some consideration. If they have not identified and measured confounders, then the results cannot be adjusted to take account of them. Second, how accurately and precisely have the confounding factors been recorded? Inaccuracy (e.g. classifying a smoker as a non-smoker) or imprecision (e.g. grouping together ages into age bands) may result in residual confounding. In other words, the confounding factor is still having an impact on the results.

2. Is it likely that there is selection bias?

For a cohort study, there is considerable overlap between the concept of selection bias and the concept of confounding. Selection bias occurs if the exposed and unexposed groups are selected in such a way that they have different risks of developing the outcome of interest (independent of any effect exposure might have). This differential risk would be mediated by a confounding factor. Women who take HRT may be healthier than women who do not take HRT for a number of reasons (e.g. smoke less; more health conscious; higher social class). This selection bias will confound any observational study looking at the health effects of HRT and disguise any adverse health effects. Although observational studies had consistently shown that HRT was associated with lower risk of coronary heart disease, randomised controlled trials have demonstrated the opposite, suggesting that the observational studies were 'severely biased' (Beral et al 2002). This is likely to be because of the selection of healthier women to take HRT, whether by doctors or self-selection by the women themselves.

Selection bias is a significant problem in case-control studies, where it is useful to consider it as a distinct phenomenon from confounding. In this instance, selection bias occurs if the cases or controls are selected in a way that is related to exposure status. There may be bias both in the selection of the control group and in the selection of the cases.

Perhaps the most difficult part of a case-control study is deciding how the controls should be selected. In essence, the purpose of the controls is to provide an unbiased estimate of the prevalence of exposure in the population from which the cases are drawn. Thus, the control patients should be drawn from the same population as the cases. One way of considering this is to ask the question: if a control patient had the outcome of interest, would they have been included in the study? For a study where the cases are identified by virtue of their admission to hospital, this can be a difficult question to answer, since hospital catchment areas do not necessarily coincide with discrete geographical areas. Often, in such a circumstance, the controls are also selected by virtue of their admission to the same hospital, but for a reason other than the outcome of interest. This is what Daly et al did in their study. The potential downside of using hospital controls is that many types of admission might be indirectly related to HRT-use. For example, HRT may protect against osteoporotic fracture (Barrett-Connor 1998), but is associated with increased risk of breast cancer (Million Women Study Collaborators 2003). Thus, if controls included patients with breast cancer, then the prevalence of exposure to HRT in the population from which the cases are drawn would be overestimated, whereas if patients with fractures were included, then the prevalence of exposure might be underestimated. Daly et al tried to avoid these pitfalls by selecting women with a diagnosis 'judged to be unrelated to HRT-use'.

Selection of cases can be a problem if there is the possibility of a diagnostic bias: are people more likely to be identified as cases simply because they have been exposed to the risk factor under study? This is sometimes referred to as Berkson's bias. For example, if general practitioners were aware that there might be an association between oral contraception and HRT, then they might be more inclined to refer women with a swollen leg to hospital if they were taking HRT. Again, this is a particular problem where the case-control study relies on hospital admission for identification of cases, and would be avoided if efforts were made to conduct a population-based case-control study where one identifies community cases as well as hospital cases. However, in this example, Berkson's bias probably would not have been a major problem as the guidance at the time was that there was no link between HRT and venous thromboembolism (British National Formulary 1995).

Another form of selection bias is that cases may be more (or less) likely than controls to participate or respond. Egger et al (2001) give the example of a case-control study looking at whether infection with Helicobacter pylori is associated with coronary heart disease. The response rate of cases was 60%, but of controls only 20%. Egger et al argue that response is likely to be related to socioeconomic status, which is also known to be related to H. pylori infection. Therefore, this selection bias might have exaggerated the association between H. pylori and coronary heart disease, since the control group will have had a higher proportion of more affluent people, who have a lower incidence of H. pylori infection than people from more deprived backgrounds.

3. Is it likely that there is information bias?

Information bias occurs when there are systematic differences in the way information is collected on exposure or outcome between cases and controls, or between the different groups in a cohort study (Hennekens & Buring 1987).

In a cohort study, potential problems occur if an exposed person is more likely to be diagnosed with the outcome of interest than an unexposed person with the same symptoms. Thus, for example, surveillance for disease may be greater in exposed people: HRT-users may see health care professionals more frequently because they are on this therapy. Similarly, doctors may be more likely to make a diagnosis of venous thromboembolism if a patient is on HRT and the study investigators may be more inclined to categorise someone as suffering from a venous thromboembolism if they are on HRT. These problems can be minimised by using objective criteria to define the presence of the disease – thus in Grodstein et al's study a positive ventilation-perfusion scan, pulmonary arteriogram or post-mortem was required for a diagnosis of pulmonary embolus to be made. If the outcome of interest is more subjective (e.g. health status) then it would be important to blind (make unaware of) the investigator to the exposure status of the individual, and the individual to the hypothesis being tested.

Another way in which information bias can creep into a cohort study is if the investigators lose contact with the study participants – referred to as losses to follow-up. This will be a particular problem if loss to follow-up is related to exposure and/or outcome occurrence. Grodstein et al report that they achieved over 90% of follow-up – which makes significant information bias through losses to follow-up less likely.

In case-control studies, problems occur if identification of exposure status is influenced by whether the participant is a case or control. Again, blinding the investigator and the participant can help reduce such bias. An elegant example of the impact of blinding in case-control studies is provided by Egger et al (2001), who showed that there was a significant association of intermittent sunlight exposure with melanoma in the pooled results of unblinded case-control studies, but this association was not found in the blinded studies. This implies that there was differential recording of past sunlight exposure between cases and controls in the unblinded studies, but not in the blinded studies. A related problem, recall bias, where cases may be more likely to remember exposure than controls, may still occur even if participants are blinded. For example, recall bias is a problem in case-control studies of congenital abnormalities, where parents of children with abnormalities may be more likely to remember exposure to possible risk factors than parents of healthy children (Swan et al 1992). One way of reducing this sort of problem is to provide prompts during the interview. Thus, the investigators in the HRT case-control study used photographs of currently available HRT preparations while interviewing participants (Daly et al 1996). An effective way of eliminating recall bias in a case-control study is to nest a case-control study within a prospective study. This is what was

Box 8.4 Is an association between exposure and disease causal?

1. How strong is the association?	How large is the odds ratio (case control study) or relative risk (cohort study)?
2. How consistent is the evidence?	Have different types of study in different places and at different times shown the same association between exposure and disease?
3. Is the temporal relationship correct?	Does exposure precede onset of the disease?
4. Is causation biologically plausible?	Does a causal link fit with what we know already from our understanding of the basic sciences such as pathology and physiology in relation to the disease process?
5. Is there a dose response relationship?	Are people who have had greater exposure at greater risk of the disease?
6. Is there evidence of reversibility?	If the risk factor is removed, does the incidence of the disease fall?
7. Might confounding still explain the association?	Is it plausible that the association is due to confounding factors that have been inadequately dealt with in the studies?

done in a second case-control study, nested within a long-term cohort study, the Oxford Family Planning Association contraceptive study (Daly et al 1996a). In this study, data on thrombo-embolic events and on HRT-use were being prospectively collected on women as part of a long-term cohort study of the health effects of oral contraception. This approach avoided recall bias, as exposure history was ascertained prior to the 'cases' having their thromboembolic event.

4. What is the size of the odds ratio/relative risk?

Having decided whether or not the results are valid, the next step is to consider what they mean. There are two aspects to this: looking at the size of the odds ratio/relative risk, and the size of the confidence interval around the odds ratio/relative risk. The higher the odds ratio/relative risk, the stronger the association between exposure and disease.

5. How large are the confidence intervals around the odds/ratio relative risk?

Having decided whether or not the results are valid, the next step is to consider what they mean. There are two aspects to this: looking at the size of the odds ratio/relative risk, and the size of the confidence interval around the odds ratio/relative risk. The higher the odds ratio/relative risk, the stronger the association between exposure and disease. The 95% confidence intervals represent the bounds within which the true odds ratio/relative risk probably[2] lies given the results of the study. If the confidence intervals include 1, then no statistically significant association between exposure and disease has been observed in the study. In the Nurses' Health Study, the adjusted relative risk was reported to be 2.1, with a 95% confidence interval from 1.2 to 3.8 (Grodstein et al 1996). This implies that there is a significant association between HRT and pulmonary embolus, and HRT may lead to as high as a fourfold or as low as a 20% increase in risk, though the best estimate from the study is that the risk is doubled.

6. Is it likely, if an association is observed, that the relationship between exposure and disease is causal?

From a clinical point of view, one wants to be able to form a judgement as to whether or not an association between exposure and disease is causal, since this would guide whether you advised patients to avoid exposure or not. Unfortunately, observational studies cannot provide definitive proof of causality, only circumstantial evidence. In order to weigh up the likelihood that an association is causal, it is necessary to consider the evidence from an observational study in the context of other evidence that is available. A classic guideline for doing this was produced by Bradford-Hill (1965). An adaptation of this guideline is shown in Box 8.4.

7. How big is the risk?

Risk can be presented in two main ways: relative and absolute. Odds ratios and relative risks are relative measures of risk, in that they tell you how much more likely it is that someone who is exposed will develop the disease as compared with someone who is not exposed. They do not tell you how big the risk is for an individual, since this is dependent on what is their underlying risk. It is not possible to derive an absolute measure of risk from a case-control study without using information fromm other sources. For example, in a case-control study of third-generation oral contraceptives and risk of venous theomboembolism (Spitzer et al 1996), the odds ratio for thromboembolism in third-generation users as compared with second generation users was 1.5. The authors estimated that this equated to an absolute risk of death from thromboembolism of 14 per million users per year in second-generation users and 20 (approximately 1.5 x 14)[3] per million

---

2 i.e. the confidence interval will contain the true value for the odds ratio/ relative risk 19 times out of 20 – or 95% of the time.

3 It is not exactly 1.5 x 14 since an odds ratio is not identical to a relative risk, though it can often be thought of as being virtually equivalent to a relative risk. Further discussion of the relationship between an odds ratio and a relative risk can be found in Chapter 8.

users per year in third-generation users. They did this by finding out what the death rates for thromboembolism were from routine national statistics, and assuming that the prevalence of exposure in the controls reflected the prevalence of exposure in the whole population. Thus, they could conclude that if one million patients were switched from third-generation to second-generation pills, this would prevent six deaths per year. In other words, 166 666 women[4] would need to switch to prevent one death. This representation of the size of the risk in absolute terms is easier to interpret when it comes to making informed choices about which pill to take. Absolute risk can be derived from a cohort study. Thus, in Box 8.1, the risk of a pulmonary embolus in someone who has never used HRT is 0.84 per 10,000 years. In other words, if you had 10 000 women who had never used HRT, you would expect one of them to suffer a pulmonary embolus over the course of a year. Multiplying this risk by 1.7 still produces a very low absolute risk of pulmonary embolus in HRT users – 1.4 events in 10 000 HRT users over the course of a year.

8. Is exposure of patients in the study similar to the exposure of your own patients?

There are a number of different formulations of HRT: oestrogen-only, oestrogen combined with progesterone, different oestrogen doses and indeed methods of administration. It is useful to know whether the formulations of HRT used in the studies are the same as that used in your own local practice. Grodstein et al did not report what types of HRT were being used in the Nurses' Health Study. Daly et al (1996), in a sub-group analysis, looked at the risks associated with different formulations, and found there was a consistently raised risk, regardless of the type of HRT being taken.

Box 8.5 Criteria for assessing validity of a cohort study giving information on prognosis

Key issues
1. Was there a representative sample of patients?
2. Were the patients at a similar point in the course of their illness?
3. Was follow-up complete?

Secondary issues
4. Was follow-up over a sufficient period of time?
5. Were the outcomes used objective and unbiased?
6. Was adjustment made for important prognostic factors?

Adapted from Laupacis et al (1994)

---

4   1 000 000 / 6 = 166 666

STUDIES ASSESSING PROGNOSIS

As mentioned at the beginning of the chapter, observational studies, and in particular, cohort studies, can be a useful source of information about prognosis. The major criteria for assessing the validity of studies describing prognosis are shown in Box 8.5 (Laupacis et al 1994). Perhaps the most important question to consider is whether the patients in the study are representative of patients in the population as a whole. For example, studies that are based on patients who are referred to specialist centres are likely to give estimates of prognosis that are worse than studies that also include patients who are managed in primary care. This is sometimes labelled referral filter bias.

It helps if the patients are at a similar point in the illness when they are entered into the study. This might be early (sometimes referred to as an inception cohort) or later in the course of the disease. If patients are entered into the study at different stages of an illness, then the results can be difficult to interpret since duration of illness is likely to be associated with outcome.

Completeness of follow-up is particularly important for prognosis studies, since it is likely that loss to follow-up will be associated with outcome. For example, patients who have a good outcome (i.e. remain well) may be less likely to attend follow-up, because it does not seem relevant to them. Conversely, it could be argued that patients with a poor outcome may be less likely to be followed up, either because it is too much effort for them to attend, or perhaps because they have died. Either way, the bigger the loss to follow-up, the less certain the reader can be that the prognosis observed in the patients followed up is truly representative of the prognosis in the whole study population.

CONCLUSION

Cohort and case-control studies play an important role in answering questions about harm and aetiology (causation). However, because they are prone to bias, in particular as a result of confounding, the conclusions that can be drawn from any one observational study tend to more circumspect than those that can be drawn from a well-designed randomised controlled trial. Therefore, such papers need to be appraised carefully and interpreted in the light of whatever other evidence is available.

References

Barrett-Connor E 1998 Hormone replacement therapy. British Medical Journal317:457-461

Beral V, Banks E, Reeves G 2002 Evidence from randomised trials on the long-term effects of hormone replacement therapy. Lancet 360:942-944

Bradford-Hill A 1965 The environment and disease: association or causation? Journal of the Royal Society of Medicine 58:295-300

British National Formulary 1995 Number 28. British Medical Association and the Royal Pharmaceutical Society of Great Britain, London

Connor R, Prorok P, Weed D 1991 The case-control design and the assessment of the efficacy of cancer screening. Journal Clinical Epidemiology 44:1215-1221

Daly E, Vessey M, Hawkins M et al 1996 Risk of venous thromboembolism in users of hormone replacement therapy. Lancet 348:977-980

Daly E, Vessey M, Painter R, Hawkins M 1996a Case-control study of venous thromboembolism risk in users of hormone replacement therapy. Lancet 348: 1027

Egger G, Davey Smith G, Schneider M 2001 Systematic reviews of observational studies. In: Egger M, Davey Smith G, Altman DG (eds) Systematic reviews in health care: meta-analysis in context. British Medical Journal Publication. London, p 211-227

Grimes D A, Schulz K F 2002 An overview of clinical research: the lay of the land. Lancet 359:57-61

Grodstein F, Stampfer M J, Goldhaber S Z et al 1996 Prospective study of exogenous hormones and risk of pulmonary embolism in women. Lancet 348:983-987

Hennekens C H, Buring J E 1987 Epidemiology in medicine. Little, Brown, Boston

Inskip PD, Tarone RE, Hatch EE et al 2001 Cellular telephone use and brain tumours. New England Journal Medicine 344:79-86

Laupacis A, Wells G, Richardson S, Tugwell P 1994 Users' guides to the medical literature V. How to use an article about prognosis. Journal of the American Medical Association 272:234-237

Mant J, Vessey M 2002 Using case-control studies for prescribing research. Journal of Clinical Pharmacy and Therapeutics 27:67-74

Million Women Study Collaborators 2003 Breast cancer and hormone replacement therapy in the Million Women Study. Lancet 362:419-427

Nichol K L, Nordin J, Mullooly J et al 2003 Influenza vaccination and reduction in hospitalisations for cardiac disease and stroke among the elderly. New England Journal of Medicine 348:1322-1332

Spitzer W O, Lewis M A, Heinemann L A J et al 1996 Third-generation oral contraceptives and risk of venous thromboembolic disorders: an international case-control study. British Medical Journal 312:83-88

Swan S H, Shaw G M, Schulman J 1992 Reporting and selection bias in case-control studies of congenital malformations. Epidemiology 3:356-63

Titan S M O, Bingham S, Welch A et al 2001 Frequency of eating and concentrations of serum cholesterol in the Norfolk population of the European prospective investigation into cancer (EPIC-Norfolk): cross-sectional study. British Medical Journal 323:1286-1288

Vandenbroucke J P, Helmerhost F M 1996 Risk of venous thrombosis with hormone replacement therapy. Lancet 348:972

Chapter 9

Systematic review

Kate Seers

INTRODUCTION

Imagine it is a usual day at work. You are working with patients and you need to make a decision about the best plan of care for one particular patient. There may be one or more parts of that care where you are not sure what the best plan would be. For example, perhaps you are planning pain management, and you think that this patient might benefit from relaxation to enhance the pain relief. Is there any evidence on which to base this decision? So you start with a clinical problem; a patient with pain, and not knowing whether relaxation might help. This then is turned into a first draft of a clinical question: is relaxation effective in reducing pain? (see Chapter 2 for more details on moving from a clinical problem to a clinical question) and the clinical question is used to direct a search for evidence that can answer this question.

You may find a mountain of research papers, and it is just not feasible to read all of them. Or the amount may be more manageable, but some of the studies you find suggest the evidence is very positive, whereas others are less clear or even negative. Or perhaps there are several small studies, but you are not sure how robust their findings are. Where does that leave you with your clinical question that needs answering so that you can give the best possible care? What do you do and how do you decide what the overall evidence shows?

This chapter will look at how you try to judge studies that search for all research on a specific question and in some way combine it. If you are interested in actually undertaking such a review, then the Centre for Reviews and Dissemination Report (2001), the Cochrane Library reviewers' handbook (Clarke & Oxman 2003) and the QUOROM statement (Moher et al 1999), are useful resources.

One way to try to get an overview of research that might answer your clinical question is to search the literature for a systematic review of the area (see Chapter 3 for searching using 'publication type'). But what exactly is a systematic review, and how is it different from any other sort of review?

You may be familiar with the narrative reviews traditionally found in many journals. Normally someone, usually an expert, looks at the evidence in a certain area. Mulrow (1987) argued that traditional reviews do not routinely use systematic methods to identify, assess and synthesise information. Thus, normally there is no methods section for the actual conduct of the review. The reader then has no way of knowing whether the review is based on a systematic review of the evidence, or on a collection of papers which the author has found in a less systematic way and thus the evidence presented may not be complete. Mulrow (1987, 1994) argues there is a need for systematic reviews of the evidence. This needs to be undertaken in just as rigorous a way as any primary piece of research, with a clear question and explicit methods for all stages of the process.

Definitions of a systematic review have identified this need to be methodical. One such definition describes a systematic review as:

> a review of a clearly formulated question that uses systematic and explicit methods to identify, select and critically appraise relevant research, and to collect and analyse data from studies that are included in the review. Statistical methods (meta-analysis) may or may not be used to analyse and summarise the results of the included studies.
>
> *Cochrane Library 2003: Glossary Version 4.1.4*

This should mean that another person could replicate the review, as the next definition highlights.

A systematic review is:

> an attempt to minimise the element of arbitrariness . . . by making explicit the review process, so that, in principle, another reviewer with access to the same resources could undertake the review and reach broadly the same conclusions.
>
> *Dixon et al 1997:157*

Three key features of such a review are:

- a strenuous effort to locate all original reports on the topic of interest
- critical evaluation of the reports
- conclusions are drawn and based on a synthesis of studies which meet preset quality criteria (Crombie & McQuay 1998:1).

When synthesising results, a meta-analysis may be undertaken. This is: 'the use of statistical techniques in a systematic review to integrate the results of the included studies' (Cochrane Library 2003: Glossary Version 4.1.4).

A meta-analysis is thus a statistical technique for combining data (or pooling data) from several studies within a systematic review. A meta-analysis in itself does not necessarily mean the review on which it is based is systematic. The Centre for Reviews and Dissemination Report (2001) suggests it may be best to pool studies on each relevant measurement of the effect of the intervention that is presented in the original studies.

WHY UNDERTAKE A SYSTEMATIC REVIEW?

There are many reasons for undertaking a systematic review, and some of these are outlined by Mulrow (1994):

- to reduce large quantities of information into smaller pieces for easier digestion
- decision-makers need to integrate critical pieces of biomedical information
- it is an efficient scientific technique
- generalisability of findings of the individual studies included can be established
- to assess consistency of relationships (e.g. same direction and same size of effect)
- explain data inconsistencies and conflicts
- increased power
- increased precision in estimates of risk or effect size
- improved reflection of reality.

Another reason for the importance of systematic reviews is outlined by Antman et al (1992). They looked at the accumulating data from randomised controlled trials (RCTs) of treatments for myocardial infarctions and the recommendations of clinical experts writing review articles and textbook chapters. They found that review articles and textbooks often failed to mention important advances and in some cases potentially harmful treatments continued to be recommended by some experts.

WHERE CAN YOU FIND SYSTEMATIC REVIEWS?

Systematic reviews have been published in a variety of journals. In addition, the Cochrane Collaboration provides an important resource in this area. Jadad et al (1998) found the Cochrane reviews tended to have greater methodological rigour and to be updated more frequently than those published in paper-based journals. The Cochrane Collaboration was founded in 1993 and is 'an international non-profit and independent organisation, dedicated to making up-to-date, accurate information about the effects of health care readily available worldwide. It produces and disseminates systematic reviews of health care interventions and promotes the search for evidence in the form of clinical trials and other studies of interventions.' (Cochrane Library 2003). It promotes and publishes the Cochrane Library, a collection of seven separate databases, one of which is the Cochrane Database of Systematic Reviews (CDSR).

In Cochrane Library 2003, Issue 4, there were 1837 completed reviews and protocols for an additional, 1344 reviews currently being undertaken. Such a review has a pre-specified protocol, where every stage of the process of undertaking the review is made explicit. The rapid rise in the number of reviews available can be seen by comparing these figures with those from 5 years ago in 1998 when there were 481 completed reviews, an additional 438 protocols in the CDSR.

Sections covered in a protocol include background, objectives, criteria for considering studies for the review (including types of participants, types of interventions, types of outcome measure, types of study), search strategy for identification of studies, study selection, methodological quality assessment, data extraction, meta-analysis, the comparisons to be made, sub-group analysis and sensitivity analysis to be undertaken. The point to note here is that all these aspects of the protocol are set out before the review is undertaken.

DIFFERENT TYPES OF SYSTEMATIC REVIEWS

Many of the systematic reviews so far completed are based on evidence of effectiveness of an intervention from RCTs. Methodologies for systematic reviews using other research designs, such as observational studies, diagnosis, prognosis, economic appraisal and qualitative research are less well developed, although there are guidelines or discussions of the issues (qualitative: Noblit & Hare 1988, Sandelowski et al 1997, 2003, Finfgeld 2003; diagnosis: Irwig et al 1994, Deeks 2001; observational studies: Egger et al 1998, 2001, Stroup et al 2000; prognosis: Altman 2001; economics: Donaldson et al 2002, Rigby et al 1996). There are also Cochrane Health Economics and Qualitative Methods Groups. The recent Centre for Reviews & Dissemination (2001) publication on undertaking systematic reviews reflects this move towards a much wider range of types of evidence being used to compile systematic reviews.

CRITICAL APPRAISAL OF SYSTEMATIC REVIEWS

If you find a systematic review, how do you assess whether or not it is any good? Most of the checklists developed relate to assessing the reporting of meta-analyses of RCTs (e.g. Moher et al's 1999 QUOROM statement). Some do apply to observational studies (Stroup et al 2000 MOOSE). Work on developing appropriate criteria for qualitative systematic reviews is ongoing (see Cochrane Qualitative Research Methods Group website http://mysite.freeserve.com/Cochrane_Qual_Method/qmmodule5.htm [accessed 1.12.03])

Heading	Subheading	Descriptor	Reported? (Y/N)	Page number
Title		Identify the report as a meta-analysis (or systematic review) of RCT's		
Abstract		Use a structured format		
		Describe		
	Objectives	The clinical question explicitly		
	Data sources	The databases (ie, list) and other information sources		
	Review methods	The selection criteria (ie, population, intervention, outcome, and study design); methods for validity assessment, data abstraction, and study characteristics, and quantative data synthesis in sufficient detail to permit replication		
	Results	Characteristics of the RCT's included and excluded; qualitative and quantitative findings (ie, point estimates and confidence intervals); and subgroup analysis		
	Conclusion	The main results		
		Describe		
Introduction		The explicit clinical problem, biological rationale for the intervention, and rationale for review		
Methods	Searching	The information sources, in detail (eg, databases, registers, personal files, expert informants, agencies, hand-searching), and any restrictions (years considered, publication status,"language of publication")		
	Selection	The inclusion and exclusion criteria (defining population, intervention, principal outcomes, and study design)		
	Validity assessment	The criteria and process used (eg, masked conditios, quality assessment, and their findings)		
	Data abstraction	The process or processes used (eg, completed independently, in duplicate)		
	Study characteristics	The type of study design, participants' characteristics, details of intervention, outcome definitions, &c, and how clinical heterogeneity was assessed		
	Quantitative data synthesis	The principal measures of effect (eg, relative risk), method of combining results (statistical testing and confidence intervals), handling of missing data; how statistical heterogeneity was assessed; a rationale for any a-priori sensitivity and subgroup analysis; and any assessment of publication bias		
Results	Trial flow	Provide a meta-analysis profile summarising trial flow (see figure)		
	Study characteristics	Present descriptive data for each trial (eg, age, sample size, intervention, dose, duration, follow-up period)		
	Quantitative data synthesis	Report agreement on the selection and validity assessment, present simple summary results (for each treatment group in each trial, for each primary outcome); present data needed to calculate effect sizes and confidence intervals in intention-to-treat analyses(eg, 2x2 tables of counts, means and SD's proportions)		
Discussion		Summarise key findings; discuss clinical inferences based on internal and external validity; interpret the results in light of the totality of available evidence; describe potential biases in the review process (eg. publication bias) and suggest a future research agenda		

Quality of reporting of meta-analyses

Figure 9.1 Meta-analysis of the effect of combined topical and systemic antibiotics as prophylaxis for respiratory tract infections in patients in intensive care units. This figure illustrates the different weights given to different studies (the different sized square boxes) and the overall effect (the diamond). The figure shows there is a strong protective effect of combined topical and systemic antibiotics in this group of patients, with an odds ratio of 0.35 (CI 0.29-0.41). Thus patients having this combination reduced their incidence of respiratory tract infection by 65%. (This figure was first published in the BMJ: D'Amico R, Pifferi S, Leonetti C et al 1998 Effect of antibiotic prophylaxis in critically ill adult patients: a systematic review of randomised controlled trials. British Medical Journal 316:1275-1285. It is reproduced by permission of the BMJ)

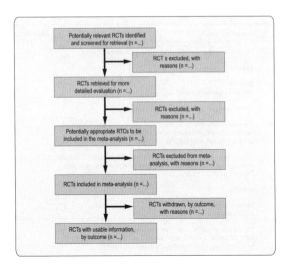

Figure 9.2

Since most work has been undertaken on systematic reviews of RCTs, this will be the focus of this section. However, systematic reviews using other types of evidence are very important and as work develops in this area, future editions of this book will be updated to include this wider range of types of evidence.

One place to start is to use a guide which suggests a structured way of looking at the systematic review. Such guides have been developed by Oxman et al (1994), Dixon et al (1997), Greenhalgh (1997) and Moher et al (1999) [QUOROM statement], amongst others. The latter publication is based on the best available evidence. Its authors suggest it can be used for planning, performing and reporting a meta-analysis, as well as during peer review of the report. The QUOROM statement 18 item checklist is reproduced in Figure 9.1 and its flow diagram in Figure 9.2. Shea et al (2001) compare the QUOROM statement with other tools and conclude that most others are missing important evidence-based items.

The Oxman et al (1994) checklist is also presented here, following reports from some students that they find it more accessible when starting to critically appraise systematic reviews for the first time.

Oxman et al (1994) break down their approach into three sections:

- are the results valid?
- if they are, what are the results?
- will the results help in my patient care?

Answers are, typically, yes, no or cannot tell.

These three sections are further sub-divided as outlined below, with the first two questions being called a primary guide (to quickly screen out unsuitable studies) and questions 3 to 11 called secondary guides because they look at the research in more detail.

ARE THE RESULTS VALID?

Primary guides

1. Did the review address a focused clinical question?

If the clinical question being addressed is not clear, Oxman et al (1994) suggest moving on to the next article. (See Chapter 2 on asking clinical questions.)

2. Were the criteria used to select articles for inclusion appropriate?

The reader needs to know what criteria were used to select the research. This should include who the study participants were, what was done and what outcomes were assessed. In addition, the methodological criteria for selecting the study should reflect the essential elements of good design in the primary study. Thus if studies included were RCTs, you would expect only studies which had randomised patients to treatments to be included. The strictness of additional elements of good RCT design should be applied, such as randomisation being adequately and appropriately described. Other criteria, such as blinding or intention to treat analysis may vary, but should be explicit.

For example, if a systematic review was undertaken looking at the use of relaxation for acute pain control, studies may be restricted to randomised studies of patients aged 18 to 65 who had no pre-existing chronic pain, and had a particular type of relaxation administered in a standardised manner. Outcomes may be only changes in pain, or might be broader and include changes in anxiety, medication use or perceptions of control.

A point to consider is that the narrower the inclusion criteria, the less generalisable are the results. In the above example, it would be difficult to know how far or whether one could apply the results of such a review to patients who had chronic pain and who were over 65. Similarly, if a different type of relaxation had been used, it would be uncertain how transferable any findings might be. However, this needs to be balanced with using very broad inclusion criteria, when heterogeneity becomes an issue. Such studies may cover a wide range of patients and/or interventions and/or outcomes and the justification for then combining these differing groups comes into question.

The importance of a clear statement of inclusion criteria is that studies should be selected on the basis of these criteria (i.e. any study that matches these criteria is included) rather than selecting the study on the basis of the results.

Secondary guides

3. Is it unlikely that important relevant studies were missed?

Here you are looking for the comprehensiveness of the search. Which databases have been searched? Have any obvious ones been missed? Have the researchers checked the reference lists of articles and of textbooks, contacted experts (to get their list of references checked for completeness, tried to find out about ongoing or unpublished research) and searched for the 'grey' (unpublished) literature? Has hand-searching been used? Search terms used are also important – has an obvious MeSH term been missed or is there another term they have not used? For example, when searching for papers looking at care of the elderly, use of the term 'senior' in the North American literature may be overlooked. Are languages other than English included? This may have important implications; for example, Dickersin et al (1994) found 20% of vision trials were not in English. Unpublished data are useful to include because Egger and Davey Smith (1998) highlight how studies with significant results are more likely to be published than studies without significant results (publication bias). One way of looking for publication bias is to use a funnel plot. This shows graphically 'the distribution of effect sizes according to sample size' (Centre for Reviews and Dissemination 2001: Stage II:17). The points on this graph should look like a funnel, and if they do not, then some studies may not have been found or published. Egger et al (1997) have proposed a graphical test to detect bias in meta-analysis.

4. Was the validity of the included studies appraised?

Was the quality of the original studies included in the review assessed? Here you are looking to see whether the design and execution of the included studies suggest likely systematic biases.

Ensuring studies of effectiveness are randomised is important. For example, Seers and Carroll (1998) found that non-randomised studies into the effectiveness of relaxation for acute pain were much more likely to show a positive result than randomised studies. Schultz et al (1995) found studies where randomisation was inadequately concealed could overestimate odds ratios by as much as 40%, and trials that were not double blind exaggerated odds ratios by 17%. However, a systematic review by Kunz et al (2003: 2) was more conservative. They concluded that whilst 'non-randomised trials and randomised trials with inadequate concealment of allocation tend to result in larger estimates of effect than randomised trials with adequately concealed allocation … it is not generally possible to predict the magnitude or even the direction of possible selection biases and consequent distortions of treatment effects'.

Whether or not one should use a quality filter to decide whether to include studies has been the subject of debate. Although Dixon et al (1997:157) argue that a systematic review 'requires … an explicit system for grading the quality of evidence obtained', the advice from the Cochrane Library reviewers' handbook (Clarke and Oxman 2003: section 6.7.2) is that 'none of the currently available scales for measuring the validity or "quality" of trials can be recommended without reservation. If reviewers … choose to use such a scale, it must be with caution.' These scales have been reviewed by Moher et al (1995), who assessed 25 scales and nine checklists. One pragmatic approach is to use some sort of quality scale, and then do a sensitivity analysis and look at the results with low-quality studies in, and then with them excluded (Sindhu 1996). This also gives an indication of the robustness of the findings of the review.

5. Were assessments of the studies reproducible?

Oxman et al (1994) point out that each decision about which studies to include, their validity and which data to extract are all subjective decisions requiring judgements which are affected by mistakes (random errors) and bias (systematic errors). They argue that having two or more people making these judgements guards against such errors. So here you are looking for more than one person reading the paper and deciding whether or not to include it.

6. Were the results similar from study to study?

In some ways this is a difficult question, because how similar is 'similar'? It is common that a variety of patients having a range of broadly similar but slightly different interventions which have been assessed using a range of outcomes are included in a systematic review. There may also be differences in study design. Is it still sensible to combine results if this is the case? One factor which may help in this decision is a test for heterogeneity. This test looks at the probability that the differences between the studies result from chance alone.

Statistical heterogeneity is when results of individual trials are to some extent incompatible with each other (Thompson 1994). It exists when there is greater variation between the results than is likely owing to chance. Thompson (1994) points out that to understand these tests, it is useful to know that the chi square statistic on which they are based has an average p value equal to its degrees of freedom. Values much larger than the degrees of freedom suggest a smaller p value and thus significant statistical heterogeneity. This means greater variation exists between the studies than is likely by chance alone. One might then conclude that the studies are so different that it makes no sense to combine them. However, this test has a lower power (Thompson 1994). Higgins et al (2003) argue it is susceptible to the number of trials in the meta-analysis. They propose a new quantity, I^2, as giving a better measure of consistency. This I^2 ranges from 0-100%, and associated confidence intervals can be calculated. It is described as measuring the degree of inconsistency across studies in a meta-analysis. The advantanges of I^2 include that it can be compared between meta-analyses which have differing numbers of studies and different types of outcome data. Higgins et al (2003) give a tentative indication of low, medium and high heterogeneity as being 25%, 50% and 75% respectively. Clinical and statistical heterogeneity need to be distinguished. Clinical heterogeneity refers to differences between settings, patients, techniques and outcomes, which might lead you to suggest it does not make sense to combine the data.s

WHAT ARE THE RESULTS?

Systematic review

7. What do the results of a systematic review mean?

Terms that you will probably come across when looking at systematic reviews include vote counting, binary or continuous data, odds ratios, relative risks, weighted mean differences, fixed and random effects, diagnostic tests and meta-regression.

Vote counting. If a systematic review does not contain a meta-analysis, the results may be presented as a simple vote count, that is, the number of studies supporting, for example, an intervention and the number not supporting it. Problems associated with vote counting need to be kept in mind when interpreting these results, such as equal weight being given to each study, regardless of size.

Binary or continuous data. The type of data will dictate what you see when you look at a meta-analysis.

1. Binary data (e.g. an event rate: something that happens or it does not – myocardial infarction, stroke, improved/not improved) is usually combined using odds ratios. Methods exist for combining relative risks and risk differences. Note that absolute risk reduction and risk differences are synonymous, as are relative risk and risk ratio. Numbers needed to treat (NNTs) can also be helpful here (see Chapter 14 on therapy for more details on NNTs). McQuay and Moore (1997) argue for systematic reviews to produce an NNT so that results from systematic reviews can be more easily applied in practice.
2. Continuous data (e.g. numbers of days, peak expiratory flow rate) are combined using differences in mean values for treatment and control groups (weighted mean differences or WMD) when units of measurement are the same (e.g. all using the same anxiety scale), or standardised mean differences when units of measurement differ (e.g. using a variety of

anxiety scales, where one numerical value could mean very different things, depending on the scale used). Here the difference in means is divided by the pooled standard deviation.

Thus when you look at a meta-analysis, you will see odds ratios and/or weighted mean differences or standardised mean differences, depending on the outcomes measures that have been used in the included studies.

Odds ratio. What are the odds and where does the ratio come into it? The odds look at how much a treatment affects an event rate. The odds of an event are the probability of it occurring compared to the probability of it not occurring. The odds ratio is the ratio of the odds of an event in the treatment (or exposed) group compared with the odds in the control (or unexposed) group (see Chapter 8). Relative risk and absolute risk reduction may also be used to express these sorts of differences between a treatment and control group. An odds ratio of 1 means no difference between the groups.

Relative risk (also known as risk ratio). 'The risk (proportion, probability or rate) is the ratio of people with an event in a group to the total in that group' (Cochrane Library 2003. Glossary version 4.1.4). A relative risk is the risk in the treatment group compared to the risk in the control group. A relative risk of 1 means there is no difference between the groups (see Chapter 14 to see how the calculation of relative risks differs from odds ratios).

Relative risk is appealing because it is easier to understand than the rather abstract notion (to non-gamblers at least!) of an odds. There is debate over whether relative risks should be used in preference to odds ratios (see Deeks 1996), but odds ratios are commonly used. In case-control studies relative risks cannot be calculated (because the disease prevalence is not known), so odds ratios are used. If an event is rare, odds ratios and relative risks will be similar. At around a 10 to 20% event rate they start becoming different and if an event is common, they can be very different with the odds ratio showing a larger effect than the relative risk.

What do these odds and relative risks mean in plain English? Let's say a study looked at the odds of getting inadequate pain relief with relaxation compared with the odds of getting inadequate pain relief without relaxation. If the odds ratio was 0.70, this would mean you had 30% reduction in the odds of having inadequate pain relief with relaxation, compared with without relaxation. If the relative risk was 0.82, this would mean patients' risk of having inadequate pain relief is 18% less if they had relaxation.

What do odds ratios used in a meta-analysis look like? See Figure 9.3. The square box or 'blob' on the Forest plot (which is sometimes known colloquially as a 'blobogram') is the individual study effect (technically referred to as the point estimate) with its associated confidence intervals as lines either side of that box (technically known as the interval estimate).

Sometimes the size of the box may vary to reflect the weight that particular study is given, with larger boxes representing higher weighting. Lower weighted studies are usually those with smaller samples and large confidence intervals. The overall or summary effect (from combining or pooling the studies) is usually depicted as a diamond. Lau et al (1998) argue that since patients may respond differently to treatment, this pooling may need to be supplanted by summarising evidence along multiple covariates of interest. They conclude that 'patients' heterogeneity should be anticipated and sought up front, not ignored in pursuit of aggregate statistical significance' (Lau et al 1998: 127). Thus, although one overall number is appealing in its simplicity, it may oversimplify a more complex situation.

An odds ratio of 1 on a linear scale means there is no difference between the experimental and control group. This value of 1 is the line down the middle of the figure (sometimes with the wording 'favours treatment' on one side and 'favours control' on the other). If the confidence interval does not cross the line, it means that there is a 95% chance that there is a true difference between the groups. That is, that there is a significant difference on that particular outcome between the intervention and control groups.

Whether this favours the treatment or control will depend on which side of the vertical line the confidence interval appears. The left-hand side is less of

Figure 9.3

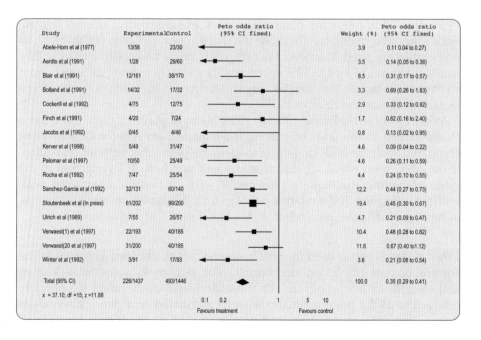

something, and the right-hand side is more of something. Whether this is 'good' or 'bad' depends on the variable. For example, fewer years alive might be 'bad' if you are aiming to improve survival, whereas fewer heart attacks might be 'good' if this was your intent. If the confidence interval does cross this vertical line labeled '1', it means that any difference in that outcome between the treatments could have occurred by chance (i.e. there are no significant differences, equal odds are plausible, there is no treatment effect). It may be that a very wide confidence interval is due to a very small sample size, and it would reduce with more people in the study. A 95% confidence interval covers likely results from a set of similar studies. It therefore provides a more realistic view of what will happen in practice than a point estimate, because it takes potential variability into account.

It is worth noting that a lack of evidence for an intervention is not the same as evidence of a lack of effect.

Odds ratios are often plotted on a log scale. This is because if we assume a desirable or good outcome of a particular treatment meant you had less of something (such as fewer strokes or fewer anxiety attacks), on a linear scale 0 to 1 would equal 'good', whereas 1 to infinity would equal 'bad'. This is clearly visually unbalanced, and using a log scale gives an equal line length for good and bad.

The other terms that are often seen in meta-analysis include the type of model used.

Fixed effects model. This ignores between-study heterogeneity and estimates treatment effect as if it were a single true value underlying all study results. That is, it assumes the treatment effect in all studies is the same and it ignores between-study variability. Any differences are described as the result of random (sampling) error within studies.

For binary data, tests used include Mantel-Haenszel method and the Peto method.

For continuous data, tests used include the weighted mean of study effects (if measures are on the same scale), or standardised mean effect sizes, or 'd-statistics' (if measures are on different scales).

Random effects model. This assumes individual study effect sizes will exhibit random variation, as they are a random sample from a population of effect sizes (Sindhu 1998). Differences between studies are thus a combination of random (sampling) error and variation between studies. This estimate is likely to be more conservative with a wider confidence interval. The Centre for Reviews and Dissemination Report (2001) suggests both are reported. Tests used in random effects are known as the DerSimonian-Laird method (DerSimonian & Laird 1986).

A Bayesian approach can also be used in meta-analysis. Cochrane Library (2003) glossary version 4.1.4 describes this as incorporating 'a prior probability distribution based on subjective opinion and objective evidence, such as the results of previous research'. This prior distribution is then updated based on the study results using Bayes' theorem, producing a posterior distribution, on which the statistical inferences are based. Since the prior probabilities are based partly on opinions, which can vary, this approach is described in the glossary as "controversial".

Diagnostic tests. Here you do not have an odds ratio. You will be looking at sensitivity/specificity, positive/negative predictive values or likelihood ratios. You might find the pictorial representation of this by Loong (2003) helpful.

Receiver-operating characteristic (ROC) curves mean several studies can be displayed (see Chapter 13 on diagnosis). The plot can show how differences in cut-off points taken can affect, for example, sensitivity and specificity, or true positive and false positive rates. The top left-hand corner represents maximum joint specificity and sensitivity or maximum true positive rate and minimum false positive rates.

Meta-regression. This is relatively new in meta-analysis. Lau et al (1998:124) describe it as an 'attempt to identify significant relations between the treatment effect … and the covariates of interest'. The unit of observation is the study or sub-group, rather than the individual patient. Lau et al (1998) argue that it may provide more insight than traditional pooling, as data can be modelled along one or multiple dimensions. However, Thompson and Higgins (2002) highlight the 'tension between the scientific rationale for using meta-regression and the difficult interpretative problems to which such analysis are prone'

8. How precise are the results?

This is asking whether there are any confidence intervals used, so the reader can see the range of values around the effect size, where one is 95% confident that the 'true' effect would lie. Clarke and Oxman (2003), section 6.1, define precision as 'a measure of the likelihood of chance effects leading to random errors. It is reflected in the confidence interval around the estimate of effect from each study … more precise results are given more weight.' Thus, the more precise the results, the narrower (smaller) the confidence interval. For example, an odds ratio of 0.35 and 95% confidence interval 0.22–0.56 shows the confidence interval does not cross the line (the value of 1) and there is a significant difference between the groups; an odds ratio of 1.12 and 95% confidence interval 0.75–1.67 clearly crosses the line (the value of 1) and the difference between groups is not significant.

WILL THE RESULTS HELP ME IN CARING FOR PATIENTS?

9. Can the results be applied to patient care?

How similar are the patients you care for to those included in the review? The wider the type of patients included in the review, the more likely you are to feel the results may apply across a range of different patients. However, it is sometimes a difficult decision to know whether, for example, something that works on men will be equally effective with women, or something that works in younger people will work in the same way in older people.

Sub-group analysis may be one way of addressing this concern, although there are concerns with this approach (e.g. Oxman & Guyatt 1992, Counsell et al 1994), especially if the study is not powered to consider sub-groups, and the sub-groups are not specified before the study starts. Sub-group analysis may be more like a fishing trip (to try to find significant results) when, in fact, the play of chance may have more to do with apparently significant results than any intrinsic differential effect of the intervention, as the Counsell et al (1994) article clearly highlighted. They looked at sub-group analysis and concluded that chance influences the outcome of clinical trials and systematic reviews much more than many investigators realise and this may lead to incorrect conclusions about the benefit of treatment. Davey Smith et al (1997) argue that you often need individual patient data for meaningful sub-group analysis. Clarke and Stewart (1997, 2001) similarly argue for the use of individual patient data to improve the reliability of meta-analysis, but also highlight the difficulties of obtaining such data.

10. Were all clinically important outcomes considered?

What is clinically important can depend on your perspective. Sometimes, whilst factors like bone density may be included in a review to assess the effectiveness of certain orthopaedic procedures, it may be some other outcome, like the ability to get to the shops, that needs to be considered and this sort of outcome may be crucial from the patient's perspective.

11. Are the benefits worth the harms and costs?

This may cover a range of factors, like benefit of early treatment following a positive cervical smear vs the harms of high anxiety. Or it may be the benefits of a chemotherapeutic agent vs its unpleasant side-effects. An economic evaluation may be included (see Chapter 10).

These criteria suggested by Oxman et al (1994) are worth considering when critically appraising a systematic review. But they can also create difficulties. When you use a set of criteria like this, you may end up with a variety of 'nos' or 'can't tells' in answer to the questions you pose. It is sometimes difficult to decide when a review is 'too bad' to give you any confidence in the findings. Perhaps one pragmatic approach would be that when you have several 'nos' or 'can't tells', you are more wary about the validity and robustness of the review's findings. What this does illustrate is that, like undertaking a systematic review, critically appraising these reviews is not an exact science, but there are many subjective decisions along the way. Just like undertaking a systematic review, making explicit your decisions in the critical appraisal is therefore very important.

It may be useful to ponder that although a systematic review can provide you with high-quality evidence, clinical experience and patient preferences are an important part of evidence-based health care (Sackett et al 1997). It may be that even high-quality evidence does not apply to a particular patient. This decision is the province of the health professional(s) in collaboration with the patient.

LIMITATIONS OF SYSTEMATIC REVIEWS AND META-ANALYSIS

Crombie and McQuay (1998) point out that it is important not to overstate potential limitations, as systematic reviews are a major advance on both the traditional review and the use of selected evidence that went before. However, there are some limitations. Crombie and McQuay (1998) raise the possibility that sometimes a review may mislead. They argue this can occur when the quality of the review is poor or when publication bias occurs. Thus a review may overestimate the effectiveness of the treatment/intervention. If the results of a review (which may combine several small trials) are compared with those of a large RCT, the results may not be the same. For example, Cappelleri et al (1996) found over 80% of 79 reviews agreed with large trials. LeLorier et al (1997) found a 65% agreement, although this article has been criticised by Naylor and Davey Smith (1998).

Eysenck (1995) argues that meta-analysis is often used to recover something from poor studies. The same article argues against combining varied treatments and end points. Petticrew (2003) concludes that uncertainty will often remain, but that systematic reviews can map what is known and where uncertainty lies.

Meta-analysis may be seen as concerned with the whole population, rather than an individual patient. However, with the shift away from a summary statistic to looking at multiple covariates that Lau et al (1998) advocate, their goal for meta-analysis of 'knowing how best to treat the individual' perhaps comes a little closer.

Acknowledgement

Many thanks to Nicola Crichton for her helpful comments on drafts of this chapter in the first edition.

References

Abele-Horn M, Dauber A, Bauernfeind A et al 1997 Decrease in nosocomial pneumonia ventilated patients by selective oropharyngeal decontamination (SPO). Intensive Care Medicine 23:187-195.

Aerdts S J A, van Dalen R, Clasener H A L et al 1991 Antibiotic prophylaxis of respiratory tract infection in mechanically ventilated patients. Chest 100:783-791

Altman D G 2001 Systematic reviews of evaluations of prognostic variables. In: Egger M, Davey Smith G, Altman DG (eds) Systematic reviews in health care. Meta-analysis in context. 2nd edn. British Medical Journal Publishing, London (Ch. 13), p 228-247

Antman E M, Lau J, Kupelnick B et al 1992 A comparison of the results of meta-analyses of randomised controlled trials and recommendations of clinical experts. Treatments for myocardial infarction. Journal of the American Medical Association 268 (2):240-248

Blair P, Rowlands B J, Lowry K et al 1991 Selective decontamination of the digestive tract: a stratified, randomized, prospective study in a mixed intensive care unit. Surgery 110:303-310

Boland J P, Sadler D L, Stewart W et al 1991 Reduction of nosocomial respiratory tract infections in the multiple trauma patients requiring mechanical ventilation by selective parenteral and enteral antisepsis regimen (SPEAR) in the intensive care [abstract]. Seventeenth Congress of Chemotherapy, Berlin, No 0465

Cappelleri J C, Ionnidis J P A, Schmid C H et al 1996 Large trials vs meta-analysis of smaller trials: how do their results compare? Journal of the American Medical Association 276:1332-1338

Centre for Reviews and Dissemination 2001 Undertaking systematic reviews of research on effectiveness. CRD's Guidance for those carrying out or commissioning reviews. CRD Report 4, 2nd edn. University of York. York

Chalmers I, Altman D (eds) 1995 Systematic reviews. British Medical Journal Publishing, London

Clarke M, Oxman AD 2003 (eds) Cochrane Reviewers' Handbook 4.2.0 [updated March 03] http://212.49.183.203/newgenMB/WebHelpSpecific/handbook.pdf (accessed 1st December 2003)

Clarke M J, Stewart L A 1997 Meta-analyses using individual patient data. Journal of Evaluation in Clinical Practice 3 (3):207-212

Clarke M J, Stewart L A 2001 Obtaining individual patient data from randomised controlled trials. In: Egger M, Davey Smith G, Altman DG (eds) Systematic reviews in health care. Meta-analysis in context. 2nd edn. British Medical Journal Publishing, London (Ch. 6), p 109-121

Cochrane Library 2003 Issue 4 . Wiley & Sons Ltd, Chichester, UK

Cockerill F R III, Muller S R, Anhalt J P et al 1992 Prevention of infection in critically ill patients by selective decontamination of the digestive tract. Annals of Internal Medicine 117:545-553

Counsell C E, Clarke M J, Slattery J et al 1994 The miracle of DICE therapy for acute stroke: fact or fictional product of sub group analysis. British Medical Journal 309:1677-1681

Crombie I K, McQuay H 1998 The systematic review: a good guide rather than guarantee. Pain 76:1-2

Davey Smith G, Egger M, Phillips A N 1997 Beyond the grand mean? British Medical Journal 315:1610-1614

Deeks J J 1996 Swots corner: What is an odds ratio? Bandolier 3(issue 25):6-7

Deeks J J 2001 Systematic reviews of evaluations of diagnostic and screening tests. In: Egger M, Davey Smith G, Altman DG (eds) Systematic reviews in health care. Meta-analysis in context. 2nd edn. British Medical Journal Publishing, London (Ch. 14), p 248-282

DerSimonian R, Laird N 1986 Meta-analysis in clinical trials. Controlled Clinical Trials 7:177-188

Dickersin K, Scherer R, Lefebvre C 1994 Identifying relevant studies for systematic reviews. British Medical Journal 309:1286-1291

Dixon R A, Munro J F, Silcocks P B 1997 The evidence-based medicine workbook. Critical appraisal for clinical problem solving. Butterworth-Heinemann, Oxford

Donaldson C, Mugford M, Vale L 2002 (eds) Evidence-based health economics. From effectiveness to efficiency in systematic review. British Medical Journal Publishing , London

Egger M, Davey Smith G 1998 Bias in location and selection of studies. British Medical Journal 316:61-66

Egger M, Davey Smith G, Altman DG 2001 Systematic reviews in health care. Meta-analysis in context. 2nd edn. British Medical Journal Publishing, London.

Egger M, Davey Smith G, Schneider M et al 1997 Bias in meta-analysis detected by a simple graphical test. British Medical Journal 315:629-634

Egger M, Davey Smith G, Schneider M 1998 Meta-analysis. Spurious precision? Meta-analysis of observational studies. British Medical Journal 316:140-144

Egger M, Davey Smith G, Schneider M 2001 Systematic reviews of observational studies. In: Egger M, Davey Smith G, Altman DG (eds) Systematic reviews in health care. Meta-analysis in context. 2nd edn. British Medical Journal Publishing, London (Ch. 12), p 211-227

Eysenck H J 1995 Problems with meta-analysis. In: Chalmers I, Altman D G (eds) Systematic reviews. British Medical Journal Publishing London (Ch 6), p 64-74

Finch R G, Tomlinson P, Holliday M et al 1991 Selective decontamination of the digestive tract (SDD) in the prevention of secondary sepsis in a medical/surgical intensive care unit [abstract]. Seventeenth International Congress of Chemotherapy. Berlin, No 0471

Finfgeld D L 2003 Meta-synthesis: the state of the art – so far. Qualitative Health Research. 13(7):893-904

Greenhalgh T 1997 How to read a paper. The basics of evidence-based medicine. British Medical Journal Publishing, London

Higgins J P T, Thompson S G, Deeks J J et al 2003 Measuring inconsistency in meta-analysis. British Medical Journal 327:557-560

Irwig L, Tosteson A N A, Gatsonis C et al 1994 Guidelines for meta-analyses: evaluating diagnostic tests. Annals of Internal Medicine 120 (8):667-676

Jacobs S, Foweraker J E, Roberts S E 1992 Effectiveness of selective decontamination of the digestive tract (SDD) in an ICU with a policy encouraging a low gastric pH. Clinical Intensive Medicine 3:52-58

Jadad A R, Cook D J, Jones A et al 1998 Methodology and reports of systematic reviews and meta-analyses. Journal of the American Medical Association 280(3):278-280

Kerver A J H, Rommes J H, Mevissen-Verhage E A E et al 1988 Prevention of colonisation and infection in critically ill patients: a prospective randomized study. Critical Care Medicine 16:1087

Kunz R ,Vist G, Oxman AD 2003 Randomisation to protect against selection bias in health care trials (Cochrane methodology review) In: Cochrane Library, Issue 4, Wiley & Sons Ltd. Chichester, UK

Lau J, Ioannidis J P A, Schmid C H 1998 Summing-up evidence: one answer is not always enough. Lancet 351:123-127

LeLorier J, Georgoire G, Benhaddad A et al 1997 Discrepancies between meta-analysis and subsequent large randomised controlled trials. New England Journal of Medicine 337:536-542

Lenhart F P, Unertl K, Neeser G et al 1994 Selective decontamination (SDD) and sucralfate for prevention of acquired infections in intensive care [abstract]. Seventeenth International Congress Chemotherapy, Vienna, K101

Loong, T W 2003 Understanding sensitivity and specificity with the right side of the brain. British Medical Journal 327:716-719

McQuay H J, Moore R A 1997 Using numerical results from systematic reviews in clinical practice. Annals of Internal Medicine 126(9):712-720

Moher D, Cook DJ, Eastwood S et al for Quorum Group 1999 Improving the quality of reports of meta-analyses of randomised controlled trials: the QUOROM statement. Lancet 354(9193):1896-1900

Moher D, Jadad A R, Nichol G et al 1995 Assessing quality of randomised controlled trials: an annotated bibliography of scales and checklists. Controlled Clinical Trials 16:62-73

Mulrow C D 1987 The medical review article: state of the science. Annals of Internal Medicine 106:485-488

Mulrow C 1994 Rationale for systematic reviews. British Medical Journal 309:597-599

Naylor C D, Davey Smith G 1998 Test meta-analyses for stability (letter). British Medical Journal 317:206

Noblit G W, Hare R D 1988 Meta-ethnography: synthesising qualitative studies. Sage, Newbury Park

Oxman A D, Cook D J, Guyatt G H 1994 Users' guides to the medical literature. VI. How to use an overview. Journal of the American Medical Association 272(17):1367-1371

Oxman A D, Guyatt G H 1992 A consumer's guide to subgroup analysis. Annals of Internal Medicine 116:78-84

Palomar M, Alvarez-Lerma F, Jorda R et al for the Catalan Study Group of Nosocomial Pneumonia Prevention 1997 Prevention of nosocomial infection in mechanically ventilated patients: selective digestive decontamination vs sucralfate. Clinical Intensive Care 8:228-235

Petticrew M 2003 Why certain systematic reviews reach uncertain conclusions. British Medical Journal 326:756-758

Rigby K, Silagy C, Crockett A 1996 Health economic reviews – are they compiled systematically? International Journal of Technology Assessment in Health Care 12 (3):450-459

Rocha L A, Martin M J, Pita S et al 1992 Prevention of nosocomial infection in critically ill patients by selective decontamination of digestive tract. Intensive Care Medicine 18:398-404

Sackett D L, Richardson W S, Rosenberg W et al 1997 Evidence-based medicine. How to practise and teach EBM. Churchill Livingstone, Edinburgh

Sanchez-Garcia M, Cambronero J A, Lopez J et al 1992 Reduced incidence of nosocomial pneumonia and shorter ICU stay in intubated patients with the use of selective decontamination of the digestive tract (SDD). A multicentric, double blind, placebo-controlled study [abstract]. European Congress on Intensive Care Medicine. Barcelona, No 0391

Sandelowski M, Barroso J 2003 Classifying the findings in qualitative studies. Qualtiative Health Research 13(7):905-923

Sandelowski M, Docherty S, Emden C 1997 Qualitative metasynthesis: issues and techniques. Research in Nursing and Health 20:365-371

Schultz K F, Chalmers I, Hayes R J et al 1995 Empirical evidence of bias. Dimensions of methodological quality associated with estimates of treatment effects in controlled trials. Journal of the American Medical Association 273(5):408-412

Seers K, Carroll D 1998 Relaxation techniques for acute pain management: a systematic review. Journal of Advanced Nursing 27:466-475

Shea B, Dube C, Moher D 2001 Assessing the quality of reports of systematic reviews: the QUOROM statement compared to other tools. In: Egger M, Davey Smith G, Altman DG (eds) Systematic reviews in health care. Meta-analysis in context. 2nd edn. British Medical Journal Publications, London (Ch. 7), p 122-139

Sindhu F 1996 Are non-pharmacological nursing interventions for the management of pain effective? – A meta-analysis. Journal of Advanced Nursing 24:1152-1159

Sindhu F 1998 Meta-analyses and systematic reviews of the literature. In: Roe B, Webb C (eds) Research and development in clinical nursing practice. Whurr, London (Ch 6), p 84-111

Stoutenbeck C P, Van Saene H K F, Little R A et al The effect of selective decontamination of the digestive tract on mortality in multiple trauma patients. Annals of Surgery (in press)

Stroup DF, Berlin JA, Morton SC et al 2000 Meta-analysis of observational studies in epidemiology: a proposal for reporting. Meta-analysis of Observational Studies in Epidemiology (MOOSE) group. Journal of the American Medical Association 283(15):2008-2012

Thompson S G 1994 Why sources of heterogeneity in meta-analysis should be investigated. British Medical Journal 309:1351-1355

Thompson S G, Higgins J P 2002 How should meta-regression analyses be undertaken and interpreted? Statistics in Medicine. 21(11):1559-1573

Ulrich C, Harinck-deWeerd J E, Bakker N C et al 1989 Selective decontamination of the digestive tract with norfloxacin in the prevention of ICU-acquired infections: a prospective randomized study. Intensive Care Medicine 15:424-431

Verwaest C, Verhaegen J, Ferdinande P et al 1997 Randomized, controlled trial of selective digestive decontamination in 600 mechanically ventilated patients in a multidisciplinary intensive care unit. Critical Care Medicine 25:63-71

Winter R, Humphreys H, Pick A et al 1992 A controlled trial of selective decontamination of the digestive tract in intensive care and its effect on nosocomial infection. Journal of Antimicrobial Chemotherapy 30:73-87

Chapter 10

Critical appraisal of methods: economic evaluation

Alastair Gray

INTRODUCTION

Economic evaluation is a burgeoning part of health technology assessment, and the methodology of economic evaluation is rapidly evolving. Although what constitutes good practice is by no means written in stone, it seems clear that many economic evaluations published in the recent past have not adhered to basic principles. For example, one study (Udvarhelyi et al 1992) looked at 77 cost-effectiveness and cost-benefit articles published during the periods 1978 to 1980 and 1985 to 1987. In the articles assessed, they found in relation to six fundamental principles of analysis that just three out of the 77 adhered to all six principles. The median number of principles adhered to was three, and there was no evidence of improvement in performance over time. Similar results have been obtained from other reviews (Gerard 1992).

Partly as a result of such studies, there has been a major effort amongst health economists to reach consensus on what principles should and should not be used, and clear guidelines on good practice now exist for the conduct of studies, for the preparation of manuscripts, and for journal referees and editors assessing submissions (CCTA 1997, Gold et al 1996, Drummond et al 1997, NICE 2001).

In Chapter 15 we will look in detail at the cost-effectiveness approach, and ask how the results of such studies can be used in evidence-based practice. But first it is necessary to establish some basic principles. Here, we set out a checklist condensed from the conclusions of the Panel on Cost-Effectiveness in Health and Medicine, which was convened at the instigation of the US Public Health Service to produce an explicit set of guidelines for the conduct of cost-effectiveness analyses (Gold et al 1996).

FRAMEWORK

1. The type of analysis being performed should be clearly stated and justified.

Economic evaluation consists of a small family of analyses, which are conceptually distinct. Figure 10.1 sets these out. The most elementary type of study is a cost analysis, in which there is no information on outcomes, or possibly where there is not even any attempt to compare alternative courses of action. The usefulness of this type of study is limited, as it gives no information on health outcome consequences. If there is information on the outcome or effectiveness of two alternatives, and they are known to be equivalent, then the main interest is in identifying and choosing the least cost option, and this is called a cost-minimisation study. Note that equivalence cannot be assumed from studies that fail to detect a hypothesised difference,

---

Box 10.1 Checklist adapted from Gold et al. (1996)

A: The framework
1. The type of analysis being performed should be clearly stated and justified.
2. The background of the problem being addressed, and the general design of the programme under investigation, including the target population, should be stated.
3. The comparator programme should be described.
4. The perspective and time horizon of the study should be stated.

B: Data and methods
5. All resources of interest in the analysis should be clearly identified, measured and valued.
6. All outcomes of interest in the analysis should be clearly identified, measured and valued.
7. Methods of obtaining estimates of effectiveness, resource use, unit costs and quality of life valuations should be given, alongside the sources of these estimates.

C: Results
8. The base case results in terms of costs, effectiveness, and incremental cost-effectiveness ratios, and the uncertainty surrounding them, should be clearly set out.
9. The results should be placed in the context of other relevant economic evaluations.

D: Discussion
10. The relevance of the study for policy questions, and any ethical or distributive implications, should be discussed.

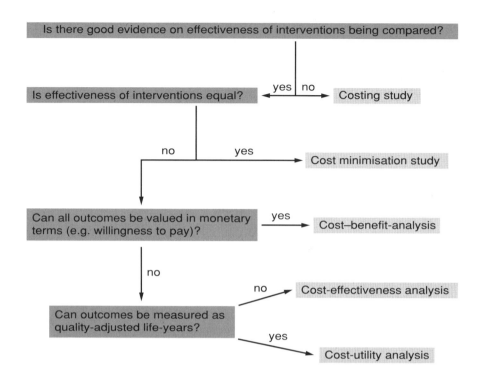

Figure 10.1 Types of economic evaluation

and can only be accepted when a properly powered equivalence study has demonstrated similar effects. However, if the outcome is known to be different, or not known to be the same, then we are in the realm of cost-effectiveness analysis. Here, we are interested in the difference in costs between a programme and a specified alternative, as a ratio of the difference in outcomes. Examples might include the cost per case detected of population screening compared with opportunistic screening; or the cost per life saved or life year gained of thrombolytic therapy following myocardial infarction. In some circumstances, the outcome may best be measured in quality adjusted life years (QALYs), a composite measure of changes in survival and quality of life. Cost-effectiveness analyses which make use of QALYs as the principle outcome measure are sometimes called cost-utility analyses, the reason being that economists are interested in measuring the value or utility derived from a state of health or health change.

Note that cost-effectiveness and cost-utility analyses are premised on the assumption that the outcome – lives saved, cases detected, and so on – is worth attaining. The only question they address is 'Given that this is a worthwhile objective, what is the most efficient way of attaining it?' But some studies (a small number at present) attempt to ask a more fundamental question: is the objective worth pursuing at all? For example, if it were possible in some way to place a monetary value on a life, then any action or intervention which saved a life for less than that value – that is, where the costs were less than the benefits – would be worthwhile, while any action which cost more than that value – where the costs were greater than the benefits – would not be worthwhile. This is cost-benefit analysis; it has the advantage of a more straightforward decision-rule, but the disadvantage is that getting agreement on monetary valuations of outcomes is very difficult.

2. The background of the problem being addressed, and the general design of the programme under investigation, including the target population, should be stated.

This is a simple but important point which many published studies unfortunately fail to comply with. Unless the background is clearly stated and the programme design and target population are clearly specified, it will be difficult to draw conclusions about the relevance of the results. Relevant aspects of the programme may include the specific technology employed, the grade and experience of staff delivering the intervention, and the physical setting, all of which may affect the costs and outcomes reported. Relevant aspects of the target population to note include their age, sex, ethnic composition and their baseline risk characteristics.

3. The comparator programme should be described.

As noted above, economic evaluation is concerned with comparing an intervention with some alternative. Consequently, the comparator that is selected is crucial to the results. If the cost-effectiveness of a new antihypertensive drug was to be calculated against the alternative of no treatment, it would undoubtedly appear as much more cost-effective than if compared with existing practice, which probably includes lifestyle advice and diuretics. So the status quo, or current practice, will usually be the appropriate comparator.

4. The perspective and time horizon of the study should be stated.

Suppose a health authority is trying to decide whether to introduce 'a hospital at home scheme' to encourage earlier discharge from medical wards. It may save hospital resources but increase primary care costs. It may mean additional informal care from families and friends, but lead to earlier recovery and a more rapid return to paid employment. Which perspective should we adopt? The health service view alone, or the impact on informal carers, or the broad impact across society as a whole? The health service decision-maker may be interested only in health care resources, and may wish to discharge patients from hospital as rapidly as possible. But from a societal point of view it would be wise to consider these wider costs, and

Table 10.1 The importance of the perspective adopted: the example of varicella-related costs with and without a projected US vaccination programme for children ($US million, 1990)

	No vaccination	Vaccination	Net cost (savings) of vaccination versus no vaccination
Medical costs:			
Vaccine and administration	0	88	88
Varicella disease costs	90	10	(80)
Total medical costs	90	98	8
Work-loss costs (savings)	439	48	(392)
Total medical + work-loss varicella-related costs (savings)	529	146	(384)

Source: Lieu T, Cochi S, Black S et al. Cost-effectiveness of a routine varicella vaccination program for US children. JAMA 1994; 271:375-81.

indeed if they are completely ignored, the treatment may be unacceptable to patients.

An illustration of this is given in Table 10.1, which is adapted from a study of the likely economic consequences of introducing varicella (chickenpox) vaccination in the USA (Lieu et al 1994). With no vaccination programme, the health care system incurs annual costs of $90m, and parents incur annual costs of $439m, mainly as a result of taking time off work to look after sick children being kept off school. If a vaccination programme were introduced, the vaccination programme itself ($88m per annum) and the residual disease costs of $10m (the vaccine being not completely effective) would fall on the health care system, so that from its perspective the annual costs would actually rise from $90m to $98m each year. However, the costs to parents would fall dramatically – from $439m to $48m each year – and society as a whole will benefit as parents' savings far outweigh the additional health care costs. So should the programme go ahead? The point is that it all depends on the perspective you adopt, but it is good practice in economic evaluations to adopt the widest perspective possible, especially if there is reason to think that different perspectives may alter the result.

The time horizon of a study should extend sufficiently far into the future to capture the main economic consequences and health outcomes. This may in practice mean that a patient's full lifetime is the appropriate horizon. For example, suppose that a trial has demonstrated that a new drug is more effective than existing therapies at lowering cholesterol over a 1-year period.

An economist would almost certainly want to consider the health outcomes of this change in terms of lower risk of fatal and non-fatal coronary events, and the longer-term cost-consequences of continuing drug therapy but also fewer coronary events. This would probably extend over a lifetime, and consequently some modelling (e.g. statistically extrapolating these effects into the future) would be required.

A final point to be made about the time horizon concerns discounting. The costs and health outcomes of a programme or service are usually spread over time, and may differ widely between programmes. For instance, the direct costs of influenza immunisation are incurred immediately, and the benefits (in terms of health effects and treatment costs avoided) are also attained more or less immediately; in contrast, the costs of a school anti-smoking health education campaign are incurred immediately, but the benefits will be attained a long time into the future. To compare these programmes at a point in time – the present – it is necessary to place the stream of future costs on a common basis of present values, by adjusting future costs and outcomes using a discount rate so that they are given less weight than present costs and outcomes.

There are two main reasons for discounting. The first is time preference: generally we prefer to receive benefits now rather than in the future, and to postpone costs to the future rather than bear them now. We value present benefits more highly than future benefits, and perceive present costs to be higher than future costs. The second concerns opportunity cost again: resources not spent now could be invested at a real rate of return, and would be worth more in real terms in the future. If the real rate of return is 5% per annum, then £100 invested now would equal £128 in 5 years, and conversely £100 in 5 years would equal £77 now. So if you knew that you would need £100 in 5 years, you could invest £77. This is the basis of pension plans. Put another way, if you were owed £100 and were offered the choice of having it now or in 5 years time, what would you choose?

The actual discount rate used has been the subject of some debate, and varies between countries. At present in the UK the discount rate recommended by the National Institute for Clinical Excellence is 6% per annum for costs and 1.5% per annum for outcomes, but it would be considered good practice to display results using a range of different discount rates, including zero and the UK Treasury-approved rate of 3.5% for costs and effects.

DATA AND METHODS

5. All resources of interest in the analysis should be clearly identified, measured and valued.

Estimating the costs of an intervention is usually done in distinct stages. First, it is necessary to identify all the resources involved in the intervention itself and any future resource consequences, such as adverse events or an altered probability of clinical events (hence the need for a clear description of the intervention). For example, the resource consequences of hormone replacement therapy include not only the drug therapy itself but also an altered future likelihood of osteoporosis, breast cancer, endometrial cancer and possibly cardiovascular and other diseases, all of which have resource consequences. Ideally, we should include not only health care resources, but also the consequences for patients, their families and society (see the discussion of the study perspective above).

Once these resource consequences have been identified, they need to be measured and then valued. The way in which they are measured will vary depending on the level of detail of the study. For example, use of hospital resources may be measured simply in terms of numbers of cases or of in-patient days, or in much more detail by documenting all the nursing and medical time, drugs and dressings, tests and consumables involved in the episode. The level of detail in turn will depend on the research question: is there reason to believe that the intensity of care in hospital may differ between interventions, for example, or is it more important simply to detect any overall difference in hospitalisation rates?

The valuation of these resources is the point at which unit costs are attached. To an economist, cost is measured in terms of the potential opportunities which are foregone when resources are committed to one purpose rather than another. The normal market price – the wage for a nurse or the price of a prescribed drug – will usually be a reasonable measure of this opportunity cost. However, prices, charges, tariffs or fees can sometimes be misleading. For example, a family planning clinic may get 'free' space in a hospital out-patient department; that is, it does not pay for it. But by using the space in this way, other potential benefits from using the space in a different way are sacrificed. So there is an opportunity cost, even though there is no charge. This distinction can become very important in areas such as informal care, where relatives and friends of patients may be sacrificing a great deal of work time or leisure time to caring for no financial reward. There is no price, but the opportunity cost may be very substantial.

6. All outcomes of interest in the analysis should be clearly identified, measured and valued.

The measure of outcome, effectiveness or benefit must always be appropriate to the intervention. For example, a measure of the effectiveness of an antidepressant drug must be capable of registering changes in those aspects of health affected by depression. If the primary purpose of a therapy is to reduce the number of days with symptoms of gastro-oesophageal reflux disease, then effectiveness can be measured in terms of symptom-free days, and hence cost-effectiveness can be measured as the cost per symptom-free day. Similarly, if the purpose is to screen for cystic fibrosis, then cost-effectiveness could be measured in terms of the cost per case of cystic fibrosis detected.

But a very disease-specific measure of effectiveness is not particularly

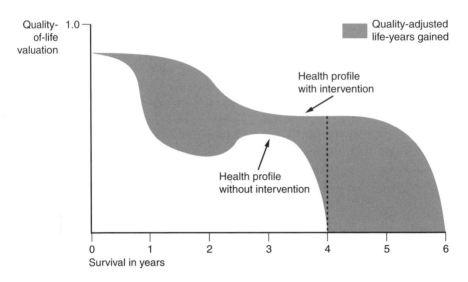

Figure 10.2 Hypothetical profiles of health related quality of life

attractive from an economic perspective as it inevitably reduces the number of comparisons it is possible to make. A more general outcome measure often used in economic evaluations is the life-year gained. With this measure, the impact of any therapy which affects mortality can be measured in the same units. Hence the cost-effectiveness of a new neonatal intensive therapy unit in comparison with the existing service could be calculated as a cost per life year gained. The cost-effectiveness of a new procedure for coronary bypass surgery in comparison with an existing procedure could also be calculated as a cost per life year gained. The two results could then be compared to see whether it would be better to expand the budget for neonatal care or cardiology.

However, many interventions are not primarily intended to affect mortality, but rather mainly affect quality of life. For example, a hip replacement operation is not mainly concerned with improving someone's survival. To measure its effectiveness in terms of life-years gained would be seriously misleading. The concept used by economists to capture these quality of life effects is the quality adjusted life-year or QALY. If we can attach weights to particular health states, we can express most health outcomes in terms of QALYs, for they combine quality and quantity of life on the same scale. Figure 10.2 shows how two profiles of ill-health could be compared in terms of QALYs. The upper line shows a gain in quality of life and an extension in life expectancy (to the right of the dotted line), so that the shaded area represents the total gain in QALYs.

We will examine different ways of calculating these values for a state of health or ill-health in Chapter 16. The key point is that the values are a numerical estimate of the value or utility which someone obtains from a health state, and therefore the study should state clearly whose values are being used (the public, patients, carers, 'experts'); the sample size; the method for eliciting values; and the mean results and the variance.

7. Methods of obtaining estimates of effectiveness, resource use, unit costs, quality of life valuations, and the sources of information.

As noted above, the process of estimating costs and effectiveness is done in steps: identification, measurement, valuation. It is important to know how these steps were taken, so that the reader can assess the methods and quality of the data used. Questions to ask include: What sample sizes were used in measuring resource use? Were the unit costs used to value these resources obtained from reliable sources? Are they generalisable? Were the effectiveness data obtained from a controlled trial or overview of trials, or from some other source? How reliable are they? If quality of life valuations were used, how and where were they obtained?

RESULTS

8. The base case results in terms of costs, effectiveness, and incremental cost–effectiveness ratios, and the uncertainty surrounding them, should be clearly set out.

The end result of an economic evaluation is usually a cost-effectiveness ratio: a cost per standard unit of outcome such as a life year. However, when reporting results it is good practice to report the actual magnitude of cost and effect differences and not just the ratio. This makes it possible to see whether the actual cost and gain in health is very small or very large: if one intervention produced an additional 10 years of life expectancy per patient at a cost of £100 000, and another produced 5 weeks of additional life expectancy per patient at an additional cost of £1000, both would have a cost-effectiveness ratio of £10 000 per life year gained, but would not necessarily be considered as equivalent by a decision-maker. One study of an adult tetanus immunization programme (Balestra and Littenberg, 1993) reported an incremental cost-effectiveness ratio of $143 138 per life year saved, but in fact this ratio was obtained from an average cost of just 91 cents per patient and an average gain in life expectancy of only 2 minutes per patient! So it is good practice to give full information on costs and outcomes, and not just a cost-effectiveness ratio. This is similar to the argument that we need more than the relative risk ratio when assessing the effectiveness of a treatment and that in addition we also need the absolute risk ratio (or the number we need to treat).

It is also crucial to note whether any reported differences in costs, effect or cost-effectiveness are statistically significant, or indeed whether the authors have reported the variance of these measures. It has become standard practice when reporting the results of clinical trials to give point estimates and their

95% confidence intervals. Similarly, information on costs should where possible report confidence intervals. Where cost estimates have not been obtained from a sample but have been modelled, or taken from the literature, or derived in some other way, the uncertainty surrounding any point estimate can still be conveyed by means of sensitivity analysis. The key assumptions can then be systematically varied to assess their impact on the results.

The same points hold with respect to the cost-effectiveness ratio, which should not be reported as a simple point estimate, but rather as a result which is subject to uncertainty concerning the cost dimension, the effectiveness dimension and the joint distribution of costs and effects. A number of methods exist for doing this: the use of ellipses on the cost-effectiveness plane, and probabilistic analysis, which can be reported using cost-effectiveness acceptability curves or other devices (van Hout et al 1994).

9. The results should be placed in the context of other relevant economic evaluations.

Cost-effectiveness is a comparative methodology, the results of which make sense only in relation to other cost-effectiveness results. Therefore, a range of other cost-effectiveness results should be quoted or referred to. This is especially important if the analyst wishes to draw a conclusion, such as the intervention being studied 'is cost-effective compared to other uses of health care resources', or 'offers good value for money'(Laupacis et al 1992). These other cost-effectiveness results should relate to areas that compete for resources with the intervention under investigation. This may be very broad, or may be confined to a specialty or age group or type of intervention. For example, if a proposed screening programme for colorectal cancer would have to be funded out of a screening budget, then it would be relevant to compare its cost-effectiveness with other screening programmes.

DISCUSSION

10. The relevance of the study for policy questions; ethical or distributive implications should be discussed.

Policymakers have to balance a whole range of considerations, including legal, ethical and humanitarian concerns as well as evidence on cost-effectiveness. Suppose that an intervention proved to be relatively cost-effective, but that it delivered most of its health gain to people who were already in very good health, or to a particular ethnic group. Or suppose it provided small health benefits to a large number of people, whereas other interventions against which it compared favourably provided large benefits to a small number of people. These implications of the intervention should be discussed.

In summary, any economic evaluation which satisfies the good practice guidelines set out above is likely to be a reliable source of information for evidence-based practice. In Chapter 16 we will consider in more detail how to interpret this evidence.

References

Balestra D J, Littenberg B 1993 Should adult tetanus immunization be given as a single vaccination at age 65? Journal of General Internal Medicine 8:405-412

Canadian Coordinating Office for Health Technology Assessment 1997 Guidelines for economic evaluation of pharmaceuticals: Canada. 2nd edn. Ottawa

Drummond MF, O'Brien B, Stoddart GL et al 1997 Methods for the economic evaluation of health care programmes. 2nd edn. Oxford University Press, Oxford

Gerard K 1992 Cost utility in practice: a policymaker's guide to the state of the art. Health Policy 21:249-279

Gold M R, Siegel J E, Russell L B et al 1996 Cost-effectiveness in health and medicine. Oxford University Press, New York

Laupacis A, Feeny D, Detsky A S et al 1992 How attractive does a new technology have to be to warrant adoption and utilisation? Tentative guidelines for using clinical and economic evaluations. Canadian Medical Association Journal 146(4):473-481

Lieu T A, Cochi S L, Black S B et al 1994 Cost-effectiveness of a routine varicella vaccination program for US children 271(5):375-381

National Institute for Clinical Excellence 2001 Guidance for manufacturers and sponsors. June 2001 Available from http://www.nice.org.uk/pdf/technicalguidanceformanufacturersandsponsors.pdf (website accessed June 2003)

Udvarhelyi I S, Colditz A, Rai A et al 1992 Cost-effectiveness and cost-benefit analyses in the medical literature. Are the methods being used correctly? Annals of Internal Medicine 116(3):238-244

Van Hout B A, Gordon G S, Rutten F F 1994 Costs, effects and C/E-ratios alongside a clinical trial. Health Economics 3(5):309-319

Chapter 11

Qualitative research

Kate Seers

Whilst reading through a recent journal, imagine you come across a piece of qualitative research that seems relevant to a clinical problem you have in your everyday practice. This article seems to throw light on something you have had in the back of your mind for some time. Perhaps the patient quotations are similar to comments you have been hearing, and you feel it could be a really useful paper.

For example, suppose you did a literature search to find out what types of medication were effective for alleviating chronic headache pain. You found several good studies that reported a specific treatment was effective. During your search, you also found a case study that looked interesting. You had not planned to use qualitative research in your review, but it caught your attention. The case study focused on one person's experience with this same pain medication that had been shown to be effective in previous studies. The article expressed a number of reservations about the treatment from the individual patient's point of view. It also gave the impression that there may be others who had similar reservations about their medication to the extent that they may not be taking it regularly. Does either study present the 'true' picture regarding the effectiveness of the medication? Could this example be typical of what other people were encountering with the treatment? Is it possible that people who were in the trials had not been taking the medication regularly because they had similar concerns?

You reread the patient's account. You notice that there are a lot of other factors you need to know about the situation. Who talked to the patient? How long had the patient been in pain? What did the patient want from the treatment? What did the patient feel about side-effects? You realise the case study suggests the need for a systematic qualitative study in this area.

What is qualitative research: how do you judge if it is any good?

This chapter will describe the various approaches to qualitative research and provide a framework for judging the quality and utility of qualitative research. If you are interested in undertaking qualitative research, suggestions for further reading are listed at the end of the chapter.

WHAT IS QUALITATIVE RESEARCH?

Qualitative research concentrates on people's experiences, attitudes and beliefs; their perceptions of a situation. It aims to generate an understanding of what is going on in an everyday setting. It can be used to generate new theory, describe a point of view, develop instruments, illustrate meanings, sensitise readers or try to understand phenomena (Forchuk & Roberts 1993). It may look at language (Silverman 1997). Qualitative research has been described as appropriate when we want to 'understand perceptions, motives and actions of individuals and organisations' (Boulton & Fitzpatrick 1997:83). Fitzpatrick and Boulton (1994) stress that it involves conceptual development and analysis of underlying patterns. It is not the opposite of quantitative research and it is not just a set of techniques for collecting descriptive data: it has a theoretical foundation (Popay & Williams 1998). This is important because this foundation is needed if knowledge generated from qualitative research is to be seen as legitimate. Qualitative research is concerned with the 'negotiation and construction of meanings in social interaction' (Popay & Williams 1998:33-34).

Qualitative research can address such issues as: What is it like to have a certain condition, diagnosis or type of care? What does it mean to the patient? For example, What is it like to have chronic pain? Qualitative research can be very good at providing the perspective of the patient and/or the health professional or other carer. The key is that the experience is explained and described by the participants, and they, not the researcher, provide the framework for what is important in that context.

Questions which can help the participant to explain their perspective might be:

- What has this experience been like?
- How has this experience made you feel?
- What do you think has helped you through this experience?
- Why do you think that happened?
- Why did you do that?

Methods used in qualitative research include interviews (often semi- or unstructured), focus groups, observation (as a participant or as a non-participant) and examination of documentary evidence.

Qualitative research is a fairly new way of generating knowledge in health care. Some health care professionals are more used to using quantitative research to inform their practice. The impetus for critically appraising quantitative research within evidence-based health care has come largely from clinical epidemiology and public health. Qualitative research has traditionally been outside that framework, and the whole process of assessing qualitative research is only just starting to be developed. However, Black (1994) argued for the value of qualitative research in health service research and Sackett and Wennberg (1997) stressed that the research question should determine the research design. The nursing profession has been publishing qualitative research for many years, and other disciplines, such as medicine, occupational therapy, physiotherapy and health psychology are increasingly recognising its place in research.

Some journals are specifically devoted to it, for example, Qualitative Health Research (http://www.ualberta.ca/~qhr/). The Cochrane Collaboration, which initially focused on quantitative research, especially RCTs, has widened its approach, and has set up a Cochrane Qualitative Methods Group (Cochrane Library 2003: Issue 4) (http:/mysite. freeserve.com/ Cochrane_Qual_Methods/index.htm). The British Medical Journal frequently publishes articles on qualitative research (47 between August 1999 and October 2003) and has published a book on this (Mays & Pope 1999). Qualitative research can provide useful information that contributes to the process of effective health care. Popay and Williams (1998) argue that barriers in the way of utilising the potential of qualitative research include the unequal social relationships of health research and the way the power and influence of different disciplines with their different views of knowledge may affect the collaboration of these disciplines. That is, the largely medical quantitative perspective is dominant and there may be a tendency to regard only knowledge generated from this approach as worthwhile knowledge. However, as qualitative research gains a higher profile in medical journals, and as a range of health professionals becomes familiar in its use and finds the knowledge it generates useful, these distinctions will very gradually become less marked. I hope that a greater understanding of a range of research methodologies, including their theoretical underpinnings and strengths and weaknesses, can only benefit patient care. This will start to happen as the wide range of clinical problems that practitioners and patients face is translated into research questions, answered using whichever research approach is most appropriate to that question.

Mutual understanding across these different approaches has not always been evident. The term 'qualitative research' just like 'quantitative research' covers a range of methodologies. Both approaches have in common the importance of asking a clear question, using a sensible methodology to answer that question, ensuring rigorous and systematic data collection and analysis and then explaining and interpreting the data and ensuring conclusions follow from the data. However, they are based on different ways of looking at the world and have different views of what constitutes valid knowledge and how it should be obtained. Thus they are based on different ways of knowing and produce different types of knowledge (epistemological differences). For example, quantitative research often produces numbers and looks at cause and effect to find out 'the truth'. Qualitative research is more likely to report on a variety of 'truths'.

Quantitative and qualitative research are also based on different ways of looking at reality or being (ontological differences). For example, quantitative research may look at very specific variables and one part of an experience, whereas qualitative research may look at the whole in context, and from the participants' perspectives. Quantitative research is often described as deductive (hypotheses are generated from theory) whereas qualitative research is described as inductive (theory is developed from the data). However, both can have elements of inductive and deductive approaches within them.

Whether qualitative research will be important to your clinical problem will depend on the question you are asking. For example, if you want to know whether relaxation is effective in reducing pain, a RCT is likely to be the appropriate design. However, if you want to know about patients' experiences of using relaxation (and this may address, for example, the barriers to using relaxation), then a qualitative approach is going to provide this sort of information. It could be that both questions are important to you, suggesting the use of both approaches.

There has been much debate about whether and how qualitative and quantitative approaches should be combined, and whether it is helpful to even use such distinctions. However, since they are commonly used, it may be helpful to look at how they can be used in a complementary way. Morgan (1998) points out that there are four basic combinations:

1. preliminary qualitative methods in a quantitative study
2. preliminary quantitative methods in a qualitative study
3. follow-up qualitative methods in a quantitative study
4. follow-up quantitative methods in a qualitative study.

It is also often appropriate to run the two approaches concurrently in one study, to illuminate different perspectives within that study. There are many different types of qualitative research, and an introductory text such as Burns and Grove (2001) can provide a useful overview. Very briefly, approaches you may come across in your reading include:

Phenomenology

This has its roots in a philosophical approach and looks at how people see their world. The term used is 'the lived experience'. Key early figures in this area include Husserl (1931) and Heidegger (1962). These texts are not easy going, and Koch (1995), Benner (1994) and Dreyfus (1991) offer more accessible accounts.

An example of a study in this area is Gravelle (1997) who looked at parents' experiences of caring for a child with progressive illness. This study found that parents reported successive hardships and challenges, and they experienced cycles of defining and managing adversity, which were repeated with each important progressive change. This knowledge could be incorporated into the care of these children and their parents, to help them through these stages.

Another example is Edwards et al (2001) who studied experiences of patients with rheumatoid arthritis admitted to hospital. They found five inter-related themes.(1) uncertainty during the first admission (2) becoming an experienced patient (3) positive and negative effects of other patients (4) knowledge and experience of staff and (5) loss of privacy. Having an understanding of these experiences should enhance the ability of health care professionals to deliver sensitive and tailored care to these patients.

Grounded theory

This comes from sociology (specifically symbolic interactionism). Here the aim is to generate theory from the data. Pioneers in this area are Glaser and Strauss (1967). Examples of studies in this area include Barclay et al (1997) who looked at women's experiences of early motherhood. They found becoming a mother was a difficult, multifactorial process and highlighted six different categories: being overwhelmed, being unready, feeling drained, feeling alone, experiencing a feeling of loss and gaining confidence. These findings suggest how health care professionals supporting these women could help them through this challenging time of change.

Werezak and Stewart (2002), who studied learning to live with early stage dementia, identified five stages: antecedents, anticipation, appearance, assimilation and acceptance. Again, an understanding of these stages and how people were engaged in a continual process of adjustment helps when planning care.

Ethnography

This has been developed from anthropology and looks at behaviour within a culture (which can include a society or a social group). An early worker in this field was Mead (1935). Examples of ethnographic research include Barroso (1997) on becoming a long-term survivor of AIDS, and Savage (1995) who explored the notion of 'closeness' in nurse-patient relationships. Barroso (1997) found five overlapping dimensions of adapting that were normalising, focusing on living, taking care of one's self, being in relation to others and triumphing. Bouthillette (1998) argues that this suggests a possible intervention for nurses of focusing on the positive rather than the negative. It may be that being aware of these five dimensions could help you plan your discussions with similar patients. The closeness identified by Savage (1995) in nurse-patient relationships was found to be affected by adequate resources being available to support the nurses. This study has implications for the planning of care and questions the basing of nursing care on 'closeness' if the resources are not available to sustain such patient-focused care.

These approaches all try to build up a picture of what is happening.

Hermeneutics

This is a perspective that aims to create a dialogue where participants' and observers' meanings and interpretations interact, producing what Gadamer (1993) refers to as a 'fusion of horizons', or a new understanding. It aims to offer an account of both the world as understood by those participating in it, and the barriers that might prevent such an understanding being achieved. Understanding is in constant movement, from the whole to the parts and from the parts to the whole. This has been termed the 'hermeneutical circle of understanding' (Heidegger 1990). For example, Smith (1998) used a hermeneutic phenomenological approach to look at the experience of people with drinking problems, and found they described their experience of suffering as a spiralling, vicious vortex.

Critical theory

This has a different approach, as it aims specifically to increase people's understanding of their situation and through this they initiate change. Emancipation or empowerment are two words often seen in this type of research.

One influential figure in this approach is Habermas (1985) (see also Fay (1987) and Dunne (1993) for more details). Much feminist research would come into this category; see, for example, Webb (1993) for more information.

Some of the traditionally more interpretative types of the research listed above may also adopt a critical theory approach. Some action research can be described as adopting this perspective, for example, Titchen and Binnie (1993). They looked at a change from traditional, standardised nursing to patient-centred nursing via primary nursing. Their action research strategy for this change included 'working towards the democratisation of health care through the emancipation of nurses who are, traditionally, trapped in a bureaucratic nursing hierarchy and in oppressive doctor-nurse relationships' (Titchen & Binnie 1993:25). Their other strategies included introducing innovation and facilitating change; helping practitioners to research their own practice; facilitating professional learning and reflective practice, and generating and testing theory.

Some qualitative research does not use a methodological framework which fits into one of these types of design. For example, Armstrong et al (1996) conducted semi-structured interviews with general practitioners to look at their reasons for changing prescribing patterns. They reported the findings without a theoretical foundation. As discussed earlier, Popay and Williams (1998) argue that a theoretical foundation is needed if knowledge generated from qualitative research is to be seen as legitimate.

Qualitative findings, partly because they use quotations that are sometimes very powerful, are often very accessible to the reader, and it is important to ensure the same level of critical appraisal is undertaken as with any other type of research design.

COMMON CRITICISMS OF QUALITATIVE RESEARCH

Before the next section addressing 'what is a good qualitative study?', some common criticisms of qualitative research will be considered. These criticisms often stem from applying quantitative criteria to qualitative research, such as 'This research is subjective, not reliable and cannot be generalised.' This is the sort of comment you may hear when qualitative research is being discussed by those unused to this approach.

Bias

When you are appraising quantitative research, you are looking for design features that minimise bias. In a qualitative study, 'bias' is treated rather differently. The whole point of the study is usually to look specifically at the experience of the participant and this process will be influenced by the researcher's perspective. What is key here is that this perspective is clearly recorded. Since many of the decisions will be subjective, a clear, documented rationale for all decisions made is crucial. This is sometimes referred to as a decision trail. This is linked to auditability (sometimes known as trustworthiness), the qualitative term similar to reliability.

Auditability (trustworthiness)/reliability

Here you are not looking for someone else to get exactly the same results in a similar setting, because it is acknowledged that the researcher's perceptions and background influence the questions asked, the data obtained and how it is interpreted. (This influence is also quite possible in quantitative research, but is not usually acknowledged.) What is important is that someone else can follow your decision trail.

Fittingness/generalisability

Generalisability is sometimes referred to as external validity in quantitative research and as fittingness in qualitative research.

A representative sample from which one can generalise to other populations is important in quantitative research. In qualitative research, participants are not usually selected as part of a random sample, but because they have the specific characteristic(s) the researcher is interested in addressing.

Fitzpatrick and Boulton (1994) stress the need to ensure the sample contains a full range of possible observations so concepts and categories provide a reasonable conceptualisation of the subject. They describe the conceptual generalisation that takes place in qualitative research. One is looking for generalising from the findings to a theoretical body of knowledge (or creating new knowledge) rather than to a population.

Qualitative research should give a description to allow you to decide whether the findings might be relevant to people for whom you care. One of the benefits of this type of research is that you may become aware of issues you had not considered or had not had time to concentrate on, and then your increased sensitivity to these issues means you can test them out in practice. For example, if you care for people who are long-term survivors of AIDS, and you read Barroso (1997) it may be that knowing they had five dimensions of adapting (normalising, focusing on living, taking care of oneself, being in relation to others and triumphing), could help you plan your discussions with your patients.

Credibility/validity

Measuring/understanding what one thinks you are measuring/ understanding? This is known as internal validity in quantitative research and as credibility in qualitative research. Both approaches may want to maximise validity by triangulation. That is, obtaining data from a range of sources. In qualitative research, respondent validation, where the researcher checks with the participants whether they agree with the researcher's analysis, can be used, although as Fitzpatrick and Boulton (1994) point out, participants may have reasons for not agreeing with the interpretation of events, which in themselves can be revealing.

WHAT IS A GOOD QUALITATIVE STUDY?

Popay et al (1998) outline why it is important to have criteria to evaluate qualitative research.

- It may be judged as inferior by those who see RCTs as the gold standard.
- There is a need to understand lay and professional decision-making.
- Questions are proposed that cannot be explored or explained by RCTs.
- It is necessary if you want to carry out a systematic review of qualitative research.
- Researchers using qualitative research in the health service may have little or no familiarity with disciplines in which the methods were developed and the assumptions underlying them. They feel this limits the capacity to maximise the potential within these approaches.
- Calls from qualitative research (Altheide & Johnson 1994) underline the need to look at the wider methodological and epistemological context within which the methods are applied, as well as the actual methods used.

Questions to help with critical appraisal

Various different sets of questions are available for helping you to undertake a critical appraisal of qualitative research (Kuckelmann-Cobb & Nelson-Hagemaster 1987, Beck 1993, Forchuk & Roberts 1993, Miles & Huberman 1994, Mays & Pope 1996, Medical Sociology Group 1996, Boulton & Fitzpatrick 1997, Greenhalgh & Taylor 1997, CASP 1998, Locke et al 1998, Popay et al 1998, Spencer et al 2003). Spencer et al (2003) provide a list of 29 studies describing such frameworks following a systematic review of research literature looking at standards in qualitative research and a review of exisiting frameworks. They also conducted exploratory interviews with a range of stakeholders, devised and refined their own framework consisting of 18 appraisal questions, then applied it to some qualitative studies.

Their framework is based around four central principles. These are that the research should advance wider knowledge and understanding, be defensible in design (the design matches the questions posed), rigourous in conduct and credible in claim. As the authors acknowledge, these principles apply to all types of research. These are the appraisal questions in Spencer et al's 2003 framework:

Findings

1. How credible are the findings?
2. How has knowledge or understanding been extended by the research?
3. How well does the evaluation address its original aims and purpose?
4. How well is the scope for drawing wider inferences explained?
5. How clear is the basis of the evaluative appraisal?

Design

6. How defensible is the research design?

Sample

7. How well defended are the sample design/target selection of cases/documents?
8. How clear is the basis for evaluative appraisal (details of eventual sample/cases)?

Data collection

9. How well is the data collection carried out?

Data analysis

10. How well has the approach to and formulation of analysis been conveyed?
11. How well are the contexts of data sources retained and portrayed?
12. How well has the diversity of perspective and content been explored?
13. How well has the detail, depth and complexity (i.e. richness) of the data been conveyed?

Reporting

14. How clear are the links between data, interpretation and conclusions, i.e. how well can the route to any conclusions be seen?
15. How clear and coherent is the reporting?

Reflexivity and neutrality

16. How clear are the assumptions/theoretical perspectives/values that have shaped the form and output of the evaluation?

Ethics

17. How clear and coherent is the reporting? (evidence of attention to ethical issues)

Auditability

18. How adequately has the research process been documented?

In order to answer these 18 questions, Spencer et al (2003) propose a series of prompts or 'quality indicators'. A copy of this document titled Quality in Qualitive Evaluation: A framework for assessing research evidence (ISBN: 07715 04465 8), can be found on the http://policyhub.gov.uk website. These 18 questions cover factors like quality of reporting as well as the quality of the study. If you felt that you only wanted to focus on the quality of the actual study, then this well-labelled list does give you the flexibility to do this.

I hope this has provided a flavour and a few signposts for starting to critically appraise qualitative research articles. These frameworks or checklists are an ongoing development and all are subject to revision and fine tuning. As you critically evaluate qualitative research, you will start to separate the wheat from the chaff and feel comfortable that high-quality qualitative research can inform your practice. One particular clinical challenge may need to be addressed by qualitative research. Linking with a qualitative researcher and using these criteria as you design your own qualitative research may help you produce qualitative research that others will want to use.

Acknowledgement

Many thanks to Janet Harris for her helpful comments and to other colleagues who commented on drafts of this chapter in the first edition of this book.

References

Altheide D, Johnson J 1994 Criteria for assessing interpretative validity in qualitative research. In: Denzin N, Lincoln Y (eds) Handbook of qualitative research. Sage, Thousand Oaks, Ch. 30, p 485-499

Armstrong D, Reyburn H, Jones R 1996 A study of general practitioners' reasons for changing their prescribing behaviour. British Medical Journal 312:949-952

Barclay L, Everitt L, Rogan F et al 1997 Becoming a mother – an analysis of women's experience of early motherhood. Journal of Advanced Nursing 25:719-728

Barroso J 1997 Reconstructing my life: becoming a long term survivor of AIDS. Qualitative Health Research 7:57-74

Beck C T 1993 Qualitative research: evaluation of it's credibility, fittingness and audibility. Western Journal of Nursing Research 15(2):263-266

Benner P 1994 Interpretative phenomenology. Sage, Thousand Oaks

Black N 1994 Why we need qualitative research. Journal of Epidemiology and Community Health 48:425-426

Boulton M, Fitzpatrick R 1997 Evaluating qualitative research. Evidence-Based Health Policy and Management 1(4):83-85

Bouthillette F 1998 Commentary on Barroso. Evidence-Based Nursing 1(1):32

Burns N, Grove S K 2001 The practice of nursing research. Conduct, critique and utilisation, 4th edn. W B Saunders, Philadelphia

CASP (Critical Appraisal Skills Programme) 1998 10 questions to help you make sense of qualitative research. CASP, Oxford (Contact: CASP Office, Institute of Health Sciences, Old Road, Headington, Oxford OX3 7LF)

The Cochrane Library 2003 Issue 4. Chichester, UK: Wiley & Sons, Ltd

Coyne I T 1997 Sampling in qualitative research. Purposeful and theoretical sampling; merging or clear boundaries? Journal of Advanced Nursing 26:623-630

C T 1993 Qualitative research: the evaluation of its credibility, fittingness, and auditability. Western Journal of Nursing Research 15(2):263-266

Dreyfus H L 1991 Being-in-the-world. A commentary on Heidegger's Being and time, Division I. MIT Press, Cambridge, Massachusetts

Dunne J 1993 Back to the rough ground: 'Phronesis' and 'techne' in modern philosophy and in Aristotle. University of Notre Dame Press, Notre Dame

Edwards J, Mulherin D, Ryan S et al 2001 The experience of patients with rheumatoid arthritis admitted to hospital. Arthritis Care Research 45:1-7

Fay B 1987 Critical social science. Liberation and its limits. Polity Press, Cambridge

Fitzpatrick R, Boulton M 1994 Qualitative methods for assessing health care. Quality in Health Care 3(2):107-113

Forchuk C, Roberts J 1993 How to critique qualitative research articles. Canadian Journal of Nursing Research 25(4):47-56

Gadamer H G 1993 Truth and Method. Sheed & Ward, London

Glaser B G, Strauss A L 1967 The discovery of grounded theory: strategies for qualitative research. Aldine, Chicago

Gravelle A M 1997 Caring for a child with progressive illness during the complex chronic phase: parents' experiences of facing adversity. Journal of Advanced Nursing 25:738-745

Greenhalgh T, Taylor R 1997 How to read a paper. Papers that go beyond numbers (qualitative research). British Medical Journal 315:740-743

Habermas J 1985 Die neue Un,bersichtlichkeit. Suhrkramp, Frankfurt (translation in The Habermas Reader 1996 Polity Press, Cambridge)

Heidegger M 1962 Being and time. Harper & Row, New York (original publication in German 1927)

Heidegger M 1990 Being and time. Blackwell, Oxford

Husserl E 1931 Ideas. General introduction to pure phenomenology. Allen Lane, London

Koch T 1995 Interpretative approaches in nursing research: the influence of Husserl and Heidegger. Journal of Advanced Nursing 21:827-836

Kuckelmann-Cobb A, Nelson-Hagemaster J 1987 Ten criteria for evaluating qualitative research proposals. Journal of Nursing Education 26(4):138-143

Locke L F, Silverman S J, Spirduso W W 1998 Reading and understanding research. Sage, Thousand Oaks

Mays N, Pope C 1999 Qualitative research in health care. 2nd edn. British Medical Journal, London

Mead M 1935 Sex and temperament in three primitive societies. Morrow, New York

Medical Sociology Group 1996 Criteria for the evaluation of qualitative research papers. Medical Sociology News 22(1):68-71

Miles M B, Huberman A M 1994 Qualitative data analysis, 2nd edn. Sage, Thousand Oaks, Ch. 10, p 277-280

Morgan D L 1998 Practical strategies for combining qualitative and quantitative methods: applications to health research. Qualitative Health Research 8(3):362-376

Popay J, Rogers A, Williams G 1998 Rationale and standards for the systematic review of qualitative literature in health services research. Qualitative Health Research 8(3):341-351

Popay J, Williams G 1998 Qualitative research and evidence-based health care. Journal of The Royal Society of Medicine 91 (Suppl 35):32-37

Sackett D L, Wennberg J E 1997 Choosing the best research design for each question. Editorial. British Medical Journal 315:1636

Savage J 1995 Nursing intimacy: An ethnographic approach to nurse-patient interaction. Scutari Press, Harrow

Silverman D (ed) 1997 Qualitative research. Theory, method and practice. Sage, London

Spencer L, Ritchie J, Lewis J et al 2003 Quality in qualitative evaluation: a framework for assessing research evidence. National Centre for Social Research. Occasional papers series 2. Government Chief Social Researcher's Office, Cabinet Office, London. (http://policyhub.gov.uk/servlet/Menu?id=1632 – document amended 14th November 2003)

Smith B A 1998 The problem drinker's lived experience of suffering: an exploration using hermeneutic phenomenology. Journal of Advanced Nursing 27:213-222

Titchen A, Binnie A 1993 A unified action research strategy. Nursing Educational Action Research 1(1):25-33

Webb C 1993 Feminist research: definitions, methodology, methods and evaluation. Journal of Advanced Nursing 18:416-423

Werezak L Stewart N 2002 Learning to live with early dementia. Canadian Journal of Nursing Research. 34:67-85

Additional reading for those interested in finding out more about qualitative research

Bryman R 2001 Social research methods, OUP, Oxford

Burns N, Grove S K 2001 The practice of nursing research. Conduct, critique and utilisation, 4th edn. W B Saunders, Philadelphia

Denzin N K, Lincoln Y S (eds) 2000 Handbook of qualitative research. 2nd edn. Sage, Thousand Oaks

Flick U 1998 An introduction to qualitative research. Sage, London

Holloway I 1997 Basic concepts for qualitative research. Blackwell Science, Oxford

Miles M B, Huberman A M 1994 Qualitative data analysis, 2nd edn. Sage, Thousand Oaks, ch. 10, p 277-280

Patton MQ 2002 Qualitative research and evaluation methods. Sage, Thousand Oaks CA

Silverman D (ed) 1997 Qualitative research. Theory, method and practice. Sage, London

Silverman D 2000 Doing qualitative research: A practical handbook. Sage, London.

Chapter 12

Critical appraisal of clinical practice guidelines

Robin Snowball

Information overload in health care, combined with greater time pressures and the need for specialist skills, makes it increasingly harder to find, appraise and put together the best high-quality original research (or to establish its lack), to feed into complex clinical decisions based on evidence. In Chapter 3, we looked at some alternatives to finding original research, such as systematic reviews, evidence summaries, and so on, but even these, when they are available, may only partially help decision-making in certain contexts. Clinical practice guidelines hold out the promise of more than an up -to-date evidence summary: of specific and practical *recommendations* based on the best available evidence, which has been critically appraised, synthesised and summarised by experts, to provide a more direct support for clinical decisions. On the other hand, there are guidelines and guidelines! How can their claims be judged? Is the new guideline published in your specialist journal or sent to you in that avalanche of paper really going to benefit anyone? Is a 'local' guideline or a 'national' guideline all it is cracked up to be? Is a 'consensus' guideline really based on the best evidence? What is it really worth? And is anyone actually going to use it?

If we want to know how best to critically appraise a clinical trial, for instance, and to use the appraisal criteria to write a checklist or appraisal instrument, we need to know the specific purpose of a trial and the process by which it best achieves that purpose, to an agreed set of standards. Since we know that the purpose of a clinical trial is to test an intervention while minimising known kinds of bias as much as possible, and some of the methods (e.g. random allocation) which may better achieve this, we can draw up a critical appraisal checklist for clinical trials, and then set standards for conducting trials, like the CONSORT statement (Begg at al 1996). It will therefore help to clarify the essential purpose and process of clinical practice guidelines, if we wish to produce, or to understand, the rationale of critical appraisal criteria which will be valid and credible.

Clinical practice guidelines are – an oft-quoted definition – 'systematically developed statements to assist practitioner and patient decisions about appropriate health care for specific clinical circumstances' (Field & Lohr 1990). Their *purpose* is to provide guidance by making recommendations of practical use in clinical decision-making, in order, ultimately, to improve care, to reduce unnecessary variation and so on. It is widely accepted that, in order to fulfil this purpose adequately, two main conditions are necessary. First, guidelines should be based on the best available evidence, but also that they must go beyond this in some way, to make specific and clear recommendations for practice. Second, they should be as credible, authoritative, and as acceptable to – 'owned by' – as many potential users as possible, or they will not be implemented. (Third, of course, they should be disseminated widely enough to be used and evaluated by others, to save the wasteful duplication of effort which results from their invisibility.)

Many guidelines in the past have simply not been, or not explicit enough , for one to judge, 'evidence-based' by today's standards – as has been the case with reviews, where we now distinguish 'opinion-based' from 'systematic' reviews. 'Few local or national guidelines are sufficiently based upon the evidence' a review by the NHS Centre for Reviews & Dissemination (1994) has concluded. Grimshaw and Russell (1993) concluded that few guidelines in the UK at that time had been 'developed rigorously.' Grilli et al (2000) discuss the 'increasing concern about the quality, reliability and independence' of practice guidelines, using three criteria: the strategy to identify primary evidence, explicit grading of recommendations according to quality of supporting evidence, and the type of professionals and stakeholders involved in the development process: some 430 guidelines were produced by 'specialty societies' over 10 years and only 5% met all three criteria. Ward and Grieco (1996) assessed 34 Australian guidelines – produced before the 'guidelines for guidelines' were set by the Australian National Health and Medical Research Council in 1995 – using clearly defined criteria modified from a checklist from the US Institute of Medicine: applicability, validity, reproducibility, clinical flexibility, clarity, multidisciplinary involvement, documentation and scheduled review. They found none that met all the criteria, only 18% that stated expected health outcomes, and none that described the processes of retrieving or synthesising evidence.

Liberati et al (2001) use the example of screening urinalysis in children, for which they find two conflicting guidelines! They discuss the role of evidence in preventing conflicting recommendations, the grading of evidence on the basis of study type design (and its limitations in view of lack of universally agreed grading scales for different study types and other factors), and emphasise the need to be explicit about *grading* the evidence to support recommendations.

An overview of the issues of evidence-based practice and guideline development is provided by Heffner (1998), who argues for a 'formal method of guideline development' which creates 'an explicit linkage between the final recommendations and the evidence on which they are based' (p 173S). Should we not ask, first of all, therefore, as appraisers, to what extent a guideline explicitly uses and describes some systematic and bias-minimising process of finding, grading and synthesising *evidence* on which its key recommendations are based?

However, even if a guideline is 'based upon' the best available evidence, this may be necessary, but not sufficient. Hayward et al (1995), in the first part of one of the famous Journal of the American Medical Association Users' Guides to the Medical Literature on clinical practice guidelines (Wilson et al 1995), point out the 'intimidating tasks of information management' faced by clinicians in decision-making and emphasise the important distinction between an evidence overview, even a systematic review, and a clinical guideline as a set of explicit and specific recommendations for clinical practice. An overview or review can systematically locate, appraise and synthesise all available evidence 'that links options to outcomes'. Other studies can list the trade-offs between benefits and harms, or the costs of various options and so on – but this may not be enough directly to support specific clinical recommendations in specific contexts.

Clinical practice guidelines, therefore, must go beyond reviews in 'attempting to address all the issues relevant to a clinical decision and all the values that might sway a clinical recommendation' (p 571). Heffner (1998) refers to this too: the experts (which may include consumers) must 'apply a "value" structure to the evidence' (p 175S). There may be two reasons for this. First, the context may be very complex: other factors may mean that strong evidence does not necessarily imply a strong recommendation (Shekelle et al 1999), or vice versa. Cultural or other complex factors may complicate the issue, or there may even be disagreement about the nature or significance of the 'problem' as well as about interventions or options: what, for example *is* 'aggressive behaviour?' Or we may be dealing with a clinical context in which strong evidence is lacking, inconclusive or conflicting, as pointed out by so many writers in this field. So guideline developers may need to include some 'qualitative reasoning', take into account relevant contextual factors, and 'deal with matters of opinion as well as of fact' (Hayward et al 1995). There may also be more than one point of view to be accounted for, despite the evidence, which may thus need interpretation or setting into a wider context. (A treatment, for example, however effective, may be unacceptable to some professionals or patients: has the guideline made other recommendations, and on what basis?) Again, should we not ask of a guideline, as appraisers, that it makes the *reasoning* behind its recommendations clear and explicit?

Second, and this links to the second condition for guidelines achieving their purpose, a growing literature attests to the central importance of designing guidelines to ensure credibility and acceptability, as well as a wide evidence-base from the outset, as much as possible, and for as many potential users as possible. Browman et al (1998) discuss the process of obtaining practitioner feedback in guideline development, necessary 'to ensure the recommendations that emanate from published evidence are relevant to clinical practice in realistic settings' (p 1226). Guideline development can consume significant resources: these may be wasted if the guideline is not used because it is not credible, acceptable or authoritative. For this reason, formal guideline development generally includes at least some explicit method of widening *consensus* by widening involvement, from multidisciplinary involvement at local level, such as strongly argued by Gray (1997) to the kind of wide 'stakeholder' involvement used by the National Institute for Clinical Excellence (NICE) for national guidelines in the UK. Formal consensus development methods may be used: for an in-depth review of these methods, see Murphy et al (1998), who warn that consensus development is 'a process for making policy decisions, not a scientific method for creating new knowledge (p 1)' – emphasising again the distinction between an evidence summary and a clinical guideline. Should we not ask, therefore, in appraising each guideline, how widely relevant opinion and expertise was canvassed, how it was used, whether this has been made explicit, and whether possible conflicts of interest are stated?

The *process* of guideline development is of crucial importance, if the guideline is to be truly evidence-based, and if it is to be fully accepted (on this and on other grounds) by clinicians and others involved, and thus be more likely to be implemented in practice. From a clearer view of the process most likely to support the purpose of a clinical practice guideline (which must, of course, evolve in practice), we can derive a set of criteria for critically appraising would-be guidelines. This could help us in turn to hone the process further, set minimum standards for guidelines, and form a useful training and communication tool. There are numerous examples of formalising and making explicit the key steps of the development and therefore of the potential appraisal instrument. Hayward et al (1995) include a set of questions in their paper, which are, in effect, a critical appraisal instrument. Grimshaw and Russell (1993) listed some 'useful attributes' of clinical guidelines, based on work by the US Agency for Health Care Policy and Research, whose system for rating evidence quality is described by Hadorn et al (1996); Shekelle et al (1999) outline a five-step process for medical guidelines. Warner and Blizard (1998) critically appraise clinical guidelines for antidepressants, using a 10-question instrument, and using suggestions from the Journal of the American Medical Association Users' Guides by Hayward et al (1995) and Wilson et al (1995); Woolf et al (1996) give a very detailed account of the experience of the US Preventive Services Task Force in developing evidence-based guidelines; Hayward and Laupacis (1993) describe Canadian experience; Browman et al (1998) give an update of the Canadian Practice Guidelines Development Cycle; Rycroft-Malone (2001) and Duff et al (1996) discuss guideline development from a nursing point of view; Eccles et al (1998) describe the North of England evidence-based guidelines development project. Mann (1996) summarises the UK NHS Executive's approach to development, appraisal and application of clinical guidelines. And the NICE website (http://www.nice.org.nhs.uk) details its own Guideline

Development Process. (NICE also produces health technology assessments for specific health interventions (Claxton et al 2002, Sculpher et al 2001); it is not without its critics (e.g. Illman 2000, Cookson et al 2001, Dent & Sadler 2002)).

In the first edition of this primer, we reproduced the 'Appraisal Instrument for Clinical Guidelines' (Cluzeau et al 1999), which was developed and tested on 60 guidelines by the Health Care Evaluation Unit at St George's Hospital Medical School, London in collaboration with the Health Services Research Unit at Aberdeen University and the Department of General Practice at Queen Mary and Westfield College. The instrument aimed to provide a 'transparent and standardised method' for critical appraisal of existing clinical guidelines and as well as a checklist for the development of new ones. Graham et al (2001) used the instrument, which 'a systematic literature search' revealed to them to be 'the most well developed... available' (p 158), to appraise some 217 drug therapy guidelines in Canada. The instrument has now been superseded by the Appraisal of Guidelines Research and Evaluation (AGREE) Instrument, which draws largely from it and is based on similar concepts, but uses a different response scale. It has been developed and tested by researchers and guideline developers from 13 countries, and validated on 100 guidelines from 11 countries coordinated by the AGREE Collaboration (see AGREE 2003). It aims to become the internationally accepted appraisal instrument for clinical practice guidelines, and has been translated into eight languages for use in some 20 countries. In the UK, both NICE (http://nice.org.uk), responsible for producing national guidelines and technology appraisals in England and Wales, and the Scottish Intercollegiate Guidelines Network (SIGN): http://www.sign.ac.uk), Scotland's national guidelines body, approve and recommend its use.

We can reproduce it here as a checklist of statements for critically appraising clinical guidelines, with the very kind permission of Françoise Cluzeau of AGREE and the Health Care Evaluation Unit at St George's, which also kindly provided some of the background information in this paragraph. The AGREE Instrument consists of 24 statements, under seven headings, as listed below, including an overall assessment section. The guideline is appraised against each statement (about which there is much supplementary information in the text of the instrument) on a scale of 4 (Strongly Agree) to 1 (Strongly Disagree). All the statements must be used to assess a guideline, in conjunction with the instructions and scoring method as given, with a great deal of other useful information, on the AGREE Collaboration website (http://www.agreecollaboration.org).

THE AGREE STATEMENTS

Scope and purpose

1. The overall objective(s) of the guideline is (are) specifically described
2. The clinical question(s) covered by the guideline(s) is (are) specifically described

3. The patients to whom the guideline is meant to apply are specifically described

Stakeholder involvement

4. The guideline development group includes individuals from all the relevant professional groups
5. The patients' views and preferences have been sought
6. The target users of the guideline are clearly defined
7. The guideline has been piloted among target users

Rigour of development

8. Systematic methods were used to search for evidence
9. The criteria for selecting the evidence are clearly described
10. The methods used for formulating the recommendations are clearly described
11. The health benefits, side-effects and risks have been considered in formulating the recommendations
12. There is an explicit link between the recommendations and the supporting evidence
13. The guideline has been externally reviewed by experts prior to its publication
14. A procedure for updating the guideline is provided

Clarity and presentation

15. The recommendations are specific and unambiguous
16. The different options for management of the condition are clearly presented
17. Key recommendations are clearly identifiable
18. The guideline is supported with tools for application

Applicability

19. The potential organisational barriers in applying the recommendations have been discussed
20. The potential cost implications of applying the recommendations have been considered
21. The guideline presents key review criteria for monitoring and/or audit purposes

Editorial independence

22. The guideline is editorially independent from the funding body
23. Conflicts of interest of guideline development members have been recorded.

Overall assessment

24. Would you recommend these guidelines for use in practice?

This is a burgeoning field, as one would expect, but, sadly and wastefully, all too many guidelines are scattered, and not easily available to those who might need them. In the Select List of Information Resources at the end of Chapter 3, some web-based resources for finding guidelines are listed. To get a fuller flavour of the literature on guideline appraisal or development, try MEDLINE, EMBASE, or CINAHL (see also the Select List), searching, e.g. either guideline* near develop* or guideline* near apprais* to begin with. For a very useful and readable overview, try Eccles and Grimshaw (2000).

References

AGREE Collaboration 2003 Development and validation of an International Appraisal instrument for assessing the quality of clinical practice guidelines: the AGREE Project. Quality and Safety in Health Care 12:18-23

Begg C, Cho M, Eastwood S et al. 1996 Improving the quality of reporting of randomised controlled trials: the CONSORT statement. Journal of the American Medical Association 276(8):637-639

Browman G P, Newman T E, Mohide I D et al. 1998 Progress of clinical oncology guidelines development using the Practice Guidelines Development Cycle: the role of practitioner feedback. Journal of Clinical Oncology 16(3):1226-1231

Claxton K, Sculpher M, Drummond M 2002 A rational framework for decision-making by the National Institute for Clinical Excellence (NICE). Lancet 360:711-715

Cluzeau F A, Littlejohns P, Grimshaw J M et al. 1999 Development and application of a generic methodology to assess the quality of clinical guidelines. International Journal for Quality in Health Care 11(1):21-28

Cookson R, McDaid D, Maynard A 2001 Wrong SIGN, NICE mess: is national guidance distorting allocation of resources? British Medical Journal 323:743-745

Dent T H, Sadler S 2002 From guidance to practice: why NICE is not enough. British Medical Journal 324:842-845

Duff L A, Kitson A L, Seers K et al. 1996 Clinical guidelines: an introduction to their development and implementation. Journal of Advanced Nursing 23:887-895

Eccles M, Freemantle N, Mason J 1998 North of England evidence-based guidelines development project: methods of developing guidelines for efficient drug use in primary care. British Medical Journal 316:1232-1235

Eccles M, Grimshaw J (eds) 2000 Clinical guidelines: from conception to use. Radcliffe Medical Press, Abingdon, Oxon

Field M J, Lohr K N (eds) 1990 Clinical practice guidelines: directions for a new program. Committee to Advise the Public Health Service on Clinical Practice Guidelines, Institute of Medicine. National Academy Press, Washington DC

Graham I D, Beardall S, Carter A O et al 2001 What is the quality of drug therapy: Clinical practice guidelines in Canada? Canadian Medical Association Journal 165(2):157-163

Gray J A 1997 Evidence-based, locally owned, patient-centred guideline development. British Journal of Surgery 84:1636-1637

Grilli R, Magrini N, Penna A et al. 2000 Practice guidelines developed by specialty societies: the need for critical appraisal. Lancet 355: 103-106

Grimshaw J, Russell I 1993 Achieving health gain through clinical guidelines: I: Developing scientifically valid guidelines. Quality in health care 2:243-248

Hadorn D C, Baker D, Hodges J S et al 1996 Rating the quality of evidence for clinical practice guidelines. Journal of Clinical Epidemiology 49(7):749-754

Hayward R S, Laupacis M D 1993 Initiating, conducting and maintaining guidelines development programs. Canadian Medical Associaiton Journal 148(4):507-512

Hayward R S, Wilson M C, Tunis S R et al 1995 Users' guides to the medical literature: VIII. How to use clinical practice guidelines: A. Are the recommendations valid? Journal of the American Medical Association 274(7):570-574

Heffner J E 1998 Does evidence-based medicine help the development of clinical practice guidelines? Chest 113(3) Suppl:173S-178S

Illman J 2000 Britain debates validity of guideline development. Journal of the National Cancer Institute 92(5):368-369

Liberati A, Buzzetti R, Grilli R et al. 2001 Which guidelines can we trust? Western Journal of Medicine 174:262-265

Mann T 1996 Clinical guidelines: using clinical guidelines to improve patient care in the NHS. NHS Executive, Department of Health, London

Murphy M K et al 1998 Consensus development methods, and their use in clinical guideline development. Health Technology Assessment 2(3) whole issue

NHS Centre for Reviews & Dissemination 1994 Implementing clinical practice guidelines: can guidelines be used to improve clinical practice? Effective Health Care 1(8):1-12

Rycroft-Malone J 2001 Formal consensus: the development of a national clinical guideline. Quality in Health Care 10:238-244

Sculpher M, Drummond M, O'Brien B 2001 Effectiveness, efficiency and NICE. British Medical Journal 322:943-944

Shekelle P G, Woolf S H, Eccles M et al. 1999 Developing guidelines. British Medical Journal 318:593-596

Ward J E, Grieco V 1996 Why we need guidelines for guidelines: a study of the quality of clinical practice guidelines in Australia. Medical Journal of Australia 165:574-576

Warner J P, Blizard R 1998 How to appraise clinical guidelines. Psychiatric Bulletin 22:759-761

Wilson M C, Hayward R S, Tunis S R et al. 1995 Users' guides to the medical literature VIII. How to use clinical practice guidelines: B. What are the recommendations and will they help you in caring for your patients? Journal of the American Medical Association 274(20):1630-1632

Woolf S H, DiGuiseppi C G, Atkins D et al. 1996 Developing evidence-based clinical practice guidelines: Lessons learned by the US Preventive Services Task Force. Annual Review of Public Health 17:511-538

Chapter 13

Is this test effective?

Jonathan Mant

Tests are performed in health care for a variety of different reasons. They may be used to establish whether or not someone has a disease, to monitor response to therapy in someone with a disease, to inform treatment decisions in someone with known disease, to assess prognosis or to assess someone's risk of developing a disease. The criteria with which you would assess if a test is effective will depend upon the purpose for which the test is being performed. In this chapter, we shall focus on using tests to help us decide whether or not someone has a disease.

Sackett and Haynes (2002) identified four types of question about test effectiveness with regard to determining whether or not someone has a disease. These are summarised in Table 13.1. Phase I and Phase II questions are asking preliminary questions about whether a test might be of value. Phase III questions are the focus for this chapter. Phase IV questions – whether it improves patient outcomes if the test is performed – are beyond the scope of this chapter. Ideally, such questions would be addressed using a randomised controlled trial (see Chapter 5), but in practice, such studies tend to be carried out where a test is being used as a screening test in a healthy person, rather than in someone in whom a disease is suspected. Thus, the Multicentre Aneurysm Screening Study Group (2002) carried out a randomised trial to assess the impact of performing abdominal ultrasound scans to screen for aortic aneurysms in men aged 65-74. They found that the risk of aneurysm-related death was significantly lower in men who were invited for screening, so demonstrating that the screening programme has a

Table 13.1 Types of question on diagnostic test effectiveness

	Question	Comment
Phase I	Do test results in patients with the target disorder differ from those in normal people?	Preliminary study to identify whether a test is of possible diagnostic value
Phase II	Are patients with certain test results more likely to have the target disorder?	Further preliminary study to quantify possible diagnostic value of test
Phase III	Do test results distinguish patients with and without the target disorder among those in whom it is clinically sensible to suspect the disorder?	Assesses utility of test for making diagnosis in clinical setting
Phase IV	Do patients undergoing the diagnostic test fare better than similar untested patients?	Assesses clinical impact of performing test

See Sackett & Haynes (2002)

positive clinical impact. An example of a randomised controlled trial to assess the impact of a diagnostic test in patients with symptoms is Kendrick et al's (2001) study of the effect of an X-ray of the lumbar spine for patients with low back pain. They found no improvement in outcome in terms of back pain and health status in the group who were X-rayed.

DECIDING WHETHER OR NOT SOMEONE HAS A DISEASE

In an ideal world, a positive test would mean that someone has a disease, and a negative test would mean that the person does not have a disease. Unfortunately, this is not always the case. As we saw in Chapter 6, how we appraise a diagnostic test is to compare its performance with a gold standard, which aims to represent 'the truth'. When a test is carried out, there are four possible outcomes:[1]

1. The test can correctly detect disease that is present (a true positive result).
2. The test can detect disease when it is really absent (a false positive result).
3. The test can correctly identify that someone does not have a disease (a true negative result).
4. The test can identify someone as being free of a disease when it is really present (a false negative result).

---

1 To keep things simple, for the time being we are ignoring 'borderline' test results, but we will come back to these later in the chapter.

These possible outcomes are illustrated in Table 13.2. Given that a test may potentially mislead us if we get a false positive or a false negative result, we need to have some way of characterising how accurate the test really is.

HOW ACCURATE IS THE TEST?

The traditional way in which the accuracy of a test is characterised is in terms of sensitivity and specificity. The sensitivity reflects how good the test is at picking up people with disease, while the specificity reflects how good the test is at identifying people without the disease. What these terms mean can best be understood by way of an example.

Let us consider mammography as a screening test for breast cancer. In the UK, women aged 50 to 64 are invited at 3-yearly intervals for a special X-ray of the breast, called a mammogram, to ascertain whether they might have breast cancer. In one study, the sensitivity of mammography was reported as 88% and the specificity as 93% (Garvican & Littlejohns 1996). What does this mean? Well, the sensitivity of 88% means that for every 100 women with breast cancer who have a mammogram, 88 of them will have a positive (i.e. abnormal) test result. The specificity of 93% means that for every 100 women without breast cancer who have a mammogram, 93 of them will have a negative (i.e. normal) test. The derivation of sensitivity and specificity is shown algebraically in Table 13.2, and using breast cancer screening data in Table 13.3. Sensitivity may then be defined as the proportion of people with disease that have a positive test result, and specificity may be defined as the proportion of people without disease that have a negative test result.

Table 13.2 Possible outcomes of a diagnostic test

		'Truth' Disease present	Disease absent	Totals
Test result	Positive	a true positive	b false positive	a + b
	Negative	c false negative	d true negative	c + d
	Totals	a + c	b + d	a + b + c + d

Sensitivity = a/(a + c)
Specificity = d/(b + d)
Positive predictive value = a/(a + b)
Negative predictive value = d/(c + d)
Prevalence = (a + c)/(a + b + c + d)

Table 13.3 Accuracy of breast cancer screening by mammography in healthy women

		'Truth' Breast cancer present	Breast cancer absent	Totals
Mammography result	Positive	90	910	1000
	Negative	12	12,090	12,102
	Totals	102	13,000	13,102

Sensitivity = 90/102 = 88%
Specificity = 12,090/13,000 = 93%
Positive predictive value = 90/1,000 = 9%
Negative predictive value = 12,090/12,102 = 99.9%
Prevalence = 102/13,102 = 0.78%

Adapted from Garvican & Littlejohns (1996)

What does the test result mean for an individual patient?

The problem with using sensitivity and specificity as a way of summarising test accuracy is that they are difficult to interpret for individual patients. This is illustrated in a study by Steurer et al (2002). They found that the majority of doctors could define sensitivity and specificity correctly, but only a minority were able to interpret the result of a test for an individual patient correctly when supplied with the test sensitivity and specificity. What the patient wants to know, as does the health care professional, might be put something like this: 'Does this positive test mean I have breast cancer?' Or, for someone who has a normal test result: 'Does this negative test mean I do not have breast cancer?' The answers to these questions may be found by looking at Table 13.3. This shows that there were 1000 women who had a positive test. Of these, 90 actually had breast cancer, and 910 did not have breast cancer. Therefore, the chance that someone with a positive test actually has breast cancer is 90/1000, or 9%. In other words, the answer to the first question is: 'No, you probably do not have breast cancer. For every hundred women like yourself with a positive mammogram, only nine will actually turn out to have breast cancer.' This figure of 9% is referred to as the positive predictive value, and its algebraic derivation is shown in Table 13.2.

With regard to the second question, Table 13.3 shows that of 12 102 people who had a negative mammogram, 12 090 really did not have breast cancer, and only 12 did. Therefore, the chance that someone with a negative test does not have breast cancer is 12 090/12 102, or 99.9%. This is referred to as the negative predictive value. Therefore, the answer to the second question is: 'Yes, this negative test means that it is very unlikely that you have breast cancer. For every thousand women like yourself with a negative mammogram, only one has breast cancer.'

Table 13.4 Accuracy of mammography in diagnosing breast cancer in women with breast lumps

		'Truth' Breast cancer present	Breast cancer absent	Totals
Mammography result	Positive	66	8	74
	Negative	21	144	165
	Totals	87	152	239

Sensitivity = 66/87 = 76%
Specificity = 144/152 = 95%
Positive predictive value = 66/74 = 89%
Negative predictive value = 144/165 = 87%
Prevalence = 87/239 = 36%

Derived from data provided by Winchester et al. (1983)

Therefore, from the perspective of the individual, breast cancer screening seems very good at ruling out disease if the test is normal, but not very good at diagnosing disease in that 91% of people with a positive test will turn out not to have breast cancer. You get no hint of this from the sensitivity and the specificity, which both sound quite impressive. Why then, do we not use negative and positive predictive values as our standard way of reporting test accuracy, since it is these values that the patient and the health care professional really need to know?

Effect of prevalence on predictive value

The problem is that predictive value is dependent upon how common the disease is in the population that is being tested. In a population of healthy women aged 50 to 64, breast cancer is in fact fairly uncommon. You can see from Table 13.3 that in the study we referred to earlier only 102 (90 true positives and 12 false negatives) out of 13 102 women tested actually turned out to have breast cancer. This represents 0.78% of the population tested. This can be referred to as the prevalence of the disease in the population. Prevalence is defined as the proportion of people with disease in a defined population at a given point in time. The algebraic derivation of prevalence in relation to a diagnostic test is shown in Table 13.2.

Suppose we had performed mammography on a different population where we would expect a higher prevalence of breast cancer, e.g. women referred to a surgical out-patient clinic with a breast lump. Of course, mammography would not usually be used in this circumstance nowadays, but has been used in the past in this way. Table 13.4 shows the results of a study reported in 1983, which looks at mammography in women with breast

Table 13.5 The effect of prevalence on predictive value: the performance of the CAGE questionnaire in a primary care and a hospital population

		'Truth': alcoholism present			'Truth': alcoholism present		
		Yes	No	Totals	Yes	No	Totals
CAGE	Positive	32	48	80			
questionnaire	Negative	8	912	920			
	Totals	40	960	1,000	200	800	1,000

A. Primary care population
Sensitivity = 80%
Specificity = 95%
Prevalence = 4%
Positive predictive value = 32/80 = 40%
Negative predictive value = 912/920 = 99%

B. Hospital population
Sensitivity = 80%
Specificity = 95%
Prevalence = 20%
Positive predictive value = 80%*
Negative predictive value = 95%*

Notes:
In this illustration, answering yes to two or more questions in the CAGE questionnaire has been taken to be a positive result. As will be seen later on in the chapter, different definitions of 'positive' can be used.

* To see how the values for positive and negative predictive values for the hospital population are derived, see worked example 13.1 at the end of this chapter.

Data taken from King (1986) and Bush et al. (1987)

lumps (Winchester et al 1983). The prevalence of breast cancer in this population is 36%. You can see that the specificity (95%) and sensitivity (76%) of the test in this population of women are not very different from when it was performed in healthy women (Table 13.3). However, the positive predictive value has changed dramatically, and is now 89%. This is much higher than the 9% using the same test in a population with a low prevalence (Table 13.3). This demonstrates that the positive predictive value of a test is dependent upon the prevalence of disease in the population being tested. Conversely, the sensitivity and specificity of the test do not change when performed in a low prevalence (healthy women) or a high prevalence population (women with breast lumps).

This is not to say that sensitivity and specificity are always constant. It is just that they are not affected by prevalence. We will look at what sort of things might make sensitivity and specificity change later in the chapter.

This effect of prevalence on positive predictive value is further illustrated in Table 13.5, which shows how well the same test, the CAGE questionnaire for identifying alcoholism, performs in a primary care population and in a hospital population.

CAGE is a mnemonic for four simple questions. Have you ever felt the need to Cut down the amount that you drink, or are you Annoyed by people who criticise your drinking, or have you felt Guilty about your drinking, or have you ever had an Eye-opener (early morning drink) to drink off a hangover, or to steady your nerves?

In one study in primary care, the prevalence of alcoholism was 4% (King 1986), and in another study in medical and orthopaedic outpatients, the prevalence was 20% (Bush et al 1987). This higher prevalence in the hospital setting is to be expected, since alcoholism is associated with medical (e.g. liver disease, gastrointestinal haemorrhage) and orthopaedic (e.g. alcohol-related trauma) admissions. The sensitivity and specificity of the CAGE questionnaire were similar in the two settings; therefore, in Table 13.5 the sensitivity and specificity have been held constant.

The values of the individual cells in Table 13.5 can be deduced if the prevalence, sensitivity and specificity are known. In the primary care population of 1000 people with 4% prevalence, 40 people would be alcoholics. Given that the sensitivity of the CAGE questionnaire is 80%, then 32 (80% of 40) alcoholics would be correctly identified and 8 (40 – 32) would have been missed by the test. If 40 people are alcoholics, then 960 (1000 – 40) are not. With a specificity of 95%, the test will have correctly identified 912 of these (95% of 960), but have mis-identified 48 of them (960 – 912) as being alcoholics when in fact they were not. You can do exactly the same exercise to fill in the cells for the hospital population. The right-hand side of Table 13.5 has been left blank to allow you to work out what should be in each of the cells. Try it! (The answers are given in the example at the end of the chapter.)

Having filled in all the cells, we can then see that the positive predictive value of the CAGE questionnaire in the primary care population is 40% (32/80). In other words, even if someone in this population is identified as positive by the CAGE questionnaire, it is more likely than not (60% vs 40%) that they are not alcoholics. Conversely, in the hospital population, with a prevalence of 20% alcoholism, someone identified as positive by the CAGE questionnaire has an 80% chance of being a genuine alcoholic.

Therefore, it can be seen that diagnostic tests seem to work better in populations where there is more disease. A positive result in a hospital patient is more likely than not to be a true positive, whereas a positive result in a primary-care patient is more likely than not to be a false positive. This is perhaps one of the explanations for the apparent over-investigation of patients in hospital, and under-investigation of patients by general practitioners. Guidelines for investigations based on hospital populations, or patients referred to specialists will be based upon a population with a high prevalence of disease, and therefore may not translate well to a community-based setting where the prevalence of disease is low. A corollary of the better predictive value of a positive test in hospital is that the negative predictive value of a test will actually be better in the community. If you look back at Table 13.4, you will see that the negative predictive value of the CAGE questionnaire is 95% in the hospital setting and 99% in the community setting. Thus, the chance that someone who screens negative with the CAGE questionnaire is really an alcoholic is 1% (100% – 99%) in the community and 5% (100% – 95%) in hospital – in this situation probably not a clinically important difference.

The measure of test accuracy that is most useful when it comes to interpreting test results for an individual patient is something called the likelihood ratio. Unfortunately, while simple to use, these ratios can be more difficult to understand than the traditional measures of test accuracy. Therefore, we will approach likelihood ratios first of all from the point of view of how they are used, and then consider what they actually mean.

INTERPRETING RESULTS OF TESTS FOR INDIVIDUAL PATIENTS

We have seen from the discussion above that it can be difficult interpreting a result for an individual patient simply knowing sensitivity and specificity. What the health care professional needs to know is the predictive value of a test, but since this depends upon the prevalence of disease, which will vary from population to population, this has to be worked out for each different population, or indeed for each individual patient. Within a primary care population, the prevalence of breast cancer will be much lower in women without breast lumps than in women with breast lumps (see above). Thus, the predictive value of the test depends both upon how good the test is, and what is the prevalence of disease in the sort of person to whom the test is being applied. In this context, prevalence can be referred to as pre-test probability. Pre-test probability reflects the likelihood that a patient has the disease before you carry out the diagnostic test. Whereas prevalence as a term is applied to populations, pre-test probability is applied to individuals. Essentially, they both mean the same thing when it comes to interpreting diagnostic tests.

Another way of thinking about predictive value is that it reflects the likelihood that a patient has the disease after you have carried out the diagnostic test. This can be referred to as post-test probability. Thus, in Table 13.5 in the hospital population, the post-test probability of alcoholism if the test was positive was 80% (= positive predictive value), and the post-test probability of alcoholism if the test was negative was 5% (100% − negative predictive value). When thinking about individual patients, pre-test probability (i.e. probability of disease before you did the test) and post-test probability (i.e. probability of disease after you did the test) are more useful terms than prevalence and predictive value.

So, to apply a diagnostic test to an individual in your practice you need to consider how likely the disease is before you do the test (pre-test probability). Then perform the diagnostic test, and interpret the result not as a simple yes/no answer, but as a probability that the patient has the disease now that you have performed the test (post-test probability). Although this might sound complicated, you are already doing this subconsciously whenever you consider whether a patient has a diagnosis. As we saw when we worked out the contents of the individual cells in Table 13.4, we can derive post-test probabilities using sensitivity and specificity, but it is quite laborious. This is where likelihood ratios come in as a measure of test performance, since, together with a simple nomogram (Figure 13.1), they can be used to derive

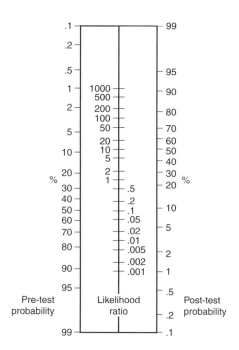

Figure 13.1 A nomogram for applying likelihood ratios (adapted from Fagan 1975 and Sackett et al. 1991)

the post-test probability from the pre-test probability and the result of the diagnostic test. Like sensitivity and specificity, likelihood ratios do not change as prevalence changes.

Examples of using likelihood ratios to interpret test results

Scenario 13.1

You are a GP. A woman, aged 54, comes to you having just been for a screening mammogram. She has just had a letter to inform her that she needs to be followed up in a specialist outpatient clinic, because the mammogram was abnormal. She wants to know whether or not this means she has breast cancer. You examine her breasts, and find no abnormality. What is the answer to her question?

You estimate the probability that she had breast cancer before the test was performed as being 0.8%. You base this on a paper you came across which evaluated a breast-screening programme (Garvican & Littlejohns 1996) (see Table 13.3). You look up the likelihood ratio for a positive test result for mammography, and find it to be 12.6. Using the nomogram, you line up with

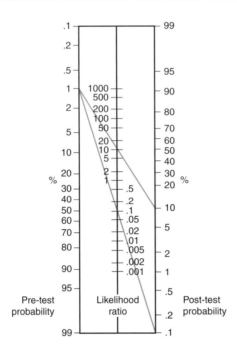

Figure 13.2 Applying a nomogram to interpret possible results of breast cancer screening

a ruler a pre-test probability of 0.8% and a likelihood ratio of 12.6, and read off the post-test probability of about 9% (Figure 13.2). Therefore, you reassure your patient that, although the test was positive, it is still unlikely that she has breast cancer, in that only nine women out of 100 in her situation will actually turn out to have breast cancer.

Scenario 13.2

Another woman, also aged 54, comes to see you. She has recently had a normal mammogram, but is worried because she recently read in a magazine that mammography could miss breast cancer, and wants to know whether it is possible that she does have breast cancer after all. On examination, her breasts are normal. What is the answer to her question?

You estimate this patient's pre-test probability as being 0.8%. You look up the likelihood ratio for a negative test result for mammography and find it to be 0.13. You use the nomogram again, this time lining up a pre-test probability of 0.8% with a likelihood ratio of 0.13 (Figure 13.2). You read off a post-test probability of 0.1%. Therefore, you reassure the patient that it is extremely unlikely that she has breast cancer at the moment in that only 1 woman out of 1000 in her situation who has had a normal mammogram really has breast cancer.

As you might have anticipated, you will see that the post-test probability in Scenario 13.1 above is the same as the positive predictive value in Table

13.3, and the post-test probability in Scenario 13.2 is the same as 100% − 99.9%, 99.9% being the negative predictive value shown in Table 13.3.

Estimating pre-test probability

It will have become clear from the examples above that you cannot use a likelihood ratio to interpret a test result for an individual patient without estimating the pre-test probability. You might view this as a weakness of the approach, but it is in fact a strength. The truth of the matter is that you cannot correctly interpret the result of a diagnostic test without considering the pre-test probability, and by using a likelihood ratio, you force yourself to do so.

So how do you estimate a pre-test probability? There are four main sources of information:

- research papers evaluating diagnostic tests
- epidemiological studies and national statistics
- audit data
- clinical experience.

Research papers in which the diagnostic test was evaluated may give valuable information, since it will be possible to derive the prevalence of the disease in the study population. If you think your patient would have been in the study, then you can use the prevalence in the study as your patient's pre-test probability. If not, then you need to decide whether your patient is likely to be at higher or lower risk of the disease than the study patients, and revise the estimate accordingly.

Epidemiological studies and national statistics that look at the incidence, prevalence and risk factors for disease can be used to inform estimates of pre-test probability. It is useful to distinguish between prevalence and incidence here. Prevalence (see above) reflects the number of cases (old and new) in a population at a given point in time. Incidence can be defined as the number of new cases in a population over a given period of time. Thus, the prevalence of breast cancer in women aged 50 to 64 is about 8 per 1000 women, whereas the incidence of breast cancer in women aged 50 to 64 is 2.5 per 1000 women per year (Office for National Statistics 1997).

In deriving pre-test probability, both can be useful depending upon the type of disease being tested for. You will need to decide on which is most appropriate depending upon what you are testing for. If you are testing for sudden onset of a new disease, such as say emergency investigation of chest pain to diagnose myocardial infarction, incidence is what is needed. If, on the other hand, you are seeking to diagnose chronic heart failure, then prevalence is likely to be more relevant. If you are considering a diagnosis of cancer, then national statistics may be of some use, since most countries have cancer registration data from which incidence rates for cancer are derived.

Data from epidemiological studies and from national statistics can be useful in estimating pre-test probabilities in healthy patients who are screened for disease, but they are of limited use in estimating pre-test probabilities in patients who present with specific complaints. The incidence of a disease will be much higher in people with symptoms than in people who are symptom-free. Most epidemiological studies will use as their denominator the whole population rather than simply the population with symptoms. For example, in Denmark, which is considered to have a high incidence of inflammatory bowel disease, the incidence of Crohn's disease was found to be 5.4 per 100 000 women per year (Fonager et al 1997). The denominator includes all women. The incidence of Crohn's disease in women with a relevant symptom (e.g. diarrhoea) would be much higher, and it is this incidence that would be relevant for a general practitioner considering whether to request colonoscopy in such a patient. Unfortunately, such data are not usually available.

The pre-test probability should be derived from all the information that the health care professional has to hand, including the history, clinical examination findings, and any diagnostic tests already carried out. Such an individualised estimation of pre-test probability cannot come from research papers, though it may be informed by them. For example, you might have a lower threshold for doing a chest X-ray in someone who smokes with a persistent cough than a non-smoker with the same symptom. Instead, the health care professional must rely on local audit data and clinical experience. This may sound a bit of a cop-out for evidence-based health care, but interpretation of diagnostic tests is an area where integration of 'individual clinical expertise with the best available external clinical evidence from systematic research' comes into its own (Sackett et al 1996).

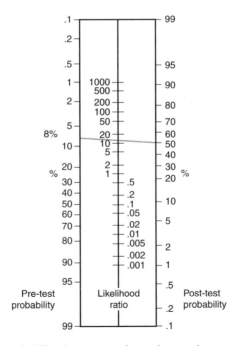

Figure 13.3 Pre-test probability: how wrong do you have to be to get the interpretation of a test result wrong?

Experienced health care professionals will intuitively take account of pre-test probability in interpreting diagnostic test results, even if (as is quite likely!) they have never heard of the term, or of likelihood ratios. An attraction of the pre-test probability and likelihood ratio approach to the interpretation of diagnostic tests is that it makes explicit something that has been done implicitly for a long time.

You may be put off by the imprecision of the way in which pre-test probability can be estimated, but it is important to keep things in context. Often, you can be quite a long way off in terms of your pre-test probability, but still come up with the correct interpretation of the test. Going back to the example of mammography and breast cancer, the best estimate of pre-test probability of 0.8% in a middle-aged woman without a palpable breast lump gives a post-test probability of 9% if she has a positive mammogram (i.e. breast cancer unlikely). How high would your estimate of pre-test probability have had to have been, for you to misinterpret this positive result? If we take misinterpreting the test as believing that breast cancer was more likely than not in this patient (i.e. post-test probability of >50%), we can work out using a nomogram what our pre-test estimate of probability would have had to have been. Lining our ruler up against a post-test probability of 50%, and a likelihood ratio of 12.6, we can see that the pre-test probability would need to have been at least 8% (Figure 13.3). This is a 10-fold overestimation of the true pre-test probability.

What is a likelihood ratio?

So far, we have shown how to use likelihood ratios to interpret the results of diagnostic tests, but we have skirted around saying what a likelihood ratio actually is, and why you need a nomogram to interpret it.

Likelihood ratios come from a mathematical theorem, called Baye's theorem, which states that:

pre-test odds x likelihood ratio = post-test odds.

In other words, if you multiply the pre-test odds of disease by the likelihood ratio of the test, you get the post-test odds of disease. You will see that Baye's theorem is expressed in terms of odds rather than probabilities, which is a little unfortunate because generally speaking we tend to find probabilities easier to understand than odds.

Gamblers amongst you will, however, be quite familiar with odds. If we say that the odds that a horse will win a race is 1:3, we mean that for every time the horse wins the race, there will be three times that it does not win the race. In other words, the probability that the horse will win the race is actually 1/4, or 25% (not 1/3!). In the probability of 1/4, the one represents the one time that the horse will win the race and the four represents the three times the horse will not win the race, plus the one time that it will.

The nomogram allows us to use the likelihood ratio while working in probabilities rather than odds. If we did not have a nomogram, we would either have to work in odds (which can be very confusing!), or alternatively,

Table **13.6** Likelihood ratios associated with different responses to the CAGE questionnaire

CAGE score	Likelihood ratio	Post test probability
0	0.14	7%
1	1.5	45%
2	4.5	72%
3	13	88%
4	100	98%

Data from Buchsbaum et al. (1991)

convert our pre-test probability to an odds, then multiply that odds by the likelihood ratio to derive a post-test odds, which we can then convert back to a probability. While this is mathematically reasonably straightforward, as long as you understand the relationship between odds and probability, it is easier to forget all this, and simply use the nomogram!

But what does a likelihood ratio actually mean? Those of you who have done any simple algebra will recognise that the formula for Baye's theorem given above could equally be written as

$$\text{likelihood ratio} = \frac{\text{post-test odds}}{\text{pre-test odds}}$$

Thus, the likelihood ratio is a ratio of the post-test odds to the pre-test odds. Therefore, it reflects how much the odds of disease will change after the test has been carried out. If the likelihood ratio is greater than 1 (i.e. the post-test odds are greater than the pre-test odds – a positive test), then the likelihood of disease after the test is greater than it was before the test. If the likelihood ratio is less than 1 (i.e. the post-test odds are less than the pre-test odds – a negative test), then the likelihood of disease after the test is less than it was before the test. The higher the likelihood ratio for a positive test, the better the test is at diagnosing disease; the lower the likelihood ratio for a negative test, the better the test is at diagnosing non-disease. As a rule of thumb, diagnostic tests with positive likelihood ratios greater than 10 and/or negative likelihood ratios less than 0.1 can be thought of as fairly powerful tests. A likelihood ratio of 10 means, literally, that the odds of disease are 10 times greater than they were before the test was performed. A likelihood ratio of 0.1 means that the odds of disease are one-tenth what they were before the test was performed.

Diagnostic odds ratios

Another way in which test accuracy is sometimes described is in terms of a diagnostic odds ratio. This is not a useful statistic when it comes to considering the interpretation of a test for an individual patient, but has value as a single measure of overall test accuracy, as opposed to needing to quote sensitivity and specificity or positive and negative likelihood ratios. The diagnostic odds ratio can be defined in many different ways, but the simplest way is to think of it as the positive likelihood ratio divided by the negative likelihood ratio. Thus, the diagnostic odds ratio for mammography is 12.6/0.13, or 96.9. You can see that the higher the positive likelihood ratio and the lower the negative likelihood ratio, the higher the diagnostic odds ratio (and thus, the better, or more accurate, the test). You may come across diagnostic odds ratios in systematic reviews, as they can be used to combine results from different studies in meta-analysis (Deeks 2001).

What about tests which do not give yes/no answers?

Of course, many tests do not actually give simple positive or negative answers. There may be borderline results, there may be several categories of result, or indeed, the results may be continuous, e.g. blood glucose. This can be illustrated by going back to the CAGE questionnaire for diagnosing alcoholism. In Table 13.5, two answers of 'yes' to the four questions was taken to indicate a positive result. However, we have lost a lot of information by summarising the data in this way. Among the 'negative' results, someone who answers 'no' to all four questions is less likely to be an alcoholic than someone who answers 'no' to three questions. Similarly, among the 'positive' results, someone who answers 'yes' to all four questions is more likely to be an alcoholic than someone who answers 'yes' to two of the questions. This is shown in Table 13.6, which gives the likelihood ratios for each level of response to the CAGE questionnaire in a study performed in patients attending a general medical clinic (Buchsbaum et al 1991). In this particular population, the pre-test probability of alcoholism was 36%. Using the likelihood ratios in Table 13.6 and the nomogram in Figure 13.1, the post-test probabilities (also shown in Table 13.6) can be derived (try it!). Thus, likelihood ratios can be quoted for any value of a test result, rather than simply reducing it to 'positive' or 'negative'. Using the CAGE questionnaire, a 'positive' result of 4/4 is associated with a likelihood ratio of 100, whereas a 'positive' result of 3/4 is associated with a likelihood ratio of 13.

Sometimes, evaluations of diagnostic tests that have multiple or continuous results can be represented as a receiver operating characteristic (ROC) curve. This is essentially a graphical representation of what happens to test sensitivity and specificity as the definition of a 'positive' test is changed. For example, there is a screening test for prostate cancer which involves analysis of blood for prostate specific antigen (PSA). PSA is present in the blood in varying amounts in different people, but men with high PSA levels are more likely to have prostate cancer than men with low PSA levels.

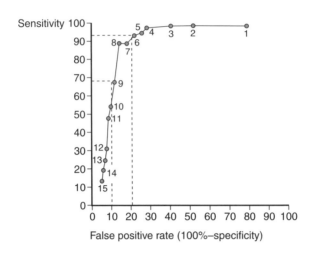

Figure 13.4 ROC curve for PSA values in prostate cancer. Numbers on the graph represent PSA values (adapted from Morgan et al. 1996)

An ROC curve for serum PSA in prostate cancer is shown in Figure 13.4 based on data from Morgan et al (1996). The range of possible values of PSA is from 1 to 15. If an 'abnormal' PSA is taken to be relatively low, say 6 or above, then it can be seen from Figure 13.4 that the sensitivity of PSA for prostate cancer would be high (about 94%), but the false positive rate would also be quite high (21%). The false positive rate is the proportion of people who do not have prostate cancer who test positive, and is 100% minus the specificity, which is 79% in this case.[2] Conversely, if an 'abnormal' PSA is taken to be high, say 9 or above, the sensitivity of the test has fallen to 68%, the false positive rate has fallen to 10% (and the specificity has risen to 90%). The cut-off that is chosen is a trade-off between sensitivity and specificity. If a low PSA value is taken to be abnormal, then few cases of prostate cancer will be missed, but more people who do not have prostate cancer will have an 'abnormal' test result, and so might worry unnecessarily.

Thus, ROC curves can be a useful graphical way of summarising test performance across the whole range of possible results. They can also be a useful way of comparing the value of different diagnostic tests, or the value of the same test in different groups of people. This is illustrated by Figure 13.5, which shows the ROC curves for three different hypothetical tests: a perfect test, a typical test and a useless test. The better the test, the closer the curve gets to the top left-hand corner of the figure. This can be quantified by calculating the area under the curve. A perfect test will have an area under the curve of 1. A useless test will have an area of 0.5. The better the test, the

---

[2] Using the nomenclature in Table 13.2, the false positive rate is given by b / (b+d) – the false positives divided by the true negatives plus the false positives.

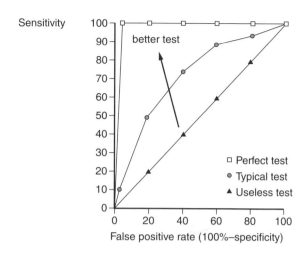

Figure 13.5 Illustrations of different ROC curves

greater the area under the curve. For example, Morgan et al (1996) found that the PSA test performed better when used in white men (area under the ROC curve: 0.94) than in black men (area under the curve: 0.91). Using an ROC curve to summarise test performance can be particularly useful in meta-analyses of studies of test performance (see Chapter 9).

What if you only know the sensitivity and specificity of the test?

Unfortunately, often studies which are published assessing the accuracy of diagnostic tests do not report likelihood ratios. It is, however, possible to calculate the likelihood ratios if sensitivity and specificity have been reported.
    A likelihood ratio for a positive test result is given by the formula:

$$\text{Likelihood ratio (+ve)} = \frac{\text{sensitivity}}{(100\% - \text{specificity})}$$

A likelihood ratio for a negative test result is given by the formula:

$$\text{Likelihood ratio (-ve)} = \frac{(100\% - \text{sensitivity})}{\text{specificity}}$$

An illustration of these calculations is shown in Table 13.7, using data that was published in a paper assessing the value of an electrocardiogram in identifying heart failure that did not report likelihood ratios (Davie et al 1996).
    However, sometimes it can be helpful just knowing sensitivity and specificity if they are very high. Table 13.8 shows data from a study assessing the accuracy of magnetic resonance imaging (MRI) at diagnosing multiple sclerosis (Mushlin et al 1993). In this case, an MRI reading of 'definite

Table 13.7 Calculation of likelihood ratios from sensitivity and specificity

In a study assessing accuracy of electrocardiogram in identifying heart failure, the sensitivity was reported as 94% and the specificity as 61%.

Likelihood ratio (+ve) = 94%/(100% - 61%) = 94/39 = 2.4
Likelihood ratio (-ve) = (100% - 94%)/61% = 6/61 = 0.1

Data from Davie et al. (1996)

Table 13.8 Diagnosis of multiple sclerosis by MRI in patients with possible multiple sclerosis – an example of a SpPin

		'Truth' Multiple sclerosis present	Multiple sclerosis not diagnosed	Totals
MRI scan result	Positive	58	2	60
	Negative	105	138	243
	Totals	163	140	303

Sensitivity = 58/163 = 36%
Specificity = 138/140 = 99%
Positive predictive value = 58/60 = 97%
Negative predictive value = 138/243 = 57%
Prevalence = 163/303 = 54%

Data from Mushlin et al. (1993)

Table 13.9 Screening for hearing loss on a special care baby unit using auditory brainstem evoked potential testing – an example of a SnNout

		'Truth' Baby is deaf	Baby is deaf	Totals
Screening result	Positive	36	44	80
	Negative	0	319	319
	Totals	36	363	399

Sensitivity = 36/36 = 100%
Specificity = 319/363 = 88%
Positive predictive value = 36/80 = 45%
Negative predictive value = 319/319 = 100%
Prevalence = 36/399 = 9%

Data from McClelland et al. (1992)

multiple sclerosis' has been taken to be a positive result, but all other readings have been counted as negative. Such a cut-off gives a test with very high specificity, but low sensitivity. You will see that the positive predictive value of such a test is very high. This is a characteristic of tests with high specificity: if the test is positive, it makes the diagnosis very likely. This can be remembered by the mnemonic – SpPin – for a test with high specificity, if the test is positive, then it rules the diagnosis in (Sackett et al 1991).

Table 13.9 shows data from a study assessing the accuracy of a screening test for hearing loss in babies admitted to a special care baby unit (McClelland et al 1992). You can see that in this example, the sensitivity is very high. In this case, the negative predictive value is 100%. In other words, if the test is negative, the diagnosis is very unlikely. This can be remembered by the mnemonic – SnNout – for a test with high sensitivity, if the test is negative, then it rules out the diagnosis (Sackett et al 1991).

ARE THE RESULTS RELEVANT TO YOUR PATIENT?

So far, we have considered how to interpret results of tests for your patients. However, it may be that you feel that the results of studies done to assess the accuracy of the test are not generalisable (or relevant) to your setting, or you may consider that it would not be helpful to your patient to perform the test.

Generalisability to your setting

One aspect to consider is whether the assessments that have been carried out of test validity are applicable to your setting. We have already seen how predictive value is dependent upon prevalence, so the predictive value of a test in one setting is usually not relevant to another setting. Sensitivity and specificity (and likelihood ratios) are not dependent on prevalence, but they can vary according to the type of patients in which the test is carried out. This variation is referred to as spectrum bias. The sensitivity of a test will depend upon the severity of disease in the population being tested. The more advanced or severe the disease, the more likely the test is to identify it. For example, in an evaluation of the accuracy of a dipstick test for urinary-tract infection, the test was assessed in two groups: one group in whom the clinician thought that the diagnosis of urinary-tract infection was likely on the basis of the clinician's assessment of the presenting symptoms and signs, and one group in which the clinician thought the diagnosis was unlikely (Lachs et al 1992). Not surprisingly, the sensitivity of the dipstick test for urinary-tract infection was found to be much higher in the first group than in the second group (92% vs 56%). The first group had more prominent symptoms and signs of urinary-tract infection, which reflected more established infection which the dipstick test could readily identify.

The specificity of a test will depend upon the prevalence of other diseases in the population which might lead to false positive results. The more that other diseases are present, the more likely a false positive result. This was also illustrated in the study which evaluated the dipstick test. In the first group, the investigators found that the specificity of the test was lower than in the second group (42% vs 78%). Again, this is to be anticipated since the more symptomatic group will have a higher prevalence of other diseases which might lead to false positive dipstick tests.

Thus, you will need to consider the setting of the study (e.g. hospital or primary care), and the characteristics of the patients that were included, such as their age and gender.

A second aspect to consider is whether the test is carried out the same way in your setting as it was in the study. Some diagnostic tests depend upon the skill of the person carrying out the test, and the skill of the people interpreting the test result. Tests may be carried out in different ways, and it is important to know that it is carried out the same way in your local hospital or laboratory as it was in the study which evaluated the test. This will include checking what cut-offs were used for positive and negative tests, and whether the definition of disease as applied by the reference standard is the same as is used in your own setting.

Will it help your patient?

One way to think about whether or not to perform the test is whether it will influence the management of the patient or groups of patients you are likely to see. If you think that a disease is unlikely in a particular patient, it may be that if you carried out the test and it was positive, you would still think that the disease was unlikely, so it would not influence your management. Conversely, if you think that a disease is likely in a given patient, it may be that a negative test result would not stop you treating the patient, since you would still think that the disease is likely whatever the test result. Putting this in terms of pre- and post-test probabilities: in the first instance the pre-test probability of disease is so low, that even with a positive test result, the post-test probability will be less than 50%; in the second instance, the pre-test probability of disease is so high that even with a negative test result, the post-test probability will be more than 50%.

These ideas are illustrated in Figure 13.6, which shows possible diagnosis and treatment thresholds in terms of pre-test probability. What you decide is a 'low' or a 'high' pre-test probability will depend upon the nature of the disease being considered and the treatment offered. For breast cancer, the consequences of missing the disease are potentially very serious. Therefore, we screen women with a pre-test probability of breast cancer of 0.8%, i.e. in effect we classify this risk as 'intermediate'. At the other end of the spectrum, if the treatment is minor (e.g. aspirin to prevent stroke in someone who has had a transient ischaemic attack), we may initiate treatment with a relatively low pre-test probability, whereas if the treatment is major (e.g. radiotherapy for cancer), we would want a very high probability that the diagnosis was correct before we started treatment.

In practice, knowledge about the accuracy of diagnostic tests will perhaps

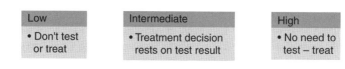

Pre-test probability of disease

Figure 13.6 Thresholds for diagnosis and treatment based on probability that patient has disease (adapted from Sackett et al. 1991)

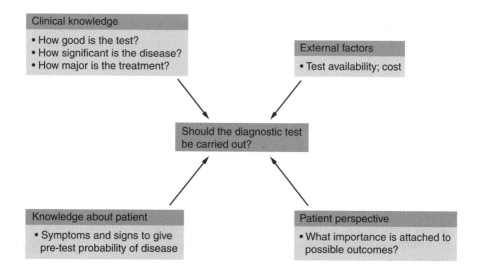

Figure 13.7 Clinical decision-making: diagnosis

be most useful when planning protocols or guidelines to manage particular groups of patients. For example, the most accurate way of diagnosing heart failure would be to use an echocardiogram. However, in general practice it may not be feasible, or indeed a good use of scarce resources, to refer all patients for this investigation with non-specific symptoms such as ankle swelling. There is a 10-fold reduction in the odds of heart failure if the patient has a normal electrocardiogram (ECG) – see Table 13.7 (Davie et al 1996). Therefore, a sensible protocol might include screening such patients with an ECG first. Only those patients with an abnormal ECG would be referred for an echocardiogram.

Any decision about carrying out a diagnostic test will be informed by four major inputs (Figure 13.7). Not only does knowledge about the patient's symptoms and signs (which informs our assessment of pre-test probability), and our knowledge (preferably in terms of likelihood ratios) about how good the test is influence the decision, but also the knowledge of external factors, such as availability of the test and its cost and the patient's perspective. The latter is particularly important. For example, one of the antenatal tests that is available for pregnant women is a blood test to screen for Down's syndrome called the triple test. If the test is positive, then the mother would be offered an amniocentesis, which carries a small (1%) risk of miscarriage, to establish whether or not the baby really had Down's syndrome. If the baby did have Down's syndrome, then the mother would be offered a termination. Whether or not it is sensible to have the test depends upon the mother's attitude to having a child with Down's syndrome, her attitude to having a termination and her attitude to the possibility that an amniocentesis will induce a miscarriage of a normal baby. Different women are going to reach different conclusions, according to the value that they attach to the different possible outcomes.

CONCLUSION

An evidence-based approach to deciding whether a test is effective for your patient involves the following steps:

1. Frame the clinical question (see Chapter 2).
2. Search for evidence concerning the accuracy of the test (see Chapter 3).
3. Assess the methods used to determine the accuracy of the test (see Chapter 6).
4. Find out the likelihood ratios for the test.
5. Estimate the pre-test probability of disease in your patient.
6. Apply the likelihood ratios to this pre-test probability using the nomogram to determine what the post-test probability would be for different possible test results.
7. Decide whether or not to perform the test on the basis of your assessment of whether it will influence the care of the patient, and the patient's attitude to different possible outcomes.

WORKED EXAMPLES

Worked example 13.1

If the prevalence of alcoholism is 20% in hospital in-patients, what might one expect the predictive value of the CAGE questionnaire to be, given that it has a sensitivity of 80% and a specificity of 95%? (see Table 13.5).

This is a relevant question, because it allows us to consider how a test evaluated in one population might perform in another population, if we assume that there is no 'spectrum bias'.

It is possible to construct a two-by-two table comparing test performance against the 'truth' if one knows the sensitivity and specificity of the test and the prevalence of the disease. From this, the predictive value can be calculated.

In this example, if we take a population of 1000 patients:

Step 1. Knowing that the prevalence of disease is 20%, then 20% of 1000 patients, i.e. 200, will have the disease. This means that 1000 – 200 (i.e. 800) patients will not have the disease. We can, therefore, fill in the column totals of our two-by-two-table:

		'Truth' Alcoholism present	Alcoholism absent	Totals
CAGE	Positive	a	b	
questionnaire	Negative	c	d	
	Totals	200	800	1000

Step 2. The sensitivity of 80% means that 80% of the 200 people who have the disease, i.e. 160, will be correctly identified by the CAGE questionnaire as having alcoholism. This can be entered into cell 'a'. If 160/200 were correctly identified, this means that 40/200 will have been incorrectly identified as 'negative' on the CAGE questionnaire. This can be entered into cell 'c':

		'Truth' Alcoholism present	Alcoholism absent	Totals
CAGE	Positive	160	b	
questionnaire	Negative	40	d	
	Totals	200	800	1000

Step 3. The specificity of 95% means that 95% of the 800 people (i.e. 760) who are not alcoholic will be correctly identified as such by the test. Into cell 'd' insert 760. If 760/800 were correctly labelled, this means that 40/800 were incorrectly labelled as alcoholic. Therefore, 40 can be entered into cell 'b':

		'Truth' Alcoholism present	Alcoholism absent	Totals
CAGE	Positive	160 (a)	40 (b)	
questionnaire	Negative	40 (c)	760 (d)	
	Totals	200	800	1000

Step 4. Now that the two-by-two table is complete, the positive and negative predictive values can be calculated:

Positive predictive value $= a/(a+b) = 160/(160+40) = 80\%$

Negative predictive value $= d/(c+d) = 760/(760+40) = 95\%$

Worked example 13.2

In a study of the accuracy of clinical assessment of deep-vein thrombosis in patients with suspected DVT, the results of clinical assessment were compared with results of a reference standard investigation, venography:

	Venography result Positive (%)	Negative (%)	Totals
Clinical assessment			
High probability of DVT	72 (85)	13	85
Moderate probability of DVT	47 (33)	96	143
Low probability of DVT	16 (5)	285	301
Totals	135 (26)	394	529

Adapted from Wells et al. (1995)

A. What is the pre-test probability of a DVT in this population before they are clinically assessed?

This is the same as the prevalence of DVT in the population of patients with suspected DVT, i.e. $135/529 = 26\%$.

B. What is the likelihood ratio for clinical assessment of high probability of DVT?

Likelihood ratio (+ve) = sensitivity / (1 – specificity).

Sensitivity is the proportion of people with DVT correctly identified by the test. This is $72/135 = 53.3\%$ (or 0.533).

Specificity is the proportion of people without DVT correctly identified as 'test negatives'. This is $(394 – 13)/394 = 96.7\%$ (or 0.967).

Therefore, likelihood ratio $= 0.533/(1 – 0.967) = 0.533/0.033 = 16.15$.

An alternative method of calculating the likelihood ratio is given in F. below.

C. What is the probability of a DVT in a patient who has been assessed as having a high probability of a DVT (i.e. the post–test probability)?

This can be approached in different ways. The post-test probability is the same as the positive predictive value, which is the proportion of people who test positive and who actually have disease. In this case, this is the proportion of people assessed as having a high probability of DVT who have a positive venogram, which is $72/85 = 85\%$.

Alternatively, knowing that the pre-test probability is 26% (see A.), and the likelihood ratio for a positive result is 16.15, then the post-test probability can be read off using the nomogram in Figure 13.1.

Alternatively, knowing that the pre-test probability is 0.26, the pre-test odds of disease are $0.26:(1 - 0.26) = 0.26:0.74 = 0.26/0.74:1 = 0.35:1$. Therefore, the post-test odds of disease are $0.35 \times 16.15:1 = 5.65:1$. This is the same as a post-test probability of $5.65/(1 + 5.65) = 5.65/6.65 = 0.85$.

D. What is the likelihood ratio for clinical assessment of low probability of DVT?

In the chapter, likelihood ratio (-ve) was given as: $(1 - \text{sensitivity})/\text{specificity}$.

This is correct where the test gives a positive or negative answer. However, where, as in this case, the test gives a graded, non-dichotomous answer, then you have to be careful how you use this formula.

In essence, clinical assessment of low probability is a 'negative' result. The specificity is given by the proportion of people who had a negative venogram who were identified as having a low probability of a DVT. This is $285/394 = 72.3\%$, or 0.723.

A 'positive' clinical assessment in this context is moderate or high probability of a DVT. Therefore, the correct sensitivity for this calculation is $(72 + 47)/135 = 88.1\%$, or 0.881.

Therefore, the likelihood ratio $= (1 - 0.881)/0.723 = 0.16$.

E. What is the probability of a DVT in someone who has been assessed as having a low probability of a DVT (i.e. the post–test probability)?

As with C. above, this can be calculated in different ways. You can apply the likelihood ratio of 0.16 to the pre-test probability of 26% using the nomogram (Figure 13.1). Alternatively, you can calculate the positive predictive value of a 'negative' result. This is $16/301$, i.e. 5%.

F. What is the likelihood ratio associated with a clinical assessment of a moderate probability of DVT?

It is more difficult with this question (though possible) to calculate what the likelihood ratio is in terms of a formula comprising sensitivity and specificity. We think of sensitivity and specificity in terms of two-by-two tables, and in this example, we have three levels of test result (high, moderate or low). We simplified things above by considering the test result as high vs moderate/low (for B.) and low vs moderate/high (for D.). It is easier, when calculating likelihood ratios for more than two levels of test result, to use an alternative definition of a likelihood ratio, which is:

For a given level of a diagnostic test result, the likelihood ratio = proportion of total patients with disease who have given level result divided by proportion of total patients without disease who have given level result.

In this example, the 'given level' is 'moderate probability'. The total number of patients with disease is 135, and the total number of patients without disease is 394. The proportion of total patients with disease who have clinical assessment of 'moderate probability' is 47/135 (0.348), and the proportion of total patients without disease assessed as having 'moderate probability' is 96/394 (0.244).

Therefore, the likelihood ratio = 0.348/0.244 = 1.4.

NB. The likelihood ratios for high and low probability clinical assessments could have been calculated in the same way:

For given level as *high* probability:
Proportion of total with disease = 72/135 = 0.533
Proportion of total without disease = 13/394 = 0.033
Likelihood ratio = 0.533/0.033 = 16.15.

For given level as *low* probability:
Proportion of total with disease = 16/135 = 0.119
Proportion of total with disease = 285/394 = 0.723
Likelihood ratio = 0.119/0.723 = 0.16.

References

Buchsbaum D G, Buchanan R G, Centor R M et al 1991 Screening for alcohol abuse using CAGE scores and likelihood ratios. Annals of Internal Medicine 115:774-777

Bush B, Shaw S, Cleary P et al. 1987 Screening for alcohol abuse using the CAGE questionnaire. American Journal of Medicine 82:321-335

Davie A P, Francies C M, Love M P et al 1996 Value of the electrocardiogram in identifying heart failure due to left ventricular systolic dysfunction. British Medical Journal 312:222

Deeks J J 2001 Systematic reviews of evaluations of diagnostic and screening tests. In: Egger M, Davey Smith G, Altman D G (eds) Systematic reviews in health care. 2nd edn. British Medical Journal Publication, London

Fagan T J 1975 Nomogram for Baye's theorem. New England Journal of Medicine 293:257

Fonager K, Sorensen H T, Olsen J 1997 Change in incidence of Crohn's disease and ulcerative colitis in Denmark. A study based on the National Registry of Patients, 1981-92. International Journal of Epidemiology 26:1003-1008

Garvican L, Littlejohns P 1996 An evaluation of the prevalent round of the breast screening programme in South East Thames, 1988-1993: achievement of quality standards and population impact. Journal of Medical Screening 3:123-128

Kendrick D, Fielding K, Bentley E et al 2001 Radiography of the lumbar spine in primary care patients with low back pain: randomised controlled trial. British Medical Journal 322:400-405

King M 1986 At risk drinking among general practice attenders: validation of the CAGE questionnaire. Psychological Medicine 16:213-217

Lachs M S, Nachamkin I, Edelstein P H et al 1992 Spectrum bias in the evaluation of diagnostic tests: lessons from the rapid dipstick test for urinary-tract infection. Annals of Internal Medicine 117:135-140

McClelland R J, Watson D R, Lawless V et al 1992 Reliability and effectiveness of screening for hearing loss in high-risk neonates. British Medical Journal 304:806-809

Morgan T O, Jacobsen S J, McCarthy W F et al 1996 Age-specific reference ranges for serum prostate specific antigen in black men. New England Journal of Medicine 335:304-310

Multicentre Aneurysm Screening Study Group 2002 The Multicentre Aneurysm

Screening study into the effect of abdominal aortic aneurysm screening on mortality in men: a randomised controlled trial. The Lancet 360:1531-1539

Mushlin A I, Detsky A S, Phelps C E et al 1993 The accuracy of magnetic resonance imaging in patients with suspected multiple sclerosis. Journal of the American Medical Association 269:3146-3151

Office for National Statistics 1997 Cancer statistics: registrations 1990 Series MBI no. 23. The Stationery Office, London

Sackett D L, Haynes R B, Guyatt G H et al 1991 Clinical epidemiology, 2nd edn, Little, Brown, Boston

Sackett D L, Rosenberg W M, Muir Gray J A et al 1996 Evidence-based medicine: what it is and what it isn't. British Medical Journal 312:71-72

Sackett D L, Haynes R B 2002 The architecture of diagnostic research. British Medical Journal 324:539-541

Steurer J, Fischer J E, Bachmann L M et al 2002 Communicating accuracy of tests to general practitioners: a controlled study. British Medical Journal 324:824-826

Wells P S, Hirsh J, Anderson D R et al 1995 Accuracy of clinical assessment of deep-vein thrombosis. Lancet 345:1326-1330

Winchester D P, Sener S, Immerman S et al 1983 A systematic approach to the evaluation and management of breast masses. Cancer 51:2535-2539

Chapter 14

Is this therapy effective?

Martin Dawes

INTRODUCTION

The aim of this chapter is to enable you to consider one or more treatments and to evaluate in a consistent way their effectiveness in reducing or preventing disease. You will find it helpful to practise these methods; I have included exercises at the end of the chapter for this purpose. The fear of interpretation of results is that it is all to do with statistics. Although the calculation of statistics can be confusing, a basic understanding of some concepts is necessary for any health care professional to assess a trial. This chapter aims at looking at trials from a user's point of view rather than from a researcher designing a trial. As such the amount of statistics is limited.

Clinical effectiveness of any procedure or intervention is directly related to the number of people who gain improvement from that procedure as well as how much they gain. It is therefore necessary to examine in detail the results of any controlled trail. The results are often presented in a way that does not make it easy for the reader to understand. This section will enable you to take information from papers and convert bare facts into more meaningful and clinically useful information.

Health care professionals are continually being informed about details of 'effective' new treatments. This may come from, among other sources, the lay press, medical companies, educational meetings or patients. The difficulty is deciding whether the treatment is likely to be clinically effective (or harmful) in our patients. 'Effective' is itself an emotive word implying some strong property. An important question to ask is 'What is meant by effective?' Is the condition cured while the patient suffers severe side-effects or is the pain relieved but the condition deteriorates?

Sometimes, a new treatment is so obviously effective that there is no difficulty in making that decision. An example of this is the use of a new anaesthetic gas. On October 16, 1846, William T.G. Morton demonstrated in public the value of ether for surgery at Massachusetts General Hospital.

Dr Fraser, who had witnessed this demonstration, left Boston on December 1, 1846, in a wooden paddle steamer. He arrived in Liverpool and reached his mother in Dumfries, Scotland, on December 17. Two days later, his surgical friends Drs M'Lauchlan and Scott administered ether to a patient there in Dumfries. That same Royal Mail steamer, Acadia, carried a letter and the Boston Daily Advertiser story to Dr Boott at Gower Street, London. Robinson etherised Dr Boott's niece for a molar extraction on December 19, 1846.

By the end of the year, ether was being used throughout Europe. This history indicates that sometimes, if a medication is dramatically effective for serious conditions that occur frequently, little needs to be done about publication as it will become general knowledge very quickly. However, streptokinase (alone or in association with aspirin) is a clinically very effective treatment for acute myocardial infarction producing an important improvement in survival, if used soon after the onset of symptoms. Only 20 patients need to be treated to save one life (Midgette et al 1990). It took many years before this important discovery was put into everyday practice (Fibrinolytic Therapy Trialists' (FTT) Collaborative Group 1994). Identifying whether the proposed new treatment is really effective is central to good care. Evaluation of the evidence within clinical research papers describing these therapies is part of that process.

In any clinical therapeutic study there are three explanations for the observed effect:

1. The effect of the treatment
2. Chance variation between the two groups
3. Bias (see Chapter 4)

Good research will explicitly endeavour to reduce the effects of chance and bias by using special designs.

NATURAL HISTORY OF A DISEASE

Many factors can affect the course and severity of a disease in an individual. We may underestimate anxiety provoked by the fear of illness and similarly

> **Box 14.1 Factors that may affect efficacy of treatment**
>
> - Age at diagnosis
> - Duration of treatment
> - Employment
> - Explanation about treatment
> - Explanation of disease
> - Fear of diagnosis
> - Health of family
> - Knowledge about diagnosis
> - Knowledge of expected outcomes
> - Knowledge of side effects
> - Pharmacological efficacy of the treatment
> - Previous history of disease
> - Social aspects
> - State of family relationships

the impact of reassurance on this anxiety. Treatment is not just the pharmacological impact of the drug. The knowledge of the diagnosis may be all that is needed to alleviate symptoms. Box 14.1 lists a number of items that may affect the efficacy of a treatment.

The information we give to patients when starting treatment may be critical to the effectiveness of that treatment. The background of the patient, including the social and medical history is also relevant. These factors must be taken into account when considering an article describing the effectiveness of any new treatment.

PLACEBO EFFECT

Placebo treatment is effective in its own right and may also have side-effects (Editorial 1972). The effect of placebos has been known for centuries. Doctors and quacks have used the impact of the placebo to great effect. The average relief rate from a placebo may be as high as 35% (Beecher 1950). That means that over one-third of patients with certain conditions may get better if you give them all a placebo!

The improvement seen when treating a group with an experimental drug might be because of the placebo effect and not the constituents of that drug. The controlled study will account for this effect by giving a placebo to one group and an experimental drug to the other group of patients.

It is important that the two groups (placebo (or control) and experimental) are similar in all relevant characteristics. Otherwise any difference in treatment effect may not be due to chance or the drug, but some other characteristic of the placebo group that differs from the experimental treatment group. For example, the treatment group may have been younger and, therefore, more likely to recover spontaneously. This difference between the treatment and placebo group is one type of bias.

This does not mean that patients in all placebo-controlled trials are not having any active therapy. There are many trials where a new treatment is added to conventional treatment. That conventional treatment is given to both the experimental and control group. The experimental group gets, in addition, the new drug, while the control group gets the placebo.

BASIC DESIGNS OF CLINICAL TRIALS

The discovery of the effect a drug has may occur by chance or design. Once safety and pharmacological tests about dosage have been performed, the drug will be tested on volunteer patients. The randomised control trial is regarded by many as the cornerstone of research design in evaluating the therapeutic effectiveness of a new therapy. Two groups of patients are compared before and after treatment. They are randomly allocated either to one of two experimental drugs or to an experimental drug and a placebo. The placebo drug should be similar in shape, size and colour and have no effect on the problem being treated.

Sometimes patients are given the placebo and the experimental treatments being studied, one following the other. Using the same patients in control and treatment groups one eliminates bias that arises from differences between patients and the design has several statistical advantages. This is called a 'cross-over design'. Occasionally, studies will not allocate patients to control or placebo groups. This is usually in diseases where the outcome without treatment is commonly or always fatal.

DID THE TREATMENT WORK?

After bias has been excluded as much as possible, there are two reasons for a difference occurring between the two groups. The drug may be causing the effect or the effect may be occurring by chance. How does one assess this when reading the article? Normally, an article should describe the statistical test used to determine whether the difference occurred by chance. Frequently, a paper will describe a difference and then add a P value. These P values are to be found liberally sprinkled through most quantitative research articles. It shows the probability of getting a result as, or more, extreme than the one observed if the difference was entirely due to chance alone. This calculation of p is, therefore, of great importance in evaluating whether chance is responsible for the observed difference. By excluding chance and bias you are left with the last explanation: that the drug was responsible.

WHAT DO WE MEAN BY AND HOW DO WE DESCRIBE RISK?

We use many terms to describe the risk of an event: risk, chance, danger, gamble, hazard, jeopardy, peril, possibility, uncertainty and venture. We use these terms with adjectives in front of them: high risk, great peril, small chance and little possibility. These phrases are used very commonly and show how accustomed we are to estimating the chances of events occurring in everyday life. What we are not used to is quantifying these chances in any uniform way. We often express chances using comparisons to common or rare events. Winning the lottery was described as less likely than being struck by lightning. In the UK National Lottery six numbers are drawn at random from the set of integers between 1 and 49, which means there are 13 983 816 combinations (the draw order does not matter). This means that the jackpot chance is approximately 1 in 14 million.

Lightning kills 100 people each year in the USA. This is approximately one death per 2.5 million people. This is what we accept as an uncommon or rare event. We are not used to talking about percentage probabilities and do not relate well to these terms. The risk of lightning killing a US citizen is 0.00004% probability ([1 / 2 500 000] which is equivalent to 100 per annum).

The risk of a 40-year-old, non-smoking male with no previous history of heart disease, normal blood pressure, normal cholesterol, and not diabetic, developing coronary heart disease (CHD) over the next 10 years is 2% (Anderson et al 1991). Another way of expressing this is to say that two out of 100 men with the same characteristics will develop CHD. This still may not be high enough for the man to worry about unduly.

We respond to risk depending on our appreciation of the impact of the event. For a 20-year-old man, death is a remote event not necessarily feared greatly. An 85-year-old man may be more likely to appreciate the risk of a fatal event more keenly but it will still depend on individuals as to how they rate their risk. The outcome is the same but the fear, and therefore the reaction to risk of death or disease, varies from individual to individual. This applies to people reading articles. The young researcher reading an article about fractured hips will feel that it is a remote possibility and, therefore, a large reduction in events would be needed before the researcher felt that the treatment was effective. An older person may feel that, as the personal risk is quite high a smaller benefit of treatment is needed before treatment is clinically effective. This awareness to individual appreciation of risk in specific contexts is important when discussing results with others. Instead of using risk or the reduction of risk to describe the effectiveness of a therapy, an alternative approach may be used.

NUMBERS NEEDED TO TREAT

This can be worked out by addition, subtraction and division. No statistics are needed – not even a calculator.

We are often faced with extremely ambitious claims by authors of research on the effect of the intervention. This may be because of the fact that the intervention is indeed very effective. However, the authors will have invested a lot of time in the research and will want to emphasise positive results. Once the effect has been established statistically, they will often feel that this is also clinically significant. Unfortunately, this is not always the case. The authors will want to put forward the best possible arguments for the use of their intervention and so may use figures that help their argument while omitting figures that are perhaps not so favourable.

The most common approach is to describe the effect of a drug in terms of the risk reduction. The risk is usually of continuing to have, for example, pain or an event such as a stroke or heart attack.

When evaluating an article on a therapeutic manoeuvre, it is possible to establish its clinical effectiveness by determining the proportion of patients receiving treatment who gain benefit. At this stage it is useful to consider an example. A trial was designed to assess the effect of a specialist nurse in the care of patients discharged from hospital with chronic heart failure. The nurse made planned home visits of decreasing frequency supplemented by telephone calls. Patient education about heart failure and its treatment as well as closer disease monitoring and self-medication were the main aim of this intervention. The reduction in readmission for heart failure was 57%. You are told about this by a colleague who says: 'Home visiting by a nurse halves readmission rates for patients with heart failure, you know!'.

At this stage you decide to look further and find the article on the British Medical Journal website (Blue et al 2001).

You are happy with the quality of the study (Chapter 5) and now want to determine for yourself the clinical effectiveness.

From Table 14.3 in the paper, the results in Table 14.2 are drawn.

This is one of the hardest steps. Identifying the key data should be easy but one has to check that the data is the correct way around and from the correct row. It is easy to be confused by the results table and only by careful checking are mistakes avoided. However, this step is vital – one needs to see the raw numbers of the events by the control and experimental groups.

From this table it can be seen that there were a total of 38 readmissions for heart failure: 26 occurred in the control group and 12 in the experimental treatment group.

Twenty-six out of 81 treated with control had a readmission for heart failure. This may be presented as a percentage $(26/81) \times 100 = 32.1\%$.

However, in the experimental treatment group there were 12 readmissions in 84 people (14.3%).

The absolute risk is that 32.1% of individuals in the control group had a readmission. Also, 14.3% of the experimental group had a readmission.

The difference between the two should give us some measure of how effective the treatment was.

32.1%-14.3% = 17.8%

There is a 17.8% difference between the control group and the experimental group. If 100 people were given the experimental drug instead of the control, then there would be 17 (rounded down from 17.8) fewer individuals readmitted. This is because we are working in percentages.

Finally, we are getting near the numbers needed to treat. To prevent 17.8 individuals getting readmitted 100 must be treated; therefore, to prevent one

Table 14.1 Results of the treatment of alendronate sodium for preventing hip fracture

	Placebo (control)	Experimental treatment	Total
Hip fracture	22	11	33
No hip fracture	983	1011	1994
Total	1005	1022	2027

Data from Black et al. (1996)

Table 14.2 Examples of NNTs

Problem	Outcome	Intervention	EER	CER	RRR (CI)	ARR	NNT (CI)
Otitis media	Pain at 2-7 days	Antibiotics	10.0%	14.3%	36% (18-50)	4.3%	24
Bell's palsy	Complete recovery	Steroid therapy	77%	68%		9%	11 (6-117)
Acute asthma	Reduce relapse rate	Steroid therapy	8%	16%	58% (21-78)	8%	14 (8-68)

EER, experimental event rate; CER, control event rate; RRR, relative risk reduction; ARR, actual risk reduction; NNT, numbers needed to treat; CI, 95% confidence interval. For more NNTs, see Bandolier 50th issue

individual being readmitted $100 \div 17.8 = 5.6$ (let us call it 6 individuals) must be treated. This is the number needed to treat (NNT) to prevent one readmission for worsening heart failure in this case.

Stepping back a bit, the difference between the control event rate (CER) and the Experimental Event Rate (EER) is called the Absolute Risk Reduction (ARR).

However, you will find that a lot of articles prefer to use Relative Risk (RR) and Relative Risk Reduction (RRR). The relative risk of having a readmission in the treatment group compared with the control group is calculated by dividing the rate in the treatment group by the rate in the control group.

$$RR = \frac{EER}{CER} = \frac{14.3}{32.1} = 44\%$$

The relative reduction in risk (RRR) of having a readmission can be calculated by subtracting this relative risk from 100%, or by using the following simple calculation:

$$\text{Relative Risk Reduction (RRR)} = \frac{\text{CER - EER}}{\text{CER}} = \frac{32.1 - 14.3}{32.1} = 55\%$$

The RRR is expressed as a percentage (55%) and means that the treatment reduced the risk of readmission by 55% relative to that occurring in this control population. You can see already that this statement conceals the fact that the risk itself is 32%.

If the risk was 3.2% for controls and 1.4% for experimental the relative risk and relative risk reduction would still be 44% and 55%, respectively. What would be the numbers needed to treat (NNT)?

$$\frac{100}{3.2 - 1.4} = \frac{100}{1.8} = 55$$

So the relative risk reduction and relative risk can seem very impressive but conceal the fact that the NNT is very large because of the low event rate.

The relative risk reduction for stroke achieved by treating patients with mild-to-moderate hypertension is 50% over 5 years. This means that if patients with mild or moderate hypertension are treated, one can expect a 50% reduction in stroke compared with the group that does not get treatment. Taken on its own these figures are very impressive and likely to persuade anyone that treatment should be used. It suggests that the treatment is clearly of benefit and should therefore be used. In younger age groups the risk of stroke on treatment is 0.552% (0.00552), over 5 years, compared with a risk without treatment of 1.2% (0.012). These rates are very low. The absolute risk reduction is $0.012 - 0.00552 = 0.00648$. The reciprocal of this is $1/0.00648 = 154$. That means that you would have to treat 154 patients with mild-to-moderate hypertension for 5 years to prevent one stroke.

There is no 'good' NNT nor is there a 'bad' NNT. They are simply numbers to give you an idea of what to expect from a therapy.

Some other examples of numbers needed to treat can be found at the Bandolier site http://www.jr2.ox.ac.uk/bandolier/band50/b50-8.html

PITFALLS IN CALCULATING NUMBERS NEEDED TO TREAT

It is very important to identify the current numbers from articles. Although the calculation of numbers needed to treat is desirable, many articles do not clearly produce the data in an easily identifiable manner. It is important to have the numbers of all people who were started on treatment and, within those, the number of people who benefited. Some studies report the numbers of patients who benefit without stating clearly how many patients were started in the study.

An NNT has a confidence interval (see below) around it. The calculations for this are at the end of the chapter. For the example of readmission, the 95% confidence interval is 3 to 19. So we may only need to treat three patients or may need to treat 19 patients to prevent one patient not needing readmission. It is easier to put the numbers into software to calculate this.

They can be found on the web by entering the searching for 'NNT calculator'.

A word of caution and encouragement. It is not easy to deal with all the arithmetic and it can easily become confusing. It is not the arithmetic that is difficult. It is identifying the correct information to take from the paper. Papers are still not written consistently and this makes it confusing when trying to identify for instance the numbers of patients that benefited from treatment compared with those who did not. Yet you would think that this was the essence of the article and so necessarily should be obvious to the reader. The most frequent confusing factors are identifying how many patients the authors are talking about.

FURTHER ISSUES ON NUMBERS NEEDED TO TREAT

The NNT calculation is being used more and more as a method of assessing clinical effectiveness but still has drawbacks that you should be aware of. Assuming the quality of the research that generated the NNT is good and that the calculations are appropriate, what other problems exist?

Time of follow-up is critical to your evaluation of the effectiveness of treatment. The study for heart failure readmission described a follow-up period of 12 months. What would have happened if you had followed the study for only 6 months or for 36 months? It would be useful to know that the longer you treated the patients the more benefit you gained as in Figure 14.1.

With the passage of time the absolute risk increases. Depending on what happens to the ratio between the placebo or control group and the treatment group, the NNT may also change with time. Where then do you draw the line for a study? Perhaps over five years a treatment may have a significantly worse effect than that seen at two years.

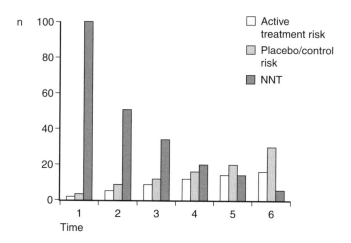

Figure 14.1 NNT and actual risk over time

NNTs are expressed in whole numbers. These numbers can hide a lot of evidence about a treatment. If the NNT was 10 and you were deciding to treat 100 people, does that mean that 90 people will gain no benefit from the treatment? If you are looking at survival then that may be the case. However, if you are looking at the relief of depression, then the answer may be very different. The calculation of the NNT may have used a predetermined threshold for a depression rating score to define depression. The way that these work is that people complete a questionnaire which is scored. This then gives a number above which one may be classed as 'depressed'. The NNT will be useful in determining how many people treated will fall below the threshold. It will not, however, tell you how many people moved towards normal.

In the treatment of high blood pressure there are several groups of drugs that act in quite different ways. These drugs have been compared: drug A will lower blood pressure in a lot of people, whereas drug B may produce the largest fall in blood pressure – but in a smaller number of patients than those receiving drug A. The NNT will only tell you how many achieved a pre-determined improvement, not the total number of people who gained any improvement.

NUMBERS NEEDED TO HARM

Similar equations can be used to identify the number of patients needed to produce harmful side-effects from treatment. An example of the need for numbers needed to harm was demonstrated a few years ago. A well-conducted study demonstrated that the risk of developing a deep-vein thrombosis (DVT) in the leg while on the oral contraceptive pill was increased in women using more recently developed pills compared with women taking pills developed earlier.

Newspaper articles described this risk as double and the result was that there was a 'pill scare'. This caused anxiety and fear in many women to the extent that there was a rise in unwanted pregnancies brought about by women stopping taking the pill without using an alternative contraceptive.

The risk of developing a DVT on the older pill was 1 per 200 000 years of oral contraceptive use (1:200 000), while the risk on the newer pills was 1:100 000.

The relative risk of developing a DVT on the newer pill was therefore:

$$\frac{1/100,000}{1/200,000} = \frac{0.00001}{0.000005} = 2$$

So the risk was double. The Department of Health was correct in alerting the public that certain pills double your risk – or were they?

The absolute increase in risk (ARR) was $0.00001 - 0.000005 = 0.000005$. The reciprocal of this is: $1/0.000005 = 200,000$. This indicates that if you treated 200 000 women for 1 year with newer oral contraceptives, you might expect one additional case of deep-vein thrombosis. This information presented at the same time might have had a less-alarming impact on the population.

INTENTION TO TREAT

This raises the issue of 'intention to treat'. How do we know a drug is going to be suitable for all patients? An analysis of the clinical effectiveness of a drug can be applied in several ways. The first is an 'intention-to-treat' analysis. In this method all patients started on the drug are considered as having taken the drug. Those who stopped because of side-effects or did not finish treatment for other reasons are then included in the analysis as treatment failures. In comparison, some analyses will only examine those patients who completed treatment regimens. The latter form of analysis is likely to show a larger benefit of the treatment than the first method. It is important to examine the results section of the article to identify which type of analysis is presented.

There are three major lines of justification for intention-to-treat analysis.

1. Intention-to-treat simplifies the task of dealing with suspicious outcomes. If there is an event that seems unrelated to the trial, e.g. if a patient dies in a motor accident in an intention-to-treat analysis that death is still counted. This may sound bizarre but it does avoid a committee-like structure deciding which death (or event) to include in the analysis.
2. Intention-to-treat reflects the way treatments will perform in the population by ignoring concordance or compliance when the data are analysed. It gives one a reflection of what would happen in the real patients.
3. Intention-to-treat preserves the baseline treatment groups achieved by randomisation. If one starts to eliminate those patients who drop out of the study then the randomisation process is lost – and one is not sure whether the difference you may see is a result of your manipulation of the data after the trial.

What now follows is some explanation to some of the statistics that you may want to know about. I have tried to stick mainly to the principles of the various statistics seen in articles discussing therapy. This next section is heavily mathematical so if you do not want to read this section why not move on to the next chapter. It does not include any material required for understanding the rest of the book.

CONFIDENCE INTERVALS

Confidence interval is a way of describing the boundaries between which one is confident that the true measure lies with a given level of certainty. It reflects both the number of observations and the amount by which each variation differs from the mean. For example, to estimate the mean systolic blood pressure of a general practice adult population, we may take the blood pressure of a random sample of patients, and find that the mean pressure is 136.2 mmHg (95%CI 134.1-138.4).

The calculation of confidence intervals is usually based on the assumption that the variable (factor being measured) is normally distributed in the population. The normal distribution curve is essential to much of statistical reasoning.

The normal distribution around a mean (normal curve) was described by Gauss and so is also known as the Gaussian distribution. This curve is symmetrical so that the mean and median (central point of distribution with equal numbers of observations on either side) are the same. The mean is usually labelled μ pronounced 'mew'.

The next characteristic of the normal distribution is the width of the distribution from the mean. This spread is described using the term 'standard deviation' labelled σ (sigma). It is calculated by working out the difference of each measurement from the mean, squaring these differences, dividing the sum of these squared differences by the number of observations, and finally taking the square root:

$$\sigma = \sqrt{\frac{(x - \mu)^2}{n - 1}}$$

where x is the individual observation. (Not a very intuitive calculation!)

As a result of the mathematical proportions of the normal curve, it was established that the probability of an observation falling within one standard deviation is 68%, and within two standard deviations 95%. Few physical, biological or social phenomena are entirely normally distributed. However, with more than 100 observations, unless the distributions are very odd, this becomes less important in terms of subsequent analysis.

Blood pressure is one of the commonest physiological measurements. This graph shown in Figure 14.2 describes the distribution of blood pressure from a cohort of patients in Oxfordshire recruited at random from general practice.

It shows the normal distribution (line) with the actual distribution behind as a histogram. There were 448 observations. The mean was 136.2, the median 133, the standard deviation 23.5. This means that there was a 68% probability

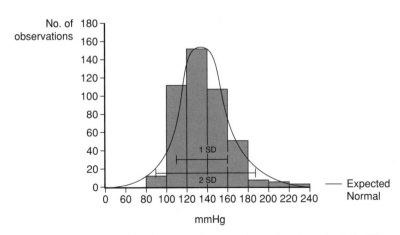

Figure 14.2 Distribution of blood pressure from a cohort of patients in Oxfordshire recruited at random from general practice

of one of these individuals having a blood pressure between 113 and 160 mmHg. In this group of people, 312 (69%) actually had a blood pressure within that range. Similarly, the number of people whose blood pressure was between 89 mmHg and 183 mmHg was 432 (96%). The standard deviation then represents the scatter of the distribution of the individuals' blood pressure. The calculation of a confidence interval represents the likelihood of this mean representing the truth. The more patients the study has, the less wide are the confidence intervals. It also includes within its formula the standard deviation so also reflects the scatter of readings.

In studies looking at the effect of a treatment, the results may then contain two means: the measurement on placebo (control) and the measurement on experimental treatment. Each may have a confidence interval in the form of a table or be represented graphically. If the confidence intervals overlap, then you cannot be sure that the difference observed did not occur through chance. More formally, you would usually test whether or not the two means were significantly different from each other by calculating the 95% confidence interval around the difference between the means. If this confidence interval included 0, then you would conclude that the observed difference between the two means might have arisen as a result of chance.

In the blood pressure study the mean of systolic blood pressure in males was 142.3 (95%CI 139.4-145.3), and in females 129.4 mmHg (95%CI 126.4-132.4). The means seem very different and the upper level of the confidence interval for females (132.4) is lower than the lower level of the confidence interval for males (139.4), indicating that the difference is likely to be real.

In statistical terms one needs to identify the difference (142.3-129.4 = 12.9) and then determine the confidence interval of the difference using software such as Confidence Interval Analysis (Altman et al 2000).

An NNT has a confidence interval around it. The calculations for this are at the end of the chapter. For the example of readmission the 95% Confidence Interval is 3.3 to 20.2. So we may only need to treat three patients or may need to treat 20 patients to see one patient not need readmission.

RELATIVE RISK AND ODDS RATIO

What is the difference between relative risk and odds ratio? The answer comes in two parts. You can only calculate the relative risk if you know the baseline or control risk. In a prospective cohort study looking at the effect of smoking it is possible to compare the risk of the patients who smoke compared with the risk of the non-smokers as shown above. However, prospective cohort studies are expensive and time-consuming. It may also involve ethical problems (as in the vaccination example in Chapter 8) to randomly allocate to vaccine or non-vaccine groups for a large trial. If you had performed a case-control study as shown in Chapter 8, then your comparison population is not the real population but a matched control group.

From Table 8.1 one is unable to calculate the risk of becoming a case in the overall population whether they were vaccinated or not as the study did not measure a population but selected matched controls. The odds of someone having a disease are the number having the disease divided by the number not having the disease. For example 25 out of 100 people have a heart attack; therefore, 75 people do not have a heart attack. The odds of having a heart attack in this group of 100 people are $25/75 = 0.33$.

The risk is the number having the event divided by the total population. 25 out of 100 people have a heart attack, therefore 75 people do not have a heart attack. The risk of having a heart attack is $25/100 = 0.25$ or 25% As you can see, there is a difference between 0.33 and 25%. When the numbers of the case study get larger, what happens? Twenty-five out of 1000 people have a heart attack, 975 people do not have a heart attack. The odds now are $25/975 = 0.026$ and the risk is $25/1000 = 0.025$. As the event becomes rarer, the odds and the risk become similar.

The point is that in large, well-performed case-control studies the odds ratio is similar in meaning to the relative risk. Therefore, if the odds ratio is 3, then you are three times more likely to suffer the event if you have been exposed compared with those who have not been exposed ('exposed' is used to describe not only such things as drugs but also environmental hazards). Similarly, if the relative risk is 3, then you are again three times more likely to suffer. So you can use both odds ratios and relative risk to mean the same thing and, most of the time for practical purposes, think of them as very similar, but they are calculated differently. So beware.

P VALUES

This book is not a statistics textbook (and I use a selection of books as I need several explanations usually). It is appropriate to mention the importance of statistical significance in research generally. Box 14.2 lists some questions to ask when looking at the statistics of a paper.

This checklist will help when checking the statistical quality of the study. There are many things that can go wrong in research, from having too few patients to studying the wrong outcome measure. P values are often reported as proof of statistical significance. A convention of stating that P is less than a value of 0.05 has been developed. Why is this the case?

We all have some understanding of probability. A colleague starts tossing

---

Box 14.2 Guidelines for assessing statistics

1. How many patients? (Were there >100 patients?)
2. Was the distribution of the feature normal?
3. What was the size of the effect?
4. Could this have happened by chance?
5. Was $p < 0.05$ or were the confidence intervals separated?

Table 14.3 Probability of 'heads' being the result of a coin tossed repeatedly

Throw	Chance of heads	Cumulative chance of heads	Probability
1	1 in 2	1/2	50%
2	1 in 2	1/4	25%
3	1 in 2	1/8	12.5%
4	1 in 2	1/16	6.25%
5	1 in 2	1/32	3.125%

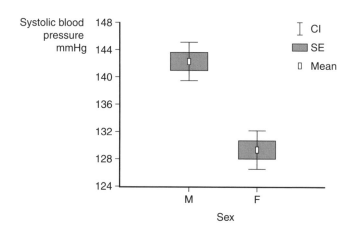

Figure 14.3 Box and whisker plot

a coin repeatedly and it comes up heads every time. At some stage in this process you will start to believe that this result is not just due to chance. If I tossed a coin now and it was heads that would be no surprise. If I do this again and it is still heads you might say 'just chance'. I do it a third time and it is still heads, 'a bit lucky'. I do it a fourth time and it comes down heads. By now, you may say that this is a bit unusual. I do it a fifth time and it is still heads. Do you suspect that something else is going on? Perhaps I am cheating? What this is demonstrating is that we accept things happening by chance until a certain level and then start to suspect that it is not just chance. In most audiences this emergence of disbelief that it is only due to chance appears after the fifth time that the coin is spun and comes up heads. What is happening in this process?

The chance of it being heads on each successive throw is shown in Table 14.3.

It has been demonstrated that when a chance occurrence is expressed in this way we start to disbelieve the phenomenon is purely due to chance at the

5% level of probability. This rather vague reason for choosing 0.05 seems very 'unscientific' but, at the same time, is very reassuring to non-statisticians that such an important feature of so many research papers should be based on the concept that this is what we as humans are 'comfortable' with.

When a difference or variation between two measurements occurs we can then describe that difference as being unlikely to have happened by chance. The converse of that is that the difference was due to the mechanism of other factors involved in the study. What it does not prove is that the factors reported by the investigators as being the cause of the variability are necessarily the major cause of that variability; that is, it still might be due to a bias, as opposed to a treatment effect.

The P level is the probability of the difference occurring purely by chance. In other words, if P is greater than 5% (0.05), then intuitively we may believe that the difference observed may have occurred by chance and not as a result of the intervention.

Another way of displaying this might be a 'box and whisker plot', showing the standard error as a box and the confidence interval as a line from top to bottom with the mean in between (Figure 14.3).

Which is best? P values or confidence intervals? P values do not give information about the size of the difference between the study groups (Gardner and Altman 1986). Both, however, give useful information and authors are now asked to provide both when submitting papers to many journals.

SAMPLE SIZE

The numbers of patients is important in determining the power of a study. Too few patients can lead to two sorts of problems. First, the intervention is shown to be effective when in reality it is not (type I error). One protects against this sort of error by calculating the P value for the results. If the P value is less than 0.05, there is a less than 5% chance that this error has occurred. With small studies, one is less likely to obtain such a P value unless the size of the difference is very large. Second, the study may show the treatment not to be effective when in reality it is (type II error). The larger the sample size, the less likely it is that this error will occur. The methods section of a paper may often specify the risk of committing a type II error. A level of 0.20 for Beta is considered adequate. In other words, this would give a 1 in 5 chance of missing a true difference. The statistical power (1-Beta, usually 80%), the Alpha level (0.05, P value) and the difference in outcome (the difference between the two means) are all included in the equation that predicts sample size (Box 14.3).

CONFIDENCE INTERVALS FOR NUMBERS NEEDED TO TREAT

There are several methods for doing this. The first I use is software from the Centre for Evidence-Based Medicine http://www.cebm.net/toolbox.asp called Dan Tandberg's confidence interval calculator. If that is not available

---

Box 14.3 Sample size calculation

Prior to using this you must specify the alpha level (usually 0.05 or 5%) and the statistical power, usually 80% (a beta level of 20%).
The equation for a sample size for a comparison of two proportions is:

$$n = \left[\frac{Z_\alpha \sqrt{2\pi_c(1 - \pi_c)} - Z_\beta \sqrt{\pi_t(1 - \pi_t) + \pi_c(1 - \pi_c)}}{\pi_t - \pi_c} \right]^2$$

where n is the number of patients for each treatment group.
Z_α = alpha level
Z_β = power
π_c = control group proportion developing disease
π_t = treatment group proportion developing disease

To compare the means from two populations based on a sample of n individuals from each population:

$$n = 2 \left[\frac{(Z_\alpha - Z_\beta)\sigma}{(\mu_1 - \mu_2)} \right]^2$$

σ = standard deviation of the variable of interest
μ = means of the two populations.

---

this is another method.

First, you calculate the absolute risk of having the undesired outcome (i.e. death) in the group of patients (N^C) taking a placebo (CER) and in those patients (N^E) having the treatment (EER). Next, you must use some arithmetic. The following equation will calculate the standard error (SE) of the absolute risk reduction:

$$SE(ARR) = 1.96 \times \left(\sqrt{\frac{CER \times (1 - CER)}{N^C} + \frac{EER \times (1 - EER)}{N^E}} \right)$$

This standard error is then subtracted and added to the ARR to give limits of standard error on either side of the ARR:

+ve SE = ARR + SE(ARR)

-ve SE = ARR − SE(ARR)

The confidence limits of the NNT are then the reciprocals of the +ve and -ve SEs.

An example may make this clearer. In the heart failure readmission prevention study the data is as follows:

CER = 32.1 , EER = 14.3

N^C = 81 , N^E = 84

$$SE(ARR) = 1.96 \times \left(\sqrt{\frac{0.321 \times (1 - 0.321)}{81} + \frac{0.143 \times (1 - 0.143)}{84}} \right)$$

= 0.126

ARR = 0.321 - 0.143 = 0.178

+ve SE = 0.178 + 0.126 = 0.304

-ve SE = 0.178 - 0.126 = 0.052

NNT = 1/ARR = 6

95% Confidence Limits = 1/0.178 = 3 and 1/0.052 = 19

The NNT can be expressed as 6 (95%CI = 3-19). Most confidence intervals have an equal amount of variation between the upper and lower levels. For example, you would have an upper confidence limit of 10 and a lower limit of 6 around a finding of 8, that is 8 (95%CI = 6-10). There is an equal distance between 8 and 10 as there is between 8 and 6. However, in confidence intervals around NNT this is not the case, because we are really calculating CIs around the ARR and then producing a reciprocal (dividing 1 by the amount). This leads to an unequal distribution.

SUMMARY

After reading all this you may be quite anxious about trying the calculations yourself. However, like most things in health care with practice and familiarity, they will become easier. The appraisal of a paper describing a therapeutic benefit can appear daunting. The arithmetic is the easy bit. Really! The hard part is getting the numbers out of the paper. So often authors use double negatives or obscure terms when describing the results. You have to search within the tables for the nuggets of information. Papers written more recently are likely to be slightly easier to appraise with information more clearly displayed.

The answer is to practise. Check your results with others. And do not be afraid to have a go. For practice, why not try articles that have been reviewed by Evidence-Based Medicine as this journal publishes the NNTs with confidence intervals.

WORKED EXAMPLES

Worked example 14.1

An article fulfils the quality checklist. You decide to work out from the data presented to calculate the NNT.
The results section states 'the proportion of children cured clinically at 1 week was 55% in the experimental group and 13% in the control.'
Work out what the NNT is to 'clinically cure' one child.

Worked example 14.2

A second article has a statement in the abstract '28 of the 260 patients on the new regime had a heart attack year compared with 48 of the 254 patients on the standard therapy'.
What is the NNT?
Try doing this yourself now before looking at the answer.

Worked example 14.3

You hear of an interesting article about duct tape for common warts (Focht et al 2002).
Of the 51 patients completing the study, 26 (51%) were treated with duct tape, and 25 (49%) were treated with cryotherapy. Twenty-two patients (85%) in the duct tape arm vs 15 patients (60%) enrolled in the cryotherapy arm had complete resolution of their warts ($P = 0.05$ by χ^2 analysis). The majority of warts that responded to either therapy did so within 1 month of treatment.
What are the NNTs and then calculate the 95% confidence interval?

ANSWERS

Worked example 14.1

This is how I approached it.
The EER was 55% and CER was 13%. The difference between the two is 42%. Roughly 100 divided by 42 is a little bit greater than 2. Therefore the NNT is about 2.

Worked example 14.2

Twenty-eight divided by 260 is 10.7% and 48 divided by 254 is 18.8%, so the ARR is 18.8 minus 10.7 = 8.1%. The NNT is therefore about 10 (I try to do the sums in my head initially and I rounded 8.1 up to 10 to make it easier so an ARR of 20% is 5, 50% is 2 etc.).

From the proper calculation the NNT is 12. The confidence interval using the calculator from the website (http://www.cebm.net/toolbox.asp) is 7 to 50.

Worked example 14.3

If we believe the percentages in the abstract the ARR is 60%-85% = minus 25% (CER-EER). The control is cryotherapy and the experimental is duct tape. This is actually a beneficial effect so the NNT is negative but don't worry.

The reason for this is that the CER is 60% had resolution compared with 85% in the experimental (duct tape) group. Now it does not matter really which way you do this – whether you subtract 60 from 85 or 85 from 60. The difference will be either minus 25% or plus 25% and the NNT will be minus 4 or plus 4. You have to put NNTs into a sentence for them to make sense, i.e. you need to treat four patients with duct tape compared with normal treatment of cryotherapy to cure one child of warts (over the period of time of the trial).

I put the figures into the calculator and came up with the 95% confidence interval of 2 to 4200. This illustrates clearly how the low numbers lead to some potentially misleading conclusions. You need to calculate not only the NNT but also the confidence interval. Notice how the P value in the abstract was significant, yet the confidence interval is very wide!

References

Altman D, Machin D et al. 2000 Statistics with confidence. British Medical Journal books

Anderson K M, Odell P M et al. 1991 Cardiovascular disease risk profiles. American Heart Journal 121(1 Pt 2):293-298

Beecher H 1950 The powerful placebo. Journal of the American Medical Association 159:1602-1606

Blue L, Lang E et al. 2001 Randomised controlled trial of specialist nurse intervention in heart failure. British Medical Journal 323(7315):715-718

Editorial 1972 Drug or placebo? Lancet 2(7768):122-123

Fibrinolytic Therapy Trialists' (FTT) Collaborative Group 1994 Indications for fibrinolytic therapy in suspected acute myocardial infarction: collaborative overview of early mortality and major morbidity results from all randomised trials of more than 1000 patients. Fibrinolytic Therapy Trialists' (FTT) Collaborative Group [published erratum appears in Lancet 1994 Mar 19;343(8899):742] [see comments]. Lancet 343(8893): 311-322

Focht D R, Spicer V et al. 2002 The efficacy of duct tape vs cryotherapy in the treatment of verruca vulgaris (the common wart). Archives of Paediatrics and Adolescent Medicine 156(10):971-974

Gardner M J, Altman D G 1986 Confidence intervals rather than P values: estimation rather than hypothesis testing. British Medical Journal Clinical Research Edition 292(6522):746-750

Midgette A S, O'Connor G T et al. 1990 Effect of intravenous streptokinase on early mortality in patients with suspected acute myocardial infarction. A meta-analysis by anatomic location of infarction. Annals of Internal Medicine 113(12):961-968

Chapter 15

Is the intervention cost-effective?

Alastair Gray

CHAPTER CONTENTS

INTRODUCTION

In Chapter 10 we set out some guidelines for good practice in economic evaluation. But why do we have to consider cost-effectiveness in the first place? And how can we use the results of economic evaluations in evidence-based practice? Until recently, the movement to improve the evidence base of medical practice has put the major emphasis on establishing the effectiveness of interventions: broadly, to ask whether there is evidence that an intervention is better than nothing, and if so, how effective it is and how it compares with alternatives. These are fundamental questions, but knowing that an intervention is effective, or even knowing that it is more effective than any alternative, is not a sufficient basis on which to provide that intervention. Already the availability of effective interventions far exceeds our capacity to purchase them all, and the technological frontier of medical science is constantly being pushed outwards, in turn pushing the potential cost upwards.

In the UK, the proportion of total national income devoted to health care has grown steadily from 4.5% in 1970 to 7.3% in 2000, and real expenditure per person per year (in 1995 £s) has risen from £339 to £1004 over the same period, yet choosing what should and should not be provided has not become any less painful. Similarly, countries which devote higher shares of national income to their health care systems, such as Germany (10.6 %) or the USA (13%) also remain locked in debate over priorities, cost-control and value for money.

These problems are very familiar to economists. Indeed, from an economic perspective health care is not fundamentally different from any other service. We live in a world of scarcity – scarce time, scarce space, scarce knowledge and skills – and, therefore, must constantly make choices about alternative courses of action. Individually, should we have the exterior of the house repainted, or put it off another year and put the money towards a summer holiday? Collectively, should we increase spending on schools or on the health service? Professionally, should we appoint another orthopaedic surgeon or expand the domiciliary chiropody service? If funding for elective surgery is suddenly reduced by 20%, who should be removed from the operating lists first? In all of these situations, we have to make a choice, which involves some comparison of the relative costs and benefits of the alternatives. By adopting the framework of economic evaluation, all we are really doing is making this comparison more explicit. Of course, explicitness can be uncomfortable and even threatening. But the advantages of explicitness over hunch and guesswork are: (a) all the relevant alternatives can be identified; (b) the viewpoint or perspective from which the choice has been made has to be stated; and (c) some attempt can be made to recognise and measure the uncertainty surrounding the choice (Eddy 1992).

So the starting point for health economics is that we have to make difficult choices concerning health care resources, and that an explicit weighing of costs and benefits surrounding these choices can lead to a better outcome, in which more health gain is obtained with the available resources.

THE COST-EFFECTIVENESS PLANE

One way of thinking about these choices in health care is by means of a simple diagram called the 'cost-effectiveness plane', which is shown in Figure 15.1.

Imagine that we wish to compare therapy A, a new drug therapy for dyslipidemia, with therapy B (the existing therapy). Along the horizontal axis we can measure whether the new therapy is more or less effective than the existing therapy, and up and down the vertical axis we can measure whether it is more or less costly. Now clearly we need to have accurate information on costs and on effectiveness in order to locate our new therapy on this diagram, a point we will return to below. But let us assume for the present that we have this information, and that the new therapy turns out to be more effective than the old therapy and less costly. It will be in Quadrant II, and we can safely assume that it will be accepted over the existing therapy: it 'dominates' the existing therapy. Conversely, if the new therapy turns out to be less effective and more expensive – Quadrant IV – it will be rejected.

Now let us imagine that the new therapy is a lot more effective and just a little bit more costly: say at point A in Quadrant I. Probably this will still be acceptable, as offering a major health gain for relatively low additional cost. But suppose the new therapy is only fractionally more effective than the existing therapy and is very much more costly: for example at point B in

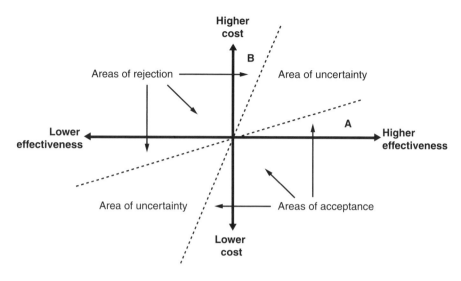

Figure 15.1 The cost-effectiveness plane (adapted from van Houtet et al 1994)

Quadrant I. Now the balance has probably tipped against the new therapy and it is adjudged to be too expensive in relation to the benefits it offers.

So at what point does acceptability turn to uncertainty and then into rejection? That will depend on many things, including the total resources available and alternative uses of those resources for other health care interventions. For example, we can easily imagine that a new therapy which is known to be more effective than the existing alternative and also more costly, could be well under the line of acceptability in the USA, in the uncertainty zone in the UK and well into the rejection zone in sub-Saharan Africa. So the judgement we reach will depend on the relative effectiveness and costs of the therapy compared with the existing alternative, but also on the resources available.

The simple but powerful logic underlying Figure 15.1 is in essence the cost-effectiveness approach. In fact the cost-effectiveness ratio is simply the slope or gradient of a line from the origin to any point in Figure 15.1. This slope is the ratio of cost to effectiveness, and cost-effectiveness can be defined as the ratio of the net difference in costs between two therapies to the net difference in effectiveness. Of course, there are many conceptual and empirical difficulties involved in this approach, but it is important to keep hold of the essential simplicity. If we can systematically measure and compare the costs and the effectiveness of health interventions, in principle, we can maximise health gain by selecting those which are most cost-effective, then the second best, then the third best, until our budget is exhausted. Any other approach will result in less health gain.

COST-EFFECTIVENESS: AN EXAMPLE

To illustrate the cost-effectiveness approach let us take a recently published economic evaluation and look at it from the point of view of the checklist we set out in Chapter 10.

A. The framework

1. The type of analysis being performed should be clearly stated and justified
2. The background of the problem being addressed, and the general design of the programme under investigation, including the target population, should be stated
3. The comparator programme should be described
4. The perspective and time horizon of the study should be stated

A number of large trials over the last 10 years have provided convincing evidence that drug therapy to lower cholesterol is effective in reducing fatal and non-fatal coronary events. One such trial, the Scandinavian Simvastatin Survival Study (4S), showed that lowering cholesterol levels with simvastatin reduces mortality and morbidity. These results were obtained in a treatment population consisting of men and women at various ages from 35 to 70 years with angina pectoris or previous acute myocardial infarction and with total cholesterol levels before treatment of between 213 and 309 mg per decilitre (4S, 1994).

However, the premise of health economics is that evidence of effectiveness is not sufficient reason to advocate the widespread use of cholesterol-lowering drugs in such patients. The cost per patient per year of such therapy would typically be around £540, and it is possible that up to 8% of all men and women aged 35-70 would fit the eligibility criteria of such trials. Treating everyone who might benefit would, therefore, be very costly: in fact, it could represent more than 20% of the existing total drug budget. So before widespread use is recommended, the cost-effectiveness of cholesterol-lowering therapy should be demonstrated.

A search of the literature would identify a large number of published cost-effectiveness analyses of cholesterol lowering therapy. But most of these are simulations or modeling exercises based on cost and effectiveness data taken from a wide range of different sources. However, an economic evaluation was performed alongside the 4S study, and used cost and effectiveness information from that trial to estimate the cost-effectiveness of simvastatin treatment, defined as the cost per year of life gained with simvastatin therapy compared with placebo (quality of life was not considered) (Johanneson et al 1997).

The perspective adopted by this study included health care system costs and the lost production costs arising from morbidity from coronary causes. The trial had a follow-up period of five years, but from an economic perspective this was not an adequate time horizon, as the differences in survival detected after five years might be expected to continue into the future. So increased life expectancy beyond the end of the trial was extrapolated from the information produced within the follow-up period on survival. Note that it is common to have to combine trial results with some modeling in this way, especially if the main outcome is survival (Buxton et al 1997).

B. Data and methods

5. All resources of interest in the analysis should be clearly identified, measured and valued
6. All outcomes of interest in the analysis should be clearly identified, measured and valued
7. Methods of obtaining estimates of effectiveness, costs and quality of life valuations, and the sources of information, should be given

The resources of interest were the drug itself, plus the treatment of coronary events, plus the time off work of patients as a result of a coronary event. The cost of the drug was the official retail price, the cost of health care resources was based on data from four hospitals with detailed accounting procedures, and the cost of time off work was based on average earnings of full-time workers. As noted above, the outcome was defined in terms of life years gained, and the data for outcomes and resource use were taken directly from the 4444 patients in the trial.

C. Results

8. The base case results in terms of costs, effectiveness, and incremental cost-effectiveness ratios, and the uncertainty surrounding these, should be clearly set out

Table 15.1 summarises the main results of the study. It can be seen that the authors show the cost, years of life gained and then the cost-effectiveness ratio, and not just the ratio itself. They also show separate results for men and women, and separate results for health care costs alone and when including work time lost. Thus for men the cost of the intervention (i.e. the drug and monitoring cost) would be $2242, but this would be offset by $718 in savings from reduced morbidity, so the net cost would be $1524. On average the gain in life expectancy would be 0.28 years, or just over 3 months, so that the cost per life year gained would be $1524/0.28 = $5400. Adding in the savings resulting from less time off work, the net cost falls to $459 and so the cost-effectiveness ratio falls to $1600 per life year gained. The authors also present results for different age groups, and for patients with different pre-treatment cholesterol levels.

Finally, the authors present the results of a sensitivity analysis, in which different base case assumptions and values are altered to assess their effect on the results. This analysis has been presented graphically here in Figure 15.2, with the base case being a 59-year-old woman with a cost per life year gained of $10 500. Thus, when the reduction in risk obtained from the therapy is set

Table 15.1 Cost effectiveness of simvastatin treatment for 5 years in 59-year-old patients with coronary heart disease and a pre-treatment total cholesterol level of 261 mg per decilitre

Variable	Analysis of direct costs only		Analysis of direct costs and production losses	
	Men	Women	Men	Women
Costs ($)				
Intervention	2,242	2,410	2,242	2,410
Associated morbidity	-718	-725	-1,783	-1,601
Net	1,524	1,685	459	809
Years of life gained	0.28	0.16	0.28	0.16
Cost per year of life gained ($)	5,400	10,500	1,600	5,100

Data from Johannesson et al. (1997)

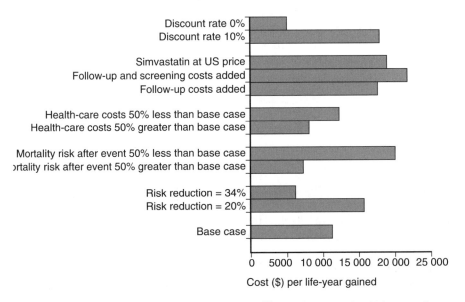

Figure 15.2 Example of a sensitivity analysis cost ($) per life-year gained, simvastatin treatment for 5 years in a 59-year-old woman with coronary heart disease and a pre-treatment total cholesterol level of 261 mg/dl

at 20%, the cost-effectiveness rises to $15 300, and when the reduction in risk is set at 34% the cost-effectiveness ratio falls to $7300. Such a sensitivity analysis allows the decision-maker to assess the robustness of the results.

9. The results should be placed in the context of other relevant economic evaluations

In discussing their results, the analysts cited four other cost-effectiveness studies published in the previous seven years, in the areas of hormone replacement therapy, screening for hypertension and cholesterol-lowering.

D. Discussion

10.   The relevance of the study for policy questions, and any ethical or distributive implications should be discussed

Based on their analysis, the authors conclude that 'the estimated cost-effectiveness ratios were well within the range that was considered cost-effective in other studies'; therefore, in patients with coronary heart disease, simvastatin therapy is cost-effective for both men and women at the ages and cholesterol levels studied.

Comments on the cost–effectiveness example

To consider this study carefully against the checklist, you would of course have to read the original article in detail. However, it should be fairly clear from the information given above that this is a well-conducted study which in most respects passes the checklist points. There are some points which you may have noticed:

- Some aspects of cost, such as costs incurred by patients in attending clinics etc. were not included. You may judge that these were unlikely to be important in this instance; but in some studies they could be significant.

- Outcome was measured in terms of survival only, and did not include quality of life. This was justified in the article on the grounds that valid weights or valuations for the health states in the study did not exist, but if quality of life was not very good (and remember all patients in this trial had a history of heart disease), then the quality-adjusted life years added by therapy could be significantly less than the life years added. Conversely, if the intervention significantly reduced the number of non-fatal events, such as angina or myocardial infarctions) as well as fatal events, and if these non-fatal events had a serious effect on quality of life, then measuring the effect only in terms of survival would tend to understate the benefits of the intervention.

- The costs reported in the article are the average costs prevailing at present. However, often in economic studies we are interested in the effect of a change at the margin, such as reducing length of stay by one day, treating more patients with cholesterol-lowering therapy, or extending a dental surgery's opening hours by three hours per week. The cost of these changes is the marginal cost, which can be defined as the change in total cost divided by the change in total output or quantity.

Suppose a dental practice was currently open from 9 a.m. until 5 p.m. with total running costs for the premises of £75 000 and total visits of 25 000 annually. Hence the average cost per visit for the premises is £3. Suppose it is now decided to extend surgery hours on two nights per week. The total cost goes up to £82 000 and the total number of visits goes up to 26 000, so the average cost has only increased fractionally to £3.08 per visit (80 000/26 000). However, if we consider the marginal cost, an additional 1000 visits are costing an additional £7000 per year, so in fact the marginal cost per visit is £7, very much more than the average cost. Indeed the difference between the average and marginal cost is so great that the practice may decide to review the decision to extend opening hours! Note, however, that marginal costs may also be lower than the average cost.

- Marginal cost refers to the consequences of expanding or contracting the size of a specific service or activity: more opening hours in a surgery, fewer beds in a ward, and so on. But often the decision is whether to expand the whole scope or coverage of a programme, for example from breast cancer screening for those aged 60 and over to breast cancer screening for those aged 50 and over. The change in cost that occurs when this happens is referred to as the incremental cost, and so the change in cost in relation to the change in outcome of such a change would be called the incremental cost-effectiveness ratio (ICER). The results are correctly reported in the article as the incremental cost-effectiveness ratio, that is, the additional costs and effectiveness compared with placebo therapy. However, a decision-maker may wish to consider other increments of therapy. For example, patients could be treated at different doses, each with different cost and effectiveness combinations.

Figure 15.3 shows some results from a different cost-effectiveness analysis of cholesterol-lowering therapy, where patients can be treated at 20 mg, 40 mg or 80 mg per day. To treat a cohort of 65-74 year old men with a 20 mg dose would have a lifetime cost of $3.6 billion, and would save a total of 348 000 life-years, giving a cost of $10 400 per life year saved. On the figure the life-years gained are plotted along the X-axis, the cost along the Y-axis, and the slope of the line to that point is the cost-effectiveness ratio of $10 400. Now increasing the dose to 40 mg would alter the total cost and the total effectiveness, so that the cost per life-year saved compared with placebo would rise to $14 800 (the line from the origin to the 40 mg point), and further increasing the dose to 80 mg would change the cost-effectiveness ratio to $25 800 per life-year saved compared with placebo. However, in order to treat someone with 40 mg it is necessary to go through treatment at 20 mg per day. Consequently, the comparison should not really be between 40 mg and 0, but between 40 mg and 20 mg: the incremental cost-effectiveness or change in costs as a ratio of the change in effectiveness of moving from 20 mg to 40 mg.

When we plot this line on the figure we get a somewhat different picture. The incremental cost per life-year gained of 40 mg is actually $26 650, and at the

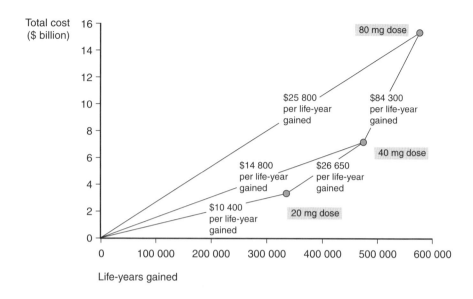

Figure 15.3 Incremental cost-effectiveness: cost ($) per life-year gained for 3 doses of cholesterol-lowering therapy (data from Goldman et al. 1991)

80 mg dose reaches $84 300 per life-year saved compared with the 40 mg dose, which appears poorer value for money. So the incremental cost-effectiveness ratio is always the appropriate basis for decision-making. The 4S study cannot be criticised for not reporting such information as the trial was not designed to identify differences between doses. However, the decision-maker may still want such information.

- In reporting their results, the authors of the 4S economic evaluation gave the actual cost and effect differences as well as the cost-effectiveness ratios, but they did not report the overall magnitude of costs in relation to the size of the eligible population. There will always be a budget constraint, and so the total cost of an intervention as well as the cost-effectiveness will always be an important piece of information.
- In looking at the sensitivity of the results to the values and assumptions used in the base case analyses, the analysts considered a number of different variables.

However, this was a one-way analysis in which each variable was altered independently whilst the others were held constant. An alternative might have been multi-way analyses in which several variables were changed simultaneously.

Figure 15.4 shows how uncertainty can affect the results of cost-effectiveness studies. In case A, the black lines represent the uncertainty

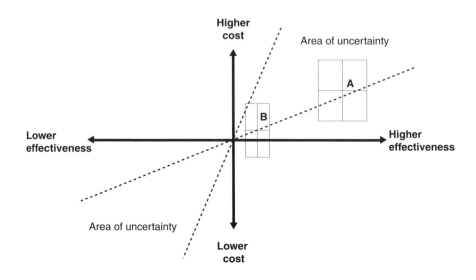

Figure 15.4 Uncertainty on the cost-effectiveness plane

surrounding effectiveness and cost, and so the box is an approximation of the area of uncertainty (in fact, a true representation of the joint uncertainty surrounding costs and effects would be elliptical). In this case, the therapy is definitely more costly and more effective than the comparator – that is, it is completely within Quadrant I of the figure, but a decision-maker could not be certain that it was within the area of acceptability. In case B, the intervention is clearly more effective than the comparator, but there is considerable uncertainty as to whether the costs are higher or lower. Consequently, the intervention could be in the area of acceptability, uncertainty or rejection.

- In reaching a conclusion about the cost-effectiveness of simvastatin, the authors refer to four other studies. This is a standard procedure, and in this case there is no reason to think that the other studies chosen were unrepresentative. However, there is always the possibility that authors could carefully choose other studies in order to show their own results in a more or less favourable light. And four studies is a small number from the hundreds which are now published each year. An alternative approach is to refer to a larger number of studies, and allow the reader to judge whether the results are good or bad within an overall distribution. For example, Figure 15.5 shows the distribution of 179 baseline incremental cost-effectiveness results extracted from published UK studies. These range across different patient groups, therapeutic categories and diagnostic/disease areas, and it should be noted that the interventions are not necessarily in routine use. It can be seen that the median value is £2911 per QALY, and the average is £26 694 (Briggs and Gray 1998). So the 4S

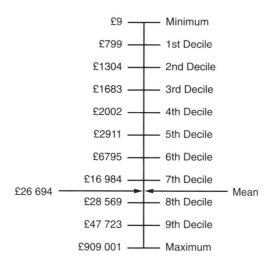

£9	Minimum
£799	1st Decile
£1304	2nd Decile
£1683	3rd Decile
£2002	4th Decile
£2911	5th Decile
£6795	6th Decile
£16 984	7th Decile
£26 694	Mean
£28 569	8th Decile
£47 723	9th Decile
£909 001	Maximum

Figure 15.5 Assessing cost-effectiveness

results are probably around the median value and well below the average, and this might be a more standardised way of reporting results.

- Finally, in discussing the results, the authors refer to cost-effectiveness 'among both men and women'. However, as the results replicated in Table 15.1 show, the cost-effectiveness was actually much better for men than for women, because they were at higher risk and, therefore, more life years were saved. This has undoubted distributive and possibly ethical implications, which the authors could have raised. Having said that, and given the complexity of these issues, perhaps it is not surprising that they decided to avoid comment!

A COST–UTILITY EXAMPLE

As noted above, the 4S economic evaluation we have been examining did not include quality of life as an outcome measure (although they did consider this hypothetically in their sensitivity analysis). So we will now look at a published cost-utility study: a study where cost-effectiveness was measured in terms of the cost per quality adjusted life year. Again we will consider this within the checklist set out earlier, under the broad headings of Framework, Data and methods, Results and discussion.

Framework

The study is a comparison of two treatments for patients at risk of recurrent depression (specifically, 35-year-old women who have experienced two previous episodes of depression within the past 4 years (Hatziandreu 1994). One is on maintenance therapy using sertraline, a fairly new class of drugs called selective serotonin reuptake inhibitors (SSRIs). The alternative treatment is episodic treatment with an older tricyclic antidepressant (TCA), dothiepin. TCAs remain the the most commonly prescribed drugs, but SSRIs are preferred by some clinicians for a variety of reasons including their non-toxicity when taken in overdose. SSRIs cost substantially more than the older classes of drugs. Depression is a major area of expenditure in the health care system.

Data and methods

The study used a decision analysis approach, in which the lifetime health care and social impact of the two treatments was simulated in a model. The outcome was measured in terms of quality adjusted life years (QALYs). Data on resource use was obtained from the expert opinion of two physician panels with experience in the area: one containing five general practitioners and the other five psychiatrists. Data on the likelihood of recurrences of depressive illness was also derived using the expert panels, which estimated the proportion of patients on each treatment who would experience a given number of recurrences, and the timing of these. Finally, data on the quality of life weight attached to depression-related health states was also obtained from the panel.

To briefly explain the background to this, imagine that we can represent our best imaginable health state by the number 1, and death by the number 0. A 75-year-old person restored to full health following a successful hip replacement operation might expect a further 10 years of life expectancy with no quality impairment, and this would be equivalent to 10 QALYs. Imagine now that the operation is not successful, and the person remains severely restricted in their mobility and is in frequent pain. If we could say that that person's quality of life had been halved, then their remaining life expectancy would be (0.5 x 10 =) 5 QALYs. Of course, the precise number or weight attached to this state of health may not be 0.5, but the point for the moment is that it is indisputably less than 1. In this study, the panel estimated that being on sertraline maintenance treatment with no recurrence of depression had a utility of 0.93, so that one year in that state was equivalent to 0.93 QALYs. Alternatively, a patient receiving dothiepin therapy who experienced a recurrence of major depression lasting three months was estimated to have a utility of 0.69 during that period.

Results

Table 15.2 gives some summary results from this study. In the base case, the lifetime costs of therapy were £3407 per patient in the sertraline group and £1648 per patient in the dothiepin group; the estimated QALYs were 14.94 per patient in the sertraline group and 14.13 per patient in the dothiepin

Table 15.2 Cost-utility of Sertraline maintenance treatment compared with Dothiepin episodic treatment for patients at risk of depressive illness

| | Sertraline maintenance treatment | | Dothiepin episodic treatment | | Comparison |
	Lifetime costs	QALYs gained	Lifetime costs	QALYs gained	Incremental cost per QALY gained
Baseline	3,407	14.94	1,648	14.13	2,172
GP utility scores	3,407	14.86	1,648	14.07	2,227
Psychiatrist utility scores	3,407	15.00	1,648	14.17	2,119
20% SSRI compliance	2,061	14.63	1,648	14.13	826
80% SSRI compliance	3,625	14.94	1,648	14.13	2,441
100% increase in SSRI cost	4,581	14.94	1,648	14.13	3,621
Equal recurrence rates	3,980	14.60	1,648	14.13	4,962

Data from Hatziandreu (1994)

group; and hence the incremental cost-effectiveness ratio was (3407-1648)/(14.93-14.13) £2172 per QALY.

This result was then subjected to a sensitivity analysis, in which compliance, utility scores, costs and recurrence rates were varied, and Table 15.2 also reports the results of this sensitivity analysis.

Discussion

The authors locate their results within a table showing 12 other cost-utility results, and conclude on this basis that '…incremental cost-utility ratios for maintenance treatment compared with episodic treatment with dothiepin for high-risk recurrent depressive patients appears to fall within a lower range than cost-utility ratios for treatment of severe hypertension and other common interventions such as estrogen replacement therapy or haemodialysis'.

Comments on the cost–utility example

As with the previous example, you would of course have to read the article carefully in order to make a full assessment of this evidence against the checklist. However, here are some points to note:

- The method used to identify, measure and evaluate the resource consequences of the therapies was entirely dependent on two panels of five physicians. Of course, if there are no large, long-term randomised controlled trials within which such information has been collected the analyst has to use other sources of information. But it is possible that case-control studies, cohort studies, observational studies or analyses of record linked or routine data could have provided some data.

- Similarly, the results of this study are crucially dependent on the panels of physicians for the estimates of likelihood of recurrences. This is very low-grade 'evidence', and a decision-maker might (should) feel uneasy about committing resources on this basis.
- Finally, the estimated quality of life weights also came from the panels. The methods section of the paper indicates that panel members `...were asked to choose between the hypothetical state and a gamble between perfect health and immediate death'. This approach is based on a standard method for estimating the value or utility of a health state, called the standard gamble.

For example, consider that you were confined to a wheelchair and in constant mild pain, and were likely to stay in that state. You are then informed of a new surgical procedure which could restore you to full health, but which carried risk of death. How much of a risk of death would you be prepared to take: 5%, 10% or 15%? The answer will depend at least in part on how bad you perceive the initial health state to be: the greater the disutility caused by the present health state, then presumably the higher the risk you would be willing to run in order to be free of it. Thus, if an individual was prepared to take a risk of 20% of death in order to be free of a particular state of ill-health, we could say that one year in that health state had a utility equivalent to 80% of full-health, which would equate to a QALY of 0.8.

An alternative approach, called the time trade-off, proceeds as follows: suppose, as above, you were in a health state which confined you to a wheelchair in constant mild pain. You are then asked which you would prefer: 10 years in that state, or some lesser period of life in a state of full health? That is, how much quantity of life might you be prepared to trade off to be restored to full health. If the response was that you would give up 3 years of life to be free of the symptoms (that is, you were indifferent between 10 years with the symptoms and seven years free of them), then the valuation of that health state is that it is equivalent to 70% of full health or a QALY of 0.7. Most standard gamble and time trade-off studies find substantial variation between individuals in their valuations of particular states, and a closer look at this paper shows the same: the valuations of a depressive episode treated with a TCA ranged from 0.35 to 0.95, and of a depressive episode treated with an SSRI ranged from 0.35 to 0.85. Therefore, in a sample of 10 the confidence intervals around these estimates would inevitably have been quite wide, and indeed there would be no statistically significant difference.

THE COST–BENEFIT APPROACH

So far, we have dealt with valuation of health states in non-monetary terms, for example, how much time one is prepared to trade-off to be free of a state of ill-health, or how much of a gamble. Cost-effectiveness and cost-utility analyses can only answer a relative question: given that we want to devote a given budget to improving health (measured in life years or quality adjusted life years), what is the most efficient way of doing so? So both approaches are concerned with efficiency, but only with what economists refer to as technical efficiency: how best to achieve a previously agreed objective? But, of course, there is a more fundamental question: is it worthwhile achieving this objective at all? Might it not be better to allocate the resources involved to some other objective altogether? This question, which concerns allocative efficiency, can only be answered if we can find some way of expressing all the costs and all the benefits of an action in money terms, and then seeing if the benefits outweigh the costs or the costs outweigh the benefits. This is what cost-benefit analysis strives to do. Although this is a widely used term, in fact it has this quite specific meaning to economists.

How might it be possible to obtain a monetary valuation of a health state or indeed of life itself? One is the human capital approach, which values survival or morbidity in terms of the value (at market prices) of the output that the person would have produced if they had not died or been ill. Time not used in market work may also be included: leisure time could be included at a market wage rate, and housework time could also be included based on the wage rate for domestic help or the opportunity wage rate: what that person could have earned. But there are many problems with this approach. First, it is difficult to value mortality and morbidity for people who have retired from the labour force. Second, its theoretical basis is rather weak. Third, health clearly does not have a value only insofar as it contributes to Gross National Income. Consequently, the human capital approach is not widely used.

A second approach is based on so-called revealed preferences, and makes use of observed individual choices concerning risk and income. For example, it is a general empirical finding that occupations with a degree of hazard attached to them have somewhat higher wages than otherwise similar jobs which do not have that element of risk. There is in effect a trade-off which employees make between the level of risk and the higher rewards. So by observing the higher risk and the wage difference it is possible to calculate the implicit valuation which individuals place on a health state. The results of such studies are fairly consistent over time and between countries: broadly, they suggest a value of life of around £4 million (OECD 1994). Of course, such valuations can only be derived under conditions of uncertainty. If you knew that the fatal accident was going to happen to you, your valuation would presumably be higher than if it was just a statistical possibility! Hence such valuations are sometimes called the value of a statistical life or VOSL.

A third method for obtaining a monetary valuation of health states is contingent valuation or willingness to pay, and is normally based on responses to hypothetical scenarios about willingness to pay to avoid certain outcomes. For example, suppose you were buying a car and could choose to have an air bag fitted at some extra cost. This would reduce the risk of death from 8 in 100 000 to 5 in 100 000. What is the most you would be prepared to pay to have the air bag fitted? If your maximum willingness to pay was £60, then your implied value of life would be (£60/3 x 10-5 = £3 million). This would imply that an intervention would be acceptable if it cost less than £3m per life saved, but would not be worthwhile if it cost more than £3m.

This is a very simplified example, but illustrates the essential features of the cost-benefit approach. Its main virtue is that it can address the fundamental question of whether something is worth doing at all. However, there are many difficulties involved in obtaining monetary values for health outcomes, and so cost-benefit studies are very rare in the health field. In fact almost all the studies published under this title are no such thing, but merely a comparison of the treatment costs and the cost savings (for example, by reducing morbidity) from a programme.

CONCLUSION: ECONOMIC EVALUATION IN EVIDENCE-BASED PRACTICE

In this chapter and the section on economic evaluation in Chapter 10 we have looked at the rationale for the economic approach; the way in which cost-effectiveness studies should be performed; and the way in which the validity of cost-effectiveness studies should be assessed. Health economists disagree on a number of things, but there is an increasing consensus on the methods to use and the guidelines to adhere to.

Until now, clinicians and other decision-makers have used methods other than cost-effectiveness analysis to make choices about health interventions, such as guidelines and recommendations devised by professional bodies. For example, in 1980 the American College of Obstetricians and Gynaecologists recommended a policy of annual smear tests for cervical cancer screening for all women from the age of 18. The same year the American Cancer Society recommended a less frequent schedule of smears, if two consecutive annual tests were negative. Then in 1988 a number of professional organisations proposed a less frequent schedule of smears if three consecutive annual tests were negative, but did not suggest an alternative screening interval. However, an economic evaluation using the same evidence available to these bodies then demonstrated that the cost per year of life saved of a four-year interval would be $10 100, but that this would increase to $184 500 at three-yearly, to $262 000 at two-yearly, and to $1 100 000 if done annually (Eddy 1992). Using this explicit information, it would seem advisable to recommend a four-year interval and then devote the resources freed up to other activities which provided more health gain.

In conclusion, cost-effectiveness analysis is an aid to making decisions about health care resources, and few economists would claim that it can be used as a complete decision-making procedure. Other values, considerations and skills will always play a part. But it does offer a powerful and explicit framework for considering information relevant to decision-making, and as the pressures on health care systems increase, so economic evaluation is likely to become a more familiar and necessary tool.

References

Briggs A, Gray A 1999 Handling uncertainty when performing economic evaluation of health care interventions. Health Technology Assessment 3(2)

Buxton M J, Drummond MF, Van Hout BA et al 1997 Modelling in economic evaluation: an unavoidable fact of life [editorial]. Health Economics 6:217-227

Eddy D M 1992 Assessing health practices and designing practice policies: The explicit approach. American College of Physicians, Philadelphia

Goldman L, Weinstein M C, Goldman P A et al 1991 cost-effectiveness of HMG-CoA reductase inhibition for primary and secondary prevention of coronary heart disease. Journal of the American Medical Association 265(9):1145-1151

Hatziandreu E J 1994 Cost-utility of maintenance treatment of recurrent depression with Sertraline vs episodic treatment with dothiepin. PharmacoEconomics 5:249-264

Johannesson M, Jonsson B, Kjekshus J et al 1997 Cost-effectiveness of simvastatin treatment to lower cholesterol levels in patients with coronary heart disease. New England Journal of Medicine 336(5):332-336

Organisation for Economic Cooperation and Development 1994 Project and policy appraisal: integrating economics and the environment. Paris 1994.

4S 1994. Randomised trial of cholesterol lowering in 4444 patients with coronary heart disease: the Scandinavian Simvastatin Survival Study (4S). Lancet 344:1383-1389

Van Houtet B, Al M J, Gordon G S et al 1994 costs, effects and C/E-ratios alongside a clinical trial. Health Economics 3(5):309-319

Further reading on health economics

Drummond M F, O'Brien B, Stoddart G L et al 1997 Methods for the economic evaluation of health care programmes. 2nd edn. Oxford University Press, Oxford

Drummond M F, McGuire A (eds) 2001 Economic evaluation in health care: merging theory with practice. Oxford University Press, Oxford

Folland S, Goodman A, Stano M 2003 The economics of health and health carwe. 3rd edn. Prentice Hall, New Jersey

Gold M R, Siegel J E, Russell L B et al (eds) 1997 Cost-effectiveness in health and medicine. Oxford University Press, New York

McGuire A, Fenn P, Mayhew K 1991 Providing health care: the economics of alternative systems of finance and delivery. Oxford University Press, Oxford

Mooney G 1994 Key issues in health economics. Wheatsheaf, Brighton

Sloan F (ed) 1995 Valuing health care: costs, benefits and effectiveness of pharmaceuticals and other medical technologies. Cambridge University Press, Cambridge

General articles

Drummond M, Jefferson T for the BMJ Economic Evaluation Working Party 1996 Guidelines for authors and peer-reviewers of economic submissions to the BMJ. British Medical Journal 313:275-283

Eddy D 1990 Clinical decision-making: from theory to practice. Series in Journal of the American Medical Association, 263:287-90, 263:877-880, 263:2239-2243, 263:2493-2505, 263:3077-3084, 264:389-391, 264:1161-1170, 264:1737-1739

Robinson R 1993 Economic evaluation and health care – a series. British Medical Journal 307:670-673, 726-728, 793-795, 859-862, 924-926, 994-996

Weinstein M C, Stason W 1977 Foundations of cost-effectiveness for health and medical practices. New England Journal of Medicine 296:716-721

Chapter 16

Context specificity: how was the study performed?

Martin Dawes

The setting in which the study takes place has a major importance when evaluating the relevance of that research. The context includes the characteristics of the patient, the medical staff involved in the study delivering clinical care and the medical facilities available to them. For example, consider a research study exploring the effectiveness of intensive insulin dosage in the treatment of diabetic patients (Reichard et al 1993). This study shows the benefit of intensive insulin dosage in achieving optimal blood sugar levels. Intensive insulin therapy also reduced the incidence of diabetic eye disease and diabetic-related nervous disease over seven and a half years.

Health professionals working within primary care reading this might want to undertake a similar approach. They may institute a similar protocol, but not see the same results. In this example, the hospital doctors may have had a more enthusiastic approach to changing insulin dosage than might be the case in primary care. The professionals working in primary care may be more wary of high doses of insulin or the use of multiple insulin regimens. The Swedish patients involved in this trial may also have been more compliant than those treated by this doctor.

ON WHOM WAS THE STUDY PERFORMED?

Many studies are carried out in secondary care where the status of the patient may be quite different from primary care. Patients with osteoarthritis treated using non-steroidal anti-inflammatory drugs (NSAIDs) at orthopaedic centres may show a benefit of a particular type of therapy (Kidd and Frenzel 1996).

This is a brief example of what may happen in such a study. All the patients have presented to their general practitioner with painful knees and reduced mobility. Some fail to respond to the practitioner's conventional treatment. These cases might then be referred to a hospital consultant rheumatologist. From this group of patients, volunteers would be sought for the trial. Patients are then randomly allocated to one of two NSAIDs. The two experimental treatments show a 50% improvement in arthritis. There was significant improvement in mobility and pain. The study was a well-performed randomised double blind study. Either drug might then be tried on patients in primary care but unfortunately produce less impressive results. Assuming the study had a large enough sample to be both clinically and statistically significant, what has happened?

The drug was tested on patients referred to orthopaedic consultants – not on all patients with painful knees in primary care. It is sometimes difficult to see how patients can be so different just because they have been referred. This difference of the characteristics of patients is extremely important in evaluating both the usefulness of a therapy and also a diagnostic or screening test. Patients usually present in primary care after the persistence of symptoms and the failure of 'over-the-counter' therapies. Yet at this stage the disease may still not be too advanced. We have to be wary about how we judge symptoms in our patients. The evidence is that we are not terribly good at matching our observation of the symptoms with those perceived by the patient (de Bock et al 1994).

WHEN WAS THE STUDY PERFORMED?

When did the study take place? The treatment of sore throats with antibiotics has been an area of considerable debate over the last 10 years. A recent meta-analysis demonstrates clearly the effect of antibiotic treatment on treating streptococcal infections associated with sore throat (Del Mar et al 2000). This meta-analysis included a study from the 1950s. It was demonstrated that the use of antibiotics in patients with streptococcal infections reduced the rate of development of rheumatic fever. However, the rate of this severe disease in developed countries has decreased considerably over the last 30 years. This improvement may have been as a result of improved housing, social and dietary conditions. Whatever the cause, the implications for this research have now changed following this reduction in the background prevalence of the disease. Therefore, this particular reason for using antibiotics in the treatment of sore throat no longer applies in these countries.

However, there are 12 million people (conservative estimate) affected by rheumatic fever or rheumatic heart disease with 400 000 deaths annually, and hundreds and thousands of disabled people, mainly among children and young adults. It remains a major public health problem in developing countries (Alwan 1993).

DIAGNOSTIC STUDIES

It is of immense importance to consider why one is undertaking a diagnostic test. This can be broken down into separate primary and secondary questions:

1. What is the probability of the disease?
2. Is the clinician trying to make a diagnosis (include the disease)?
   a. If the clinician uses this test and the result is positive will that alter the probability of the disease so much that it affects management?
3. Is the clinician trying to exclude a disease?
   b. If the clinician uses this test and the result is negative will that alter the probability of the disease so much that it affects management?

In primary care a lot of the time is spent looking after well people who are worried that they may have disease. Therefore, tests that are effective at excluding disease are routinely used. The duration of symptoms of the disease may be significant. If a child has had headache for longer than six months and it is not migrainous it is unlikely to be an aggressive brain tumour (Medina et al 2001). High sensitivities tests are most significant.

Many high-specificity tests will be used in the A&E department when one is treating a large number of patients.

It is important to understand why you or other health professionals are using tests in terms of a patient's pre-test probability of having a disease. Clearly this approach needs to be worked out in the cold light of day rather than when faced with a critically ill patient. It has led to the development and use of clinical care pathways, although the impact on patient outcomes of these pathways varies in certain settings (Johnson et al 2000, Kwan and Sandercock 2002).

Ask yourself what will be the probability of the disease if the test is negative or if the test is positive. How will this change the management of that patient in your setting? Care pathways with patients with certain symptoms are context specific. They may include the management of patients at home, in an ambulance, or in hospital. For a patient with chest pain the probability of disease varies in each of those settings; therefore, diagnostic strategies (as well as therapeutic) are accordingly adjusted. Similarly, the settings of the diagnostic study are equally important in identifying their application to your practice.

SUMMARY

It is important when considering the implementation of research findings in your own practice to consider all the changes that would need to occur to duplicate the protocol used in the study. It is therefore necessary to explore the circumstances in which the study took place. If you are considering using that therapy, can you ensure the same treatment is implemented as described in the study? Are your patients similar to those studied both in terms of disease but also general physical and social status?

References

Alwan A A 1993 Cardiovascular diseases in the eastern Mediterranean region. World Health Statistics Quarterly 46(2):97-100

de Bock G H, van Marwijk H W et al 1994 Osteoarthritis pain assessment in family practice. Arthritis Care Research 7(1):40-45

Del Mar C B, Glasziou P P et al 2000 Antibiotics for sore throat. Cochrane Database Systematic Reviews (4):CD000023

Johnson K B, Blaisdell C J et al 2000 Effectiveness of a clinical pathway for in-patient asthma management. Pediatrics 106(5):1006-1012

Kidd B, Frenzel W 1996 A multicenter, randomized, double blind study comparing lornoxicam with diclofenac in osteoarthritis. Journal of Rheumatology 23(9):1605-1611

Kwan J, Sandercock P 2002 In-hospital care pathways for stroke. Cochrane Database Systematic Reviews(2):CD002924

Medina L S, Kuntz K M et al 2001 Children with headache suspected of having a brain tumor: a cost-effectiveness analysis of diagnostic strategies. Pediatrics 108(2):255-263

Reichard P, Nilsson B Y et al 1993 The effect of long-term intensified insulin treatment on the development of microvascular complications of diabetes mellitus [see comments]. New England Journal of Medicine 329(5):304-309

Chapter 17

Changing policy and practice
Philip Davies

In most countries health care is experiencing constant challenges in terms of financial, organisational and knowledge management. The NHS has tried various ways of introducing market forces (Ham 1992, Ham & Spurgeon 1993, Robinson & Le Grand 1993) and 'customer focus' (Department of Health 2000) into a predominantly centralised, state-run service. The American health care system has undergone a major transformation in the past decade or so as it has tried to meet the increasing demands made upon it and to contain its already high costs. This has involved the development of managed care through a complex combination of health maintenance organisations, preferred provider organisations and state insurance provision such as Medicare. The dominance of the medical professions, and the knowledge base upon which they are based, is being questioned by other health professions, other academic disciplines, and the world of business administration. Health care is in a state of seemingly constant flux.

It is in this context that evidence-based health care has flourished as a means of establishing the best evidence for health care practice. Establishing best evidence, however, is not the same thing as implementing best practice, though the former does provide a basis for the latter. What is required is a process of 'transfer of information from research producers to its potential consumers' (Lomas 1993). This chapter considers this process of transfer and asks:

- what is to be changed?
- how might such change be brought about effectively and efficiently?
- how can such change be monitored and evaluated?

WHAT TO CHANGE?

Conceptual issues

Change occurs at different levels and has been written about using different types of conceptualisation. Systems theorists, e.g. Parsons 1952, Bertalanffy 1968, Cummings 1980, use biological metaphors to suggest that change occurs to social systems (such as the health service) when they respond to the demands made upon them from outside, e.g. the government, the general public, employers, etc. or from within, e.g. sub-systems, such as hospitals, professional associations, patients' groups, carers' groups, etc. They argue that there are self-adjusting 'boundary maintenance mechanisms' between social systems, sub-systems and the broader social and cultural system (i.e.'society') which brings about new social arrangements and establish a new equilibrium (homeostasis). The analogy is with the way in which the human body responds to changes in one sub-system, e.g. the vascular system or to demands that are made on it from outside (e.g. atmospheric change), to adjust in ways that make the maintenance of human life viable. One limiting feature of using this analogy for social systems is that the 'self-adjusting mechanism' of death is rarely possible, though systems theorists could argue that this accounts for the demise of cultures and societies, such as the Aztecs or certain aboriginal groups. Systems analysis tends to be deductive and 'top-down' in that it starts with a conceptual model or hypothesis of how social change occurs, and then confronts the real world to see how well it fits with the model.

Another limiting feature of the systems approach is that by objectifying social mechanisms in terms of systems, sub-systems, boundaries and the like it gives them a sense of existence and tangibility that is at best a social construction and at worst false. In doing so, systems theory can deny human agency and draw attention away from the fact that it is not systems that act and interact to produce social order and social change, but individuals and groups of individuals. Consequently, an alternative conceptual approach to social change is one which gives much more attention to the actions and interactions of individuals, and the ideas, beliefs, values, prejudices, ideologies, traditions, fads and fancies that they bring to their actions and interactions. This approach is referred to as the social interactionist approach to social change. The social interactionist approach tends to be inductive, or 'bottom up', in that it starts with the actions and interactions of individuals and groups of individuals and operates conceptual models and explanations.

The distinction between deductive and inductive methods of inquiry is seldom as pure as the above description might suggest. Systems theorists almost always have observational data (and impressionistic evidence) on human actions, interactions and agency at their disposal when they are developing conceptual models and explanatory schema. Similarly, social interactionists bring to their observations of actions and interactions ideas and conceptual models which may influence the questions they ask, and structure their perceptions, observations and interpretations of naturally occurring events and activities. Also, systems theorists talk about the collective actions of individuals and the consequences of human agency in terms of structures or institutions, even though many deny this, or camouflage the very actions, interactions and agency that brought them about. Giddens (1982, 1984) uses the term structuration to refer to the dual, hermeneutic process whereby the structures of society are created, maintained and changed by the actions and agency of individuals, and at the same time appearing independent from these actions and agency, thereby gaining them a reified and objectified status.

For health care practitioners, this degree of conceptual abstraction may seem irrelevant. However, unless those who are seeking to bring about health care change are clear as to whether they are seeking to change systems or individuals and groups of individuals, they are likely to fail in their endeavours simply by trying to do the wrong thing at the least appropriate level with the least chance of success.

Levels of change

Change can take place at the macro and the micro level of health care, at the national and the local level, at the strategic level and the operational level. The terms 'macro' and 'micro' often lack precision and specificity. Textbook and dictionary definitions refer to macro as 'long, large, large-scale' and 'any great whole', and to micro as 'small', and 'miniature' (OED 1976). In social science, macro level concerns those involving social structures, social systems and the operation of these at the aggregate level, whereas micro level analysis focuses on the more detailed processes and procedures that underlie and make up these aggregates. Nutley et al (2000) have expressed this macro/micro distinction in terms of a focus on systems change (i.e. macro approaches) and approaches that seek to change individual attitudes and behaviour.

The changes to the NHS that have been introduced by initiatives, such as Working for Patients (Department of Health 1989), Care in the Community (Department of Social Security 1989), and the NHS Plan (Department of Health 2000) are examples of macro level changes which have both a national and strategic focus. At the same time, the implementation of these health care changes, under programmes such as Shifting the Balance of Power (Department of Health 2002b), require local and micro level actions by health services personnel in front-line health care settings. Change at the macro level of health care, then, tends to involve whole populations, areas, regions or units, whereas changes at the micro level focus on smaller units, and the interactions and behaviour of individuals and groups of individuals within them.

Evidence-based health care plays a part at both the macro/national/strategic level and the micro/local/implementation level. It is important that health care practitioners clarify at the outset the level at which they are operating, the types of innovation that are appropriate and feasible at that level, and the systems, individuals and groups that they are likely, and unlikely, to be able to influence. Effective change is most likely to occur where it is focused on problem-solving and practice-based activities over which practitioners have some control or influence, and less likely to occur with activities that are more remote from practitioners' day-to-day concerns and responsibilities (Davis et al 1995, Kitson et al 1998).

Effective change involves context-sensitive practice (Greenhalgh and Worrall 1997) and integrating the best-available evidence with clinical judgment and expertise (Sackett et al 1996). This involves tacit and explicit knowledge and external evidence from systematic research and evaluation. The difference between tacit and explicit knowledge lies in the integration and experience of the person. For example, explicit knowledge is the list of signs that may be present in an ill child, whereas tacit knowledge is the ability to recognise that a child is ill. Nutley et al (2003) have suggested that this tacit knowledge is about know-how, know-who, and know-why, and that this needs to be integrated with know-about (e.g. the nature of a problem) and know-what (e.g. what works in bringing about desired outcomes).

Processes and outcomes of health care

Confusion often occurs in health care planning, organisation and change with respect to whether one is trying to influence the process of health care or the outcomes of patients and patient care. The process of health care refers to how the service is organised and run, and to its throughputs over time. Typical measures of health care process are the number of admissions and discharges to and from a hospital, the number of completed patient episodes, and various measures of waiting time. The outcome of health care involves some measure of patients' health status, such as death, survival, acute and chronic morbidity, impairment, disability and handicap, physical and social functioning, and patients' satisfaction with their state of health.

Both the processes and outcomes of health care have objective and subjective dimensions, though the objectivity of many health care measures is uncertain and subject to variable categorisation and recording practices (Robinson & Le Grand 1993, MacBeth 1996). Moreover, there is often a lack of congruence or consistency between objective and subjective dimensions of health care, which means that a successful outcome from the point of view of health care providers may not be so from the point of view of patients or their carers. Similarly, what appears to be a negative outcome of health care from a provider's points of view may be perceived as an acceptable service or state of health from the perspective of patients or carers (Davies 1996).

Models of health, illness and disablement

The focus of change is also determined by the different models of health, illness and disablement that are used in health care. The various disease/pathology models that are used in health care tend to focus on the signs and symptoms that are presented by patients, and the underlying disease and pathological processes that are causing them. This raises the question of whether one is trying to change the presenting signs and symptoms of disease/pathology, or the underlying disease/pathology itself (or both). The often uncertain relationship between signs, symptoms and pathology can make it difficult to determine what to change and how to monitor and evaluate change of health care status.

Wood and Bagley (1980) have argued that disease/pathology models of health and illness are inadequate because they treat disease and its signs and symptoms as an end point and ignore the consequences of disease/pathology for patients' overall health status. Wood and Bagley propose three distinct consequences of disease: impairment, disability and handicap, and independent systems of classifications for each (the WHO International Classification of Impairment, Disability and Handicap [ICIDH]).

Impairment refers to 'any loss or abnormality of psychological, physiological or anatomical structure or function' and is similar to the disease terms in the International Classification of Diseases in that impairments are threshold phenomena. That is to say, 'all that is involved is a judgment about whether the impairment is present or not' (Wood & Bagley 1980:14).

Disability and Handicap are treated by the ICIDH as, respectively, functional and social consequences of impairments. Unlike impairments, disabilities reflect failures in accomplishment such that a gradation in performance is to be anticipated. Handicaps are seen by the ICIDH as the disadvantages experienced by the individual as a result of impairments and disabilities, and are based not on attributes of individuals but on the circumstances in which people are likely to find themselves. These will vary from individual to individual, and from social group to social groups, and, therefore, have a contingent relationship to the underlying disabilities, impairments or diseases that individuals are experiencing.

In determining what one wishes to change, and how that change might be monitored, the evidence-based practitioner must clarify whether they are trying to change pathology, disease, signs and symptoms, impairments, disabilities or handicap. Other indicators of health status, such as activities of daily living, social functioning, and psychological and psychiatric well-being (Davies 1996) must also be considered as possible targets of change. Given that there are subjective as well as objective dimensions of each of these, and various contingent elements affecting some of them, careful and precise specification of what one is attempting to change is imperative.

A public health model often distinguishes between host, agent and the environment. The interactions between these three elements produce different types of health status which require different types of responses for health care and health policy. In the case of responding to alcohol problems, for instance, the individual becomes the focus of change if the causal mechanism is seen to be the host (the problem drinker). At this level, clinical treatment and health promotion are appropriate responses and levers of change. If the causal mechanism is seen to be the agent (i.e. alcoholic beverages) then the change process may be either the pathogens of alcohol and/or the availability and use of alcoholic beverages, e.g. licensing, taxation, supply and distribution. If the causal mechanism is seen to be environmental, e.g. the demands made by driving a car then the focus of change will be public policy that deters people from driving cars, e.g. better and more frequent public transport, fail-safe ignition systems, designated driver arrangements, safer cars and roads and so forth. The evidence-based practitioner should consider whether the host-agent-environment model is relevant to their practice, and which element(s) they should focus on for the purpose of bringing about effective change.

Clarification is also required as to whether the focus of change is the knowledge, attitudes or behaviour of individuals. Health care interventions tend to be most successful at increasing people's knowledge about health and illness, less successful about changing their attitudes, and least successful at changing their behaviour (Thorley 1985). Effective change in behaviour seems to be most likely when it is organised in socially and culturally appropriate ways (Thorley 1985), using locally based resources (Yates & Hebblethwaite 1985).

HOW TO BRING ABOUT EFFECTIVE CHANGE

Bringing about effective change in health care practice is not straightforward and there are no panaceas, or 'magic bullets' for doing so (Oxman et al 1995). Lomas (1993) has identified three models, or phases, of the transfer of evidence into clinical and professional practice. First, there is the passive diffusion model, which assumes that clinicians and other health professionals read, or hear, about research evidence and then adopt this in their practice. In the diffusion model, continuing medical education (CME) is assumed to play a key role. However, the evidence from systematic reviews, such as those by Davis et al (1995) and Oxman et al (1995), suggests that 'widely used CME-delivery methods such as conferences have little direct impact on improving professional practice' (Davis et al 1995).

A more effective way of bringing about change, and the second of Lomas's models, is the active dissemination model. This requires purposive action to promote knowledge and evidence to already busy professionals. Such action is helped by groups, such as the Cochrane Collaboration, the NHS Centre for Research and Dissemination, and the British Medical Journal, who provide high-quality syntheses and appraisals of existing evidence and disseminate them using web-based libraries and journals, as well as conferences, seminars and workshops. Even where there are good syntheses of evidence, however, it is important to recognise that 'individuals are not simply sponges, soaking up new information without filtering or processing' (Nutley et al 2003). Rather, 'new knowledge is shaped by the learner's pre-existing knowledge and experience' (ibid), much of which is tacit knowledge. Kitson et al (1998) add to this that the context and culture within which individuals work, as well as their role and position within an organisation, are important mediating factors between the existence of evidence and its effective use and implementation in practice.

Lomas acknowledges these intervening mechanisms and that local and national environments provide various sources of influence on actions and practice. A third model is proposed, the 'coordinated implementation model', in which patients and community interest groups, health care administrators, public policy makers (including third-party payers), and clinical policy makers, such as professional associations and disciplinary bodies are key players in bringing about effective change. Promoting effective change involves what Lomas calls 'product champions' from each of these groups who can prepare locally based analyses of what needs to be done and what measures need to be taken to do this. This requires a shift in culture from research into practice, where evidence is generated by people separated from those in day-to-day practice, to research in practice, in which evidence generation and professional practice are much more closely connected (Nutley et al 2003).

Evidence from successful change in health care and educational settings (Dowd 1994, Martin 1997) suggests that this requires an environment that is genuinely collaborative, cooperative, democratic, non-hierarchic and involves all stakeholder groups. Ensuring ownership of problems, as well as 'buy-in' and commitment to change by appropriate stakeholders, are also major requirements for effective change. So too is effective leadership in which delegation to others is matched by trust and confidence in their judgement, regardless of their standing in organisational hierarchies. Adequate time and technical support to participate in shared decision-making, as well as sufficient local resources to implement the proposed change, are also required. Many of these requirements are not always present in health care organisations. This will be considered further in Chapter 19.

Opinion leaders, audit and feedback and informal education

Personal contact with respected colleagues can be an important way of bringing about change (Stocking 1992), though it is imperative that these colleagues are competent in identifying and critically appraising the best available evidence. Otherwise, the use of distinguished and respected colleagues to determine professional practice may involve cherished, but unproven, ways of doing things, and may be highly resistant to effective change. Stocking has noted that patients are an important group for bringing about change by questioning existing practice and demanding new procedures and interventions. Stocking concludes that 'person-to-person contact, particularly with various givers of the message, is one of the more effective ways of changing clinical practice'.

Lomas et al 1991 found that local opinion leaders were more effective than audit and feedback activities in bringing about change amongst pregnant women who had had a caesarean section and who were targeted for vaginal delivery at subsequent births. Davis et al (1995) also found that audit and feedback techniques were less effective in changing professional practice than patient-mediated interventions, e.g. patient educational materials, patient reminders, outreach visits (including academic detailing), opinion leaders and 'multifaceted activities', i.e. more than one type of change strategy. Stocking (1992) acknowledges these findings about audit and feedback but maintains that this 'does not mean that audit in the United Kingdom cannot achieve change'. Stocking points out that change has been achieved using audit and feedback, but mainly in areas such as laboratory testing, diagnostic radiology and drug prescribing, rather than with medical or surgical practice; however, 'if audit is seen as an administrative procedure with no clear criteria about practice and no commitment to change, it is unlikely to have the desired effect'. For audit to have an effect on change it is also necessary to have the appropriate clinicians, administrators, managers, fundholders and patient groups involved as part of the change process, rather than outside of it, as passive recipients of some remote and seemingly irrelevant administrative procedure.

Opinion leaders also need to be credible individuals who are competent users of the best available evidence. They also require the skills of helping people to clearly define a problem, develop their own problem-solving skills and develop informal education activities. The latter are most effective when they are practice-based and geared at problem-solving, and opportunistic (i.e. where they fit into existing work schedules and activities) or planned, (i.e. where they are arranged for a specific learning purpose). The evidence on educational activities and teaching evidence-based practice is discussed in greater detail in Chapter 19.

Clinical guidelines

Guidelines may be considered part of the active dissemination and coordinated implementation models proposed by Lomas, though many of the thousands of guidelines published each year lack high-quality filters and standards of systematic searching and critical appraisal. It is essential, therefore, to ensure that guidelines are scientifically valid and systematically searched and appraised (i.e. are evidence-based). Even then, there is a need for clinicians and other users of guidelines to determine whether these are clinically relevant and appropriate for the task and client group in hand. Grimshaw and Russell (1994) have reviewed the literature on clinical guidelines and have concluded that whilst these can change clinical practice and achieve health gain 'the evidence available on the relative effectiveness of different strategies is still sparse'. They suggest, however, 'that if guidelines are developed internally by the clinicians who are to use them, few resources are needed to disseminate or implement them, whereas successful introduction of guidelines developed externally needs much more emphasis on dissemination and implementation' (Grimshaw & Russell 1994:50).

Financial incentives

The use of incentives and disincentives to bring about change in health care is well documented (Drummond 1984, McGuire et al 1991, Drummond & Maynard 1993). Put crudely, one way in which change can be brought about in health care is to pay health professionals to do it and to allow them to see the financial benefits of doing so. Conversely, one way of stopping health professionals from doing cherished, yet unproven, ways of doing things is to make them financially disadvantaged in doing so.

Financial incentives were an underlying feature of many of the 1989 changes to the organisation of the NHS, and of more recent initiatives. They were used, for instance, to get general practitioners to undertake more blood pressure monitoring and reach target rates for immunisation. More recent initiatives to give greater operational and financial freedom to higher performing NHS Trusts (Department of Health 2002c) are a further attempt to incentivise and reward successful health care providers, and to motivate less successful providers of health care to improve their service. The emphasis given to 'customer focus' and 'patient-centered health care' provides a further degree of incentive to change demand-led ways.

Providing incentives and resources, however, does not necessarily ensure best practice, especially where professional and financial independence is given to purchasers of health care. They may, for instance, use this independence to do what they have always done, to pursue cherished activities, or respond to the demands and wishes of patients, regardless of the evidence for and against doing so. For instance, the increased provision of physiotherapy by some fundholding GPs (under the 1990 health care reforms) appears to have been popular with patients as well as the GPs and Practice Managers who offered this service. As such it can be seen as an effective market response to patient demand, to GPs' preferences and to the suppliers of physiotherapy.

A review of the evidence on the effectiveness of physiotherapy (Davies and Hill-Perkins 1994), however, indicated that this is mixed and does not extend to all interventions and all patient groups who receive this service. Consequently, it is important that the financial resources and independence that are given to purchasers of health care are matched with the best available evidence of what is most effective, with which patients groups, at attaining which outcomes, and at what costs, including opportunity costs. Failure to include these factors in business plans will lead to inappropriate and possibly ineffective services being bought, at the expense of other services and interventions that may be more cost-effective (see Chapters 10 and 15).

Impediments to change

The converse of most of the factors reviewed above will normally serve to impede change in health care. Thus, unclear objectives of change, as well as inappropriate means, messages, media, facilitators, populations, incentives, social and cultural factors, time scales and resources, will combine with top-down, hierarchic and autocratic initiatives to work against successful and effective change. The lack of high-quality, systematically searched and appraised evidence will also impede the development of effective change. So too will the tacit knowledge of practitioners if this is too embedded, and if it acts as a barrier to engaging with explicit and empirically sound evidence (Iles & Sutherland 2001, Nutley et al 2003).

Stocking (1992) has noted that change will also be impeded if the relative advantage of introducing it is not clear; if the proposed change is incompatible with current beliefs and working practices; and if it involves knock-on effects that increase the complexity of everyday practice. Failure to see the innovation in operation ('observability') and to try it out on a limited basis ('trialability') will also work against the change process. It seems hard to conceive of any meaningful change that would not challenge current beliefs and working practices, though clearly there is an evolutionary-revolutionary balance to be worked out that will not alienate key players or motivate them to obstruct any change whatsoever. This is where the observability, trialability and demonstrable relative advantage may be crucial to the change process, and this requires careful and appropriate monitoring and evaluation of the proposed change.

MONITORING AND EVALUATING CHANGE

Types of monitoring

Monitoring is an important part of evidence-based practice and can take a variety of forms. The main objective of monitoring is to determine whether a treatment, service or programme is functioning as intended, or in accordance with some agreed standard. Rossi et al (2003) suggest that there are three principal forms of programme monitoring: Process or Implementation Evaluation; Routine Programme Monitoring and Management Information Systems; and Performance Measuring and Monitoring (sometimes called Outcome Monitoring).

Process evaluation seeks to establish whether or not an intervention or programme is delivered to the targeted recipients as intended. It can also be used to establish whether an intervention or service that in known to be effective is being delivered properly. It is less concerned with the outcomes (or impact) of the intervention than with the processes by which the intervention is being implemented.

Routine programme monitoring undertakes continual monitoring of indicators of an intervention or programme as part of the effective management of a service. Such monitoring provides 'regular feedback about how well the programme is performing its critical functions' (Rossi et al 2003:199). Performance measuring and monitoring shares with process evaluation and routine programme monitoring an interest in how well

	Baseline data	Follow-up data	
	(A) Before (T1)	(B) After (T2)	(A) Previous (T3)
Trial group	Data 1	Data 2	Data 3
Control group	Data 1	Data 2	Data 3

Figure 17.1 Single group pre- and post-test design

programmes or interventions are performing, but is much more focused on assessing their outcomes. It distinguishes between the outputs of a programme (e.g. the number of patients treated, or the contact time with patients), and its outcomes (i.e. the health status of patients treated or seen).

Whichever type of monitoring is undertaken, the full range of evaluation methods can be used. This includes qualitative methods (i.e. interviews, focus groups, participant-observation, ethnography) and quantitative methods (e.g. surveys, administrative data sets, cost-benefit estimates, experimental and quasi-experimental designs). It is sometime falsely assumed that process monitoring and evaluation uses only qualitative methods, and that routine programme monitoring and performance/outcome evaluations use only quantitative methods. All methods can be used for each of these types of monitoring and evaluation, depending on the nature of the questions being asked.

Evaluation and monitoring designs

The most rudimentary form of monitoring and evaluation, sometimes called Goals-Based evaluation, simply measures whether or not the intended goals or targets of a programme have been achieved. If they have, then a process evaluation might investigate what it was that made this successful delivery come about, thereby establishing important evidence for successful programme replication elsewhere. If these goals or targets have not been met, then a process evaluation can be used to investigate why this was the case and what factors or processes impeded successful delivery. It is also important to establish whether any unintended outcomes have been caused by the intervention, especially if these may have negative or undesirable consequences.

A more ambitious and powerful type of monitoring uses some form of comparative method to establish the net effect or net impact of an intervention, compared with some other intervention, or doing nothing at

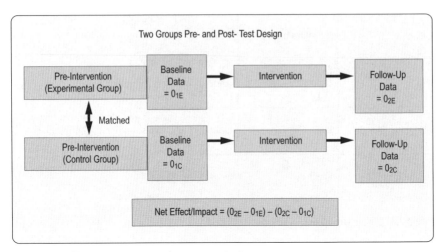

Figure 17.2 Two groups pre- and post-test design

all (some form of counterfactual). The simplest comparative method is the single group before and after (pre- and post-test) design.

A major weakness of the single group pre- and post-test design is that it cannot control what would have happened to this group of people anyway, (i.e. in the absence of the intervention) and, therefore, can give a distorted (or biased) measure of the true net impact of the intervention. One way of dealing with this is to use a matched comparison, or control group in which no intervention is introduced, and to compare the differences in outcomes in both groups before and after the intervention. The comparison group might be a similar unit, such as a hospital, health centre, school or an area, e.g. a housing estate or nearby street.

The main weakness of the two groups (pre- and post-test design) is the difficulty in matching the experimental and control groups on the variables appropriate to the anticipated outcomes. In the absence of such matching, the influence of external factors other than the intervention (known as confounds) is unknown, thereby resulting in unaccountable bias. Propensity Score Matching (Rosenbaum & Rubin 1985) is one method of achieving such matching, but it is a complicated procedure and probably beyond the capacity of many health care practitioners and researchers. Expert advice from a statistician or a researcher with experience of experimental designs should be sought if matched samples are to be achieved.

The most rigorous and robust way of monitoring the net impact of an intervention or programme is the randomised controlled trial (see Chapter. 5). The design of a randomised controlled trial is similar to that of the two groups pre- and post-test design, except that people (or units, or areas) are randomly allocated to the experimental or control groups, rather than by being matched. The randomised controlled trial design is as follows:

Although the design of randomised controlled trials is appealingly simple,

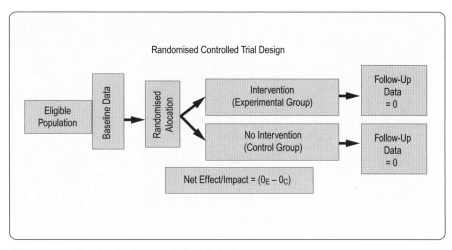

Figure 17.3 Randomised controlled trial design

their implementation and execution can be complex and requires sufficient sample sizes to ensure a minimal detectable effect. Consequently, they may also be beyond the capacity and resources of many health care professionals, and should only be considered with the assistance of an experienced evaluator. Other types of evaluation design that can be used to monitor change include regression discontinuity designs, and interrupted-time series designs. Regression discontinuity designs (RDD) work in a similar way to randomised controlled trials, except that instead of allocating people to experimental and control groups on a random allocation basis, they are allocated (or assigned) according to a cut-off point on a quantifiable pre-test measurement (e.g. some measure of health status). The assignment variable can be a pre-test on the dependent variable, or can be totally unrelated to the outcome variable. It is important, however, that the assignment variable cannot be caused by the intervention, i.e. it must be independent of the intervention. The regression discontinuity design is most powerful when the cut-off is placed at the mean of the assignment variable (Shadish et al 2002:209). For each participant in the trial the value of the first measure is plotted on the horizontal axis and the value of the second measure is plotted on the vertical axis. If there is an effect of the intervention or programme it will be detected by a shift (or discontinuity) in the regression line representing the pre-test and post-test scores (see Figure 17.4).

Interrupted-time series designs investigate repeated observations of a constant variable over time and look for 'interruptions' to the series or sequence of observations (see Figure 17.5). Such interruptions might be attributed to an intervention, though they could also be a random blip in the series of observations (not likely in the example in Figure 17.5 where the interruption was continual). There are different types of change to a time series sequence of observations; changes in the level and in the slope of the

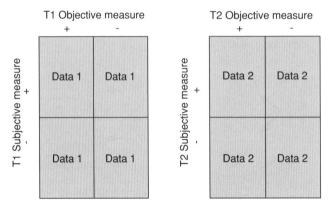

Figure 17.4 Regression discontinuity design.

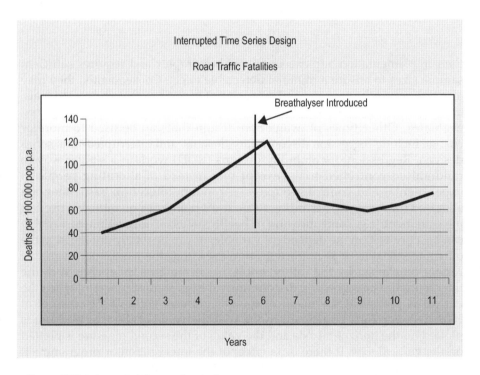

Figure 17.5 Interrupted time series design.

curve, the degree of permanency of the effect (as in Figure 17.5), and the type of impact (immediate or delayed).

In order to attribute the interruption in the time series of observations to a particular intervention, it is important to know the specific point (e.g. the date) when the intervention was introduced. This must, of course, have been before the interruption in the observations if causality is to be inferred. If this is the case, it is then necessary to consider, and rule out, any other reasonable explanations for why the interruption occurred. In the case of the clear interruption to the time series data on traffic accident fatalities, Figure 17.5, this would include ruling out, for instance, that there had been a fuel shortage after year six; that a major new tax had been introduced on road usage (or petrol); or that there had been a national alcoholic beverages strike; the price of alcoholic beverages had increased significantly, and so on. Assuming that none of these alternative explanations is accepted, we can infer that the noticeable reduction in road traffic accident fatalities was almost certainly attributable to the introduction of the breathalyser.

It is also important when working with interrupted time series designs to establish that the variable(s) being measured are constant over time. Where definitions and counting practices change frequently over time (e.g. unemployment statistics) it is more difficult, and sometimes impossible, to use such data as valid measurements, or to establish any causal significance to an interruption in the time series.

Planning the monitoring of change

Perhaps the most important principle of monitoring and evaluating change is that it is seen as an integral part of the change process and is not an optional extra. As such, it must be considered and planned at the outset of the change process and before any change is initiated. Appropriate feedback mechanisms and information need to be determined ahead of time and built into the proposed monitoring exercise. The factors that have been considered in this chapter should be made explicit and considered carefully before changes are introduced so that a clear change strategy is developed and the variables to be monitored are known ahead of time. This might include the following:

- what do you want to change?
- what do you hope to achieve by the proposed change?
- over what timescale?
- at what cost (i.e. what resources will be involved)?
- is there any existing evidence that the proposed change has worked/not worked elsewhere?
- what is the status of that evidence and what variables/measures were used in it?
- what evaluation design will be used to monitor any anticipated change?
- what process and outcome measures will be used to determine whether the change has been successful?
- what feedback mechanisms and information will be required and how will these be built into the monitoring exercise?
- what other aspects of practice will be affected by the proposed change (people, resources, timetabling)?
- what other people (health professionals, patients, administrators, etc) will be affected by the proposed change, and are they cooperative?
- what are the ethical implications of introducing the proposed change (and

have these been approved by the local health care ethics committees)?
- do you have command of the necessary personnel, resources and timetabling of professional practice to introduce and maintain the proposed change?
- is the proposed change feasible?

By systematically working through this checklist of questions, the parameters of the monitoring process will be clearer. This will also help determine which type of evaluation design is appropriate for monitoring the anticipated change, what sorts of data will need to collected and analysed, and how extensive the monitoring exercise can be given the available resources.

Gray (1997) has advised that those monitoring changes in health care should not embark on large-scale data-gathering without a rigorous review of the aims, objectives and methods of the change strategy, and not to let data gathering become an end in itself. In addition, good monitoring requires planning ahead of time for feedback of data to professional and clinical colleagues as well as to the academic community for scientific advice, interpretation and dissemination. The dissemination and publication of negative findings is as important as the reporting of positive effects of change.

Further details of the evaluation designs and methods outlined above can be found elsewhere in this book (see Chapter 5) and in Sackett et al (1991), Shadish et al (1993, 2001), Gray (1997), Rossi et al (1998), Weiss (1998), Denzin and Lincoln (2000). Online guidance on evaluation designs can be found in the Cabinet Office Magenta Book at www.policyhub.gov.uk.

CONCLUSIONS

Evidence-based health care provides considerable opportunities to change professional practice and to make health care more effective and efficient. In order to do so health care practitioners need to be able to formulate a strategy for implementing and monitoring effective change. This chapter has reviewed some of the basic principles of establishing and monitoring change in health care, as well as the evidence on effective change. It concludes that both implementation and monitoring require explicit clarification at the outset of what it is one wishes to change; what end state one wishes to accomplish; what sorts of outcomes will be involved; which health care systems and individuals (lay and professional) will be involved in the change and monitoring process; what costs and resources will be involved; and what organisational and administrative arrangements will need to be made. A key feature of successful and effective change is that it requires the cooperation of all people and groups that are likely to be involved, and their involvement in the planning and implementation process. Change from within is invariably more successful than that which is imposed or initiated from outside. At the same time, key people who are competent evidence-based practitioners are required to provide leadership, act as opinion leaders, help overcome resistance to change and ensure that inertia does not set in. The monitoring of change must be seen as an integral part of the change process and not an optional extra. As such, it must be part of the overall change strategy.

References

Bertalanffy L 1968 General system theory: Foundations, development, applications. Braziller, New York

Cummings T G (ed) 1980 Systems theory for organisation development. Wiley, New York

Davis D A, Thomson M A, Oxman AD et al 1995 Changing physician performance: a systematic review of the effect of continuing medical education strategies. Journal of the American Medical Association 274(9):700-705

Davies P T 1996 Sociological approaches to health outcomes. In: MacBeth H M (ed) Health outcomes reviewed: biological, social and economic perspectives. Oxford University Press, Oxford

Davies P T, Hill-Perkins V 1994 The education and training of rehabilitation therapists. Report to the Oxford Regional Health Authority, Oxford

Denzin N K, Lincoln Y S 2000 Handbook of qualitative research. Sage Publications, Thousand Oaks, California

Department of Health 1989 Working For Patients, White Paper. HMSO, London

Department of Health 2000 The NHS Plan: a plan for investment, a plan for reform. HMSO, London

Department of Health 2002b Shifting then Balance of Power. HMSO, London

Department of Health 2002c NHS Performance Ratings and Indicators. HMSO, London

Department of Social Security 1989 Care in the Community, White Paper. HMSO, London

Dowd S B 1994 Education as a strategy for allied health, Technical Report. Lincoln Land community College, Chicago, Illinois

Drummond M F 1984 Essentials of health economics. Northern Health Economics, Aberdeen

Drummond M F, Maynard A 1993 Purchasing and providing cost-effective health care. Churchill Livingstone, Edinburgh

Giddens A 1982 Profiles and critiques in social theory. MacMillan, London

Giddens A 1984 The constitution of society. Polity Press, Cambridge

Gray J A 1997 Evidence-based health care: how to make health policy and management decisions. Churchill Livingstone, Edinburgh

Greenhalgh T, Worrall J G 1997 From EBM to CSM: the evolution of context-sensitive medicine. Journal of Evaluation in Clinical Practice 3(2):105-108

Grimshaw J M, Russell I T 1994 Achieving health gain through clinical guidelines: II. ensuring guidelines change medical practice. Quality in Health Care 3:45-52

Ham C 1992 Health policy in Britain: The politics and organisation of the National Health Service, MacMillan, London

Ham C, Spurgeon P 1993 The development of the purchasing function: In: the new face of the NHS. Longman, Harlow

Iles V, Sutherland K 2001 Managing change in the NHS: Organisational change, NHS service delivery and organisation. London School of Hygiene and Tropical Medicine. London

Kitson A, Harvey G, McCormack B 1998 Enabling the implementation of evidence≠ based practice: a conceptual framework. Quality in Health Care 7:149-158

Lomas J 1993 Retailing research: increasing the role of evidence in clinical service for childbirth. The Milbank Quarterly 71(3):439-475

Lomas J, Enkin M W, Anderson G M et al J 1991 Opinion leaders vs audit and feedback to implement practice guidelines: delivery after previous caesarean section. Journal of the American Medical Association 265:2202-2207

MacBeth H M (ed) 1996 Health outcomes reviewed: biological and social aspects. Oxford University Press, Oxford

Martin E M 1997 Conditions that facilitate the school restructuring process. Paper presented at the southern educational research association meetings, Austin, Texas, January 1997

McGuire A, Fenn P, Mayhew K 1991 Providing health care: The economics of alternative systems of finance and delivery. Oxford University Press, Oxford

Nutley S, Davies H T, Tilley N 2000 Getting research into practice. Public Money and Management 20(4):3-6

Nutley S, Walter, I, Davies H T 2003 From knowing to doing: A framework for understanding the evidence-into-practice agenda. Evaluation 9(2):125-148

OED 1976 The concise Oxford English dictionary. Oxford University Press, Oxford

Oxman A D, Thomson M A, Davis D A et al 1995 No magic bullets: a systematic review of 102 trials of interventions to improve professional practice. Canadian Medical Association Journal 153(10):1423-1431

Parsons T 1952 The social system. Free Press, New York

Robinson R, Le Grand J 1993 Evaluating the NHS reforms. King's Fund Institute, London

Rosenbaum P R, Rubin D B 1985 Constructing a comparison group using multivariate matched sampling methods that incorporate the propensity score. The American Statistician 39:33-38

Rossi P H, Freeman H E, Lipsey M W 2003 Evaluation: A systematic approach. Sage Publications, Thousand Oaks

Sackett D L, Haynes R B, Guyatt G H et al 1991 Clinical epidemiology: A basic science for clinical medicine. Little, Brown, Boston

Sackett D L, Rosenberg W, Gray J M et al 1996 What evidence-based medicine is and what it is not. British Medical Journal 312:71-72

Shadish W R, Cook T D, Leviton L C 1993 Foundations of program evaluation: theories of practice. Sage Publications, Thousand Oaks, California

Shadish W R, Cook TD, Campbell D T 2002 Experimental and quasi-experimental designs for generalised causal inference. Houghton Mifflin Co, Boston

Stocking B 1992 Promoting change in clinical care. Quality in Health Care 1:56-60

Thorley A 1985 The role of mass media campaigns in alcohol health education. In: Heather N, Roberston I, Davies P T (eds) The Misuse of Alcohol: Current Concepts and Controversies. Croom Helm, London

Weiss C H 1998 Evaluation. 2nd edn. Prentice Hall, Upper Saddle River, New Jersey

Wood P, Bagley E 1980 International classification of impairment, disability and handicap. World Health Organisation, Geneva

Yates F, Hebblethwaite D 1985 Using natural resources for preventing drinking problems. In: Heather N, Robertson I, Davies P T (eds) The misuse of alcohol: current concepts and controversies. Croom Helm, London

Chapter 18

Evaluating change
Martin Dawes

How do we establish that change has occurred? The process of evidence-based practice is one that requires change to be monitored. After the effort of identifying the problem, formatting the question, searching for, finding and appraising the evidence, you do not want to leave it at that. The aim is to improve care. Clearly the question asked might have been: 'Am I doing the right thing to the right people at the right time?' If the answer from your search of the literature was yes, then you could sit back, pat yourself on the back and think of answering the next question.

AUDIT

But what if you were not doing the right thing, or doing it to the wrong people at the wrong time? To establish this would have meant collecting the information in the first place. The very fact that you are reading this indicates that you are likely to have heard of, and to have used audit. That is all this chapter is about. But there really is no mileage in knowing the evidence if it is not being applied. If you have done any audit, you will already know that surprising information can be revealed during this process.

The audit cycle (Figure 18.1) is very familiar and contains few surprises in itself; the main difficulty though is completing it (Lawrence 1992). It is easy to collect the data; the hard part involves setting standards.

It is the collection and appraisal of the evidence that lets you set evidence-based standards that apply in your clinical situation. This requires a decision by all those involved in the application of the process to be involved. Clearly it is not going to be an effective change if the receptionists making the appointments are not made aware of the change. Take for example the

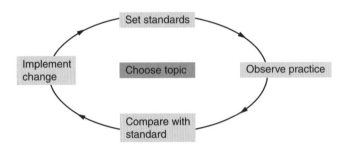

Figure 18.1 The audit cycle

implementation of a cardiac secondary prevention programme in general practice (Dalal & Evans 2003). The evidence for this programme is evaluated and the practice decides to implement a programme.

The clinicians may be agreed about the process and protocol, but the practice nurses are not, and the programme is likely to fail. Many practices only book appointments up to three months ahead. If the cardiac prevention programme requires a six-monthly visit, then the receptionists are likely to advise the patient to ring up at a later date to make that appointment. If that is the case, then it is equally likely that the patient will forget and the follow-up part of the programme will fail. For this reason it is important to identify each stage of the programme's process and the key individuals who are responsible for that stage. If each individual identified is involved, then the process is more likely to succeed.

To ensure that the audit is likely to take place it needs one or two individuals to be primarily responsible for it. They will undertake to initiate the audit, collate the results, and present it to the team on a date specified in advance when the programme was initiated. Only in this way can the team be sure that the audit will really be undertaken. So often, if the task is left unallocated and no deadline date set, the audit will be relegated to the bottom of the tray and forgotten.

It is important to identify and audit all the important parts of the process. Some of these may be harder to measure than others but be more important to individual patients. For example, in the cardiac secondary prevention programme the patients' understanding of why they are taking the cholesterol-lowering drugs is as important as the fact that a prescription has been issued (O'Connor et al 2001). The identification of the number of prescriptions issued is simply obtained from the computer system (in UK practice). The knowledge of the patient is much harder to determine and may require face-to-face interviews or questionnaires. The team members should therefore identify what their priorities are and audit the correct information.

The work done identifying and learning to use the tools to measure the patients' understanding of their disease or problem can be used with other disease audits.

The data needs to be represented to the team when the information has been collected. This should be the responsibility of one or two members of the team. It also requires the team to set aside a time when the results will be presented. This should be arranged at the beginning of the audit process so that there is a deadline for completion of the audit. Otherwise the process will be started and then forgotten. Worse, the people who have invested the time to prepare the audit will not have the opportunity to present their work or establish whether changes need to be made.

Finally, the process must establish whether change is needed. If change is to follow, then where in the process of care is that change going to have to occur? This question requires the whole process of care to be examined. Do patients find the appointment system inconvenient, or is it the doctors not telling them about the need for further appointments?

This examination of the process should occur before any suggestions about implementing change are made. It is all too easy to suggest that what is needed is an additional receptionist, whereas the process for making appointments rests more on the problem with remembering to contact the practice on the phone.

Once the process has been examined by all involved, changes can be suggested. What is important is that following the implementation of the changes a review audit of the care is performed.

These systems have now been integrated into clinical or integrated care pathways (ICP). These pathways frequently involve several teams and are usually based on firm evidence, for example, National Strategic Frameworks from the NHS. Where the health professional disagrees with the pathway and decides not to follow the pathway she/he must describe the reasons for the deviation. These pathways may lead to improvement in care in many areas of practice (Sulch & Kalra 2000, Cringles 2002, Fowell et al 2002, Onslow et al 2003). However, randomised controlled trials of ICP have not yet demonstrated large benefits and there is continuing debate over their use.

References

Cringles M 2002 Developing an integrated care pathway to manage cancer pain across primary, secondary and tertiary care. International Journal Palliative Nursing 8(5):247-255

Dalal H, Evans P 2003 Achieving national service framework standards for cardiac rehabilitation and secondary prevention. British Medical Journal 326(7387):481-484

Fowell A, Finlay I et al 2002 An integrated care pathway for the last 2 days of life: Wales-wide benchmarking in palliative care. International Journal Palliative Nursing 8(12):566-573

Lawrence M 1992 Medical audit in general practice. British Medical Journal 305(6848):314

O'Connor A, Stacey D, Entwistle V et al 2001 Decision aids for people facing health treatment or screening decisions. Cochrane Database Systematic Review (3). In: The Cochrane Library (2). John Wiley, Chichester

Onslow L, Roberts H et al 2003 An integrated care pathway for fractured neck of femur patients. Professional Nurse 18(5):265-268

Sulch D, Kalra L 2000 Integrated care pathways in stroke management. Age Ageing 29(4):349-352

Chapter 19

Teaching, learning and evidence-based health care

Philip Davies

If evidence-based health care (EBHC) has even a fraction of the importance for clinical practice, resource allocation and health care management as is claimed in this book, then it is important that its principles and practices are used by as wide a population as possible. This means that there is an educative function for health care trainers, providers and users to develop effective and efficient ways to learn about evidence-based practice and its potential for affecting clinical and lay behaviour.

This educative dimension can benefit from what is known about how people learn, and especially how adults learn. Also, it is important to understand the barriers to this learning process, and how these barriers might be overcome. These are the main themes of this chapter. Before we embark on a review of the evidence on adult learning and effective teaching, however, it is important to consider what constitutes evidence in educational and social science research. This will also serve to demonstrate that the knowledge base of competent health care practitioners and users must be much broader than that of natural science, experimental design and randomised controlled trials (RCTs) alone. As important as these approaches to knowledge and understanding are, and they are very important in the quest for valid, reliable and relevant evidence, they represent only a part of the intellectual armoury that is necessary for the competent health care practitioner and user.

TEACHING, LEARNING AND EVIDENCE

A range of methodological approaches is used in educational research and practice. As with other areas of social inquiry, educational research uses experimental and quasi-experimental research designs, as well as quantitative and qualitative methods, in controlled and naturalistic settings. Educational research also uses the research techniques of economic evaluation (cost analysis, cost-effectiveness analysis, cost-benefit analysis, and cost-utility analysis (see Chapter 10), and the analytical approaches of philosophy and ethics to establish the ethical probity of educational interventions and practice. Systematic reviews and meta-analysis also play an important role in establishing evidence for educational policy and practice.

EXPERIMENTAL AND QUASI–EXPERIMENTAL EVIDENCE

Experimental and quasi-experimental research methods are used extensively in educational research. The Campbell Collaboration maintains the Social, Psychological and Educational Controlled Trials Register (C2-SPECTR), which contains over 10 000 randomised and 'possibly randomised' trials in education, crime and justice and social welfare. A significant number of the experimental and quasi-experimental studies registered with C2-SPECTR come from educational research. Experimental and quasi-experimental methods are appropriate for answering questions such as 'does teaching method x have a better outcome than teaching method y in terms of achieving outcome z'.

One limitation of RCTs in any area of research is that it is often not possible to have control over the stock and flow of people in schools, hospitals or geographical areas, thereby making their random allocation into an experimental or control group very difficult. Another problem is the ethical issue of either exposing people in the experimental group to a potentially harmful intervention or, alternatively, making people in the control group forgo the possible advantages of the experimental intervention (Illsley 1980). Randomised controlled trials can also be expensive and difficult to run properly in terms of obtaining an adequate sample size and analytical power, and avoiding cross-over between experimental and control groups.

Some of these problems can be overcome by quasi-experimental methods, such as studies involving matched comparisons of cases and controls or of different cohorts. The principle of exposing one group to an intervention, and not exposing another group to the same intervention remains. Both groups are assessed before and after the intervention using identical pre- and post- tests. The difference between such studies and RCTs is that the allocation to experimental or control group is not done randomly. Consequently, the possible effects and biases of confounding factors cannot be confidently calculated. Nonetheless, quasi-experimental studies are used extensively in educational research. 'The randomisation of students into educational programmes is the essence of the classical experimental design' and 'is the only method of research that can test for cause and effect relationships, quasi-experimental methods are often essential in educational research because of the ethical considerations which prevent researchers from assigning humans to different artificial treatments (Anderson 1998).

Interrupted time series studies and correlational research using methods, such as simple and multiple correlation, regression analysis and analysis of variance are also used extensively in educational research. Such studies can give strong suggestions of cause and effect, but generally lack ways of dealing adequately with confounding factors, thereby making causal inferences unsound.

QUALITATIVE EVIDENCE

There are questions about teaching and learning (and about health care) that are less concerned with direct cause and effect, or the effectiveness of different teaching and learning methods, for which valid and reliable evidence is required. These are questions about the processes by which educational activities are undertaken, and about why, how and under what conditions teaching and learning can be effective. The meanings that teaching and learning have for different stakeholders (e.g. teachers, learners, educational managers, governors, etc.) are also of interest to educational researchers. The consequences that educational activities have on the social and self-identity of individuals, and groups of individuals, attract the interest of educational research. These types of question require qualitative and 'naturalistic' research methods, such as ethnography, detailed observation and face-to-face interviews (Davies 2000a).

Qualitative methods seek evidence of a more descriptive and interpretive nature than that found in experimental and quasi-experimental studies. Naturalistic studies tend to work inductively by generating hypothesis from detailed observations of activities, people, objects and events. Polgar and Thomas (2000:6) suggest that 'induction involves asserting general propositions about a class of phenomena on the basis of a limited number of observations of select elements.' Glaser and Strauss (1967) famously coined the term 'grounded theory' to capture the process of theory building based on detail observations of everyday activities.

Educational research also gathers evidence about the patterns and structures of interaction, conversation and discourse by which teaching and learning are accomplished. Such questions focus on naturally occurring classroom interactions between teachers and learners (Mehan 1977, Spindler 1982, Fetterman 1984, Cazden 1988, Hammersley 1990,1999, Hammersley and Atkinson, 1995, Mehan et al 1996, Walford 2001) and use methods, such as participant-observation, ethnography, in-depth interviews and case studies.

PHILOSOPHICAL AND ETHICAL EVIDENCE

Educational research, like health care research, seeks evidence on whether or not it is right or warrantable to undertake some educational activity or process. Each of the methodological approaches mentioned above may inform these debates, but none will resolve them without additional considerations concerning the moral and ethical issues of universal versus selective action, informed choices, resource prioritisation, the values underlying educational activity and the like. There is a considerable literature on the ethics of research and professional practice in both education (Adair et al 1985, Frankel et al 1987, Kimmel 1988) and health care (Weiss 1982, Gillon 1985, Brazier 1987, Veatch 1989, Fulford 1990). The competent practitioner needs to consider this literature when establishing appropriate evidence for good practice.

SYSTEMATIC REVIEWS AND META-ANALYSIS

The contribution of systematic reviews and meta-analysis to establishing evidence of good practice in health care is dealt with elsewhere in this book, and in the research literature (Chalmers et al 1989, Antman et al 1992, Egger et al 2001). Systematic reviews are one form of research synthesis which contribute to evidence-based policy and practice by identifying the accumulated research evidence on a topic or question, critically appraising it for its methodological quality and findings, and determining the consistent and variable messages that are generated by this body of work. Systematic reviews of the existing research evidence also help identify what is not known about a topic or question and, thereby, direct new primary research in areas where there is a gap in the evidence base.

Systematic reviews and meta-analysis had their origins in educational research with the pioneering work of Glass (Glass et al 1980). The role of systematic reviews and meta-analysis in educational research, policy and practice is discussed elsewhere (Davies 2000b, 2003a), and is a major focus of the work of the Campbell Collaboration (Davies & Boruch 2001, Davies 2003b, http://campbellcollaboration.org). Glass (1976) used the term 'meta-analysis' to refer to 'the statistical analysis of a large collection of analysis results from individual studies for the purpose of integrating the findings'. Meta-analysis is a specific type of systematic review that seeks to aggregate the findings of comparable studies and 'combines the individual study treatment effects into a "pooled" treatment effect for all studies combined, and/or for specific subgroups of studies or patients, and makes statistical inferences' (Morton 1999). In the two decades or more since Glass's original meta-analytic work on class size (Glass & Smith 1979, Glass et al 1980, 1982), and on psychotherapy (Smith, Glass & Miller 1980), meta-analysis has developed considerably in terms of the range and sophistication of data-pooling and statistical analysis of independent studies (Kulik & Kulik 1989, Cook et al 1992, Cooper & Hedges 1994, Egger et al 2001).

HOW ADULTS LEARN

For the most part teaching the principles and practices of evidence-based health care involves the teaching of, and learning by, adults. Our knowledge of how adults learn has been enhanced by the theoretical and empirical work of what is sometimes called the 'constructivist' school of learning, as well as by empirical evidence from the educational and evidence-based health care literature. The constructivist school of learning refers to those writers who propose, and in some cases have demonstrated empirically, that individuals do not learn by the passive association of ideas and symbols, or responses to stimuli, but by actively constructing knowledge and understanding in and through their daily activities. Central to the constructivist school of learning is the role of problem-solving. This suggests that learning occurs most effectively when it takes place in the context of solving a problem, or finding a solution to a situation, that is of immediate relevance to the needs and interest of the learner. A further principle of learning by problem-solving, or problem-based learning as it is often known, is that the acquisition of new knowledge requires the activation of prior knowledge. Furthermore, knowledge is said to be best remembered in the context in which it is learned. Consequently, the role of experience is very important in how adults and children, learn.

Piaget (1926, 1952, 1964, 1970, 1977) argued from empirical observations that babies and children learn developmentally through their daily interactions with others and their environment. For Piaget, learning and conceptual thinking arise from trial and error and are achieved by children's manipulation of their everyday overt activities. Piaget referred to this as learning by developing a 'logic in action', a development which takes the infant from the sensorimotor stage to the stage of concrete operations, and finally on to the stage of formal operations. A hallmark of the conceptual abstraction that is possible in the latter two stages is the ability to transfer learning from one situation to another and to carry out reversible mental actions (i.e. go back and start again). The cognitive abilities of transfer and reversibility are also important elements of how adults learn.

Bruner (1969) argued that 'the first object of learning is that it should serve us in the future' and that this involves the transfer of underlying principles and attitudes already learned. Consequently, Bruner also stressed the importance of individuals' experience in the process of learning. Bruner (1961, 1966) contrasted hypothetical learning with expository learning and argued that the former leads to learners engaging in acts of discovery.

> In expository learning the decisions concerning the mode and pace and style of exposition are principally determined by the teacher as expositor; the student is the listener... In the hypothetical mode, the teacher and the student are in a more cooperative position...The student is not a bench-bound listener, but is taking part in the formulation and at times may play the principal role in it.
>
> (Bruner 1961:126, cited in Knowles 1990:91)

The importance of learning as an active, participatory process in which the existing knowledge and prior experience of learners are fully utilised, was also central to the educational philosophy of Dewey (1938). In the book

Experience and Education, Dewey argued that individuals learn from their own needs and interests, rather than by the imposition of knowledge from above. For Dewey, learning should be a 'free activity' in the sense that it necessitates free inquiry and discipline from within the learner rather than external discipline from the teacher or elsewhere. This principle underlies what is more commonly referred to as self-directed learning. Self-directed learning does not mean, or imply, an unstructured, *laissez-faire*, or disorganised approach to learning, but does mean that learners should be able to take responsibility for their own learning, its direction, and its relevance to their everyday lives, needs and interests. Self-directed learning is often, if not usually, undertaken with the guidance of a teacher or fellow-learner who provides a 'scaffolding' (Vygotsky 1978, 1986) to the learner until full understanding and self-direction is achieved. Indeed, the term scaffolding is used by Vygotsky to refer to the support a teacher provides a learner to perform a task.

There are other construction metaphors that are used by Vygotsky, such as 'bridging' and 'structure', to express the support that learners often need in order to develop independent problem-solving, as opposed to the guided problem-solving of others. Scaffolding is an attractive metaphor for learning in that it connotes a temporary structure or support that is provided by the teacher during the learning process and the transfer of responsibility from what Vygotsky calls 'other regulation' to 'self-regulation'. Once the latter state has been reached, the 'scaffolding' can be removed and the learner is able to operate on his or her own. The gap between what a learner can do alone, and what he or she can do only with the support of a teacher, is referred to by Vygotsky as the 'Zone of Proximal and Development' (ZPD), and by others (e.g. Newman et al 1989) as the 'Construction Zone'. There is considerable literature on scaffolding and the zone of proximal development, much of it using other terms, such as 'cognitive apprenticeship' (Collins et al 1989), 'guided participation' (Rogoff 1990), 'reciprocal teaching' (Brown & Campione 1990), 'assisted performance' (Tharp & Gallimore 1991), 'appropriation' (Newman et al 1989) and 'contingent learning' (Wood 1991, Wood & Wood 1996).

Despite the attraction of scaffolding as a metaphor, there are some real limitations on its use and effectiveness in teaching. Hobsbaum and colleagues (1996) have noted that in the context of language recovery, programmes for young learners 'scaffolding can take place only in one-to-one teaching situations because contingent responding requires a detailed understanding of the learner's history, the immediate task and the teaching strategies needed to move on.' Tharp and Gallimore (1991) have also noted 'with large classrooms it is difficult for teachers to know all the children well and so provide the sensitive and accurate assistance that challenges but does not upset the learners'. Mehan et al (1996), however, talk of 'institutional scaffolds' which provide structural and interactional supports to hitherto underachieving students in order to develop an academic identity and build bridges between high school and college. This involves what Mehan et al refer to as 'social scaffolding' to refer to the 'engineering of instructional tasks so that students develop their own competencies through interactions with more capable peers or experts ... groups of students are learning about school culture, assisted by groups of experts or more capable peers (op cit., pp 78-79). This was especially important for Mehan and his colleagues in the context of 'untracking' low-achieving students in American schools and preparing them for college education. The relevance of scaffolding for adults, including health professionals learning the principles and practices of evidence-based health care, is no less significant given the diversity of professional and disciplinary backgrounds within health services and the varying degrees of knowledge and experience of evidence-based practice.

Another principle that runs through the constructivist school of learning is that effective learning takes place in democratic environments. This usually refers to structures and environments of learning that are egalitarian, non-hierarchic and non-authoritarian. This is not to deny differentials in the knowledge or skills of teachers and learners but does deny that such differentials warrant a paternalistic, top-down model of learning in which the teacher is active and the learner is passive. A democratic approach to learning also acknowledges that learning is a two-way process between teacher and learner and that there is a 'parity of esteem' between them. The notion of definitive knowledge being handed down by the teacher to the learner is antithetical to a democratic conception of learning. The term 'fellow learners' is sometimes used to express the ideal of a democratic relationship between teacher and learner.

There is a further dimension to a democratic model of learning, expressed most explicitly in the work of Dewey (1938), which is that teaching and learning should involve the preparation of learners for their active participation as citizens in the democratic business of the state. This requires education to go beyond merely teaching instrumental knowledge and skills for the demands of the workplace, or the everyday environments of learners, and to develop critical thinking and analytical ability.

The principles of the constructivist school of learning have been drawn upon, and expressed most eloquently, in the work of Knowles (1990) on The Adult Learner. Knowles offers an andragogical model of learning, i.e. a theory of adult learning, in contrast to a pedagogical model (the teaching of children). Knowles characterises the latter as a model that 'assigns to the teacher full responsibility for making all decisions about what will be learned, how it will be learned, when it will be learned, and if it has been learned. It is teacher-directed learning, leaving to the learner only the submissive role of following a teacher's instructions.' By way of contrast, Knowles argues that adult learning is driven by the need to know (purposive behaviour), the learner's self-concept (self-direction), the learner's experience (what they bring to learning), a readiness to learn (developmental appropriateness), an orientation to learning (task-centred or problem-based learning) and by motivation. Knowles acknowledges his indebtedness to the earlier writing of Lindeman (1926), who offered the following model of adult learning:

In short, my conception of adult education is this: a cooperative venture in non-authoritarian, informal learning, the chief purpose of which is to discover the meaning of experience; a quest of the mind which digs down to the roots of the preconceptions which formulate our conduct; a technique of learning for adults which makes education coterminous with life and hence elevates living itself to the level of adventurous experiment.

(Lindeman 1926:166)

The contrast that Knowles makes between an andragogical and a pedagogical model of education is rather too polemic, and it is acknowledged that during the 1970s 'a number of teachers in elementary and secondary schools and colleges reported that they were experimenting with applying the andragogical model and that children and youths seemed to learn better in many circumstances when some features of the andragogical model were applied' (Knowles 1990:63). Certainly, those aspects of primary and secondary education in the British National Curriculum that involve project work, problem-solving, students' directed activities and coursework assessment (as opposed to examinations) conform to the andragogical model of learning promoted so effectively by Knowles. Knowles adds that 'in practice ... educators now have the responsibility to check out which assumptions are realistic in a given situation [and that] if a pedagogical assumption is realistic for a particular learner in regard to a particular learning goal, then a pedagogical strategy is appropriate, at least as a starting point' (ibid.). This provides Knowles with the warrant to approve of didactic instruction in situations where the 'learners are indeed dependent, when they have had no experience with a content area, when they do not understand the relevance of a content area to their life tasks or problems, when they need to accumulate a given body of subject matter in order to accomplish a required performance, and when they feel no internal need to learn that content' (ibid). The complementary role of didactic instruction and participatory learning has been documented in a review of 19 experimental studies of explicit teaching (ET) and reciprocal teaching (RT) (Rosenshine & Meister 1991).

TEACHING AND LEARNING IN HEALTH CARE

The principles of the constructivist approach to learning, and of adult learning, have been applied in various health care education settings. Bruhn (1992) has advocated problem-based learning as a means of educating health practitioners for the future, and has characterised this approach in terms of:

- curricular organisation around problems rather than disciplines
- an integrated curriculum rather than one separated into clinical and theoretical components
- an inherent emphasis on cognitive skills as well as on knowledge.

Bruhn goes on to suggest, somewhat contentiously, that 'long-term advocates of problem-based learning (PBL) stress that it is the only known method for preparing future professionals to be able to adapt to change, learning how to reason critically, enabling a holistic approach to health, and attaining integrated, cumulative learning.'

There is a very large literature on PBL in health care, of which only a small part can be cited here (Barrows & Mitchell 1975, Barrows & Tamblyn 1976,1977, Neufeld et al 1981, Schmidt 1983, 1993, Neufeld & Chong 1984, Norman et al 1985, 1990, Premi 1988, Verma et al 1988, Hollis 1991, Norman & Schmidt 1992). Much of this is associated with, and has been developed by, the Faculty of Health Sciences at McMaster University, Canada for the education and training of doctors, nurses and, more recently, physiotherapists and occupational therapists. The education and training courses for these professions are distinct and separate but they share common goals and an educational approach built around self-directed and problem-based learning. The learning methods consist of problem-based tutorials, clinical skills laboratories, inquiry seminars, clinical education, independent study and interprofessional education.

The Curriculum Guide for the Bachelor of Health Sciences Degree Programmes in Occupational therapy and Physiotherapy at McMaster University, for instance, suggests:

> The more active they (students) are in determining their own needs and learning goals, the more effective their learning is likely to be. Within broad guidelines, students should determine their own learning needs, how they will best set and achieve objectives to address those needs, how to select learning resources, and whether their learning needs have been met.

The McMaster Curriculum Guide goes on to point out that:

> Although the programmes stress the importance of self-directed learning, it should be noted that this is not a self-paced programme. Attendance and participation in tutorials, laboratories and inquiry seminars is required. It is necessary to demonstrate by self, peer and faculty evaluation that satisfactory progress has been achieved.

Problem-based learning on the McMaster University degree course is centred around:

> A variety of problems carefully designed and selected for each curriculum block. These problems may be used in tutorials, clinical skills laboratories, inquiry seminars or clinical education. The problem scenarios promote the exploration of the underlying biological, physiological, behavioural and environmental determinants of health and the role of health care professionals. The problem scenarios also require the integration of previous learning with the acquisition of new knowledge, skills and attitudes. The problems are designed to provide a context that resembles future professional contexts as closely as possible. Problem-based learning incorporates self-directed learning, clinical reasoning and critical appraisal of related literature.

The use of problem-based, self-directed learning is also reported elsewhere in the world. Jacobs and Lyons (1992) have reported its use in the training of occupational therapists in Newcastle, New South Wales, Australia. Students develop problem-solving skills and 'an attitude to therapy which encourages them to focus on each client as an individual, living and working within their specific environment'. The authors add that 'the reductionist view of intervention does not seem to be compatible with the self-directed, problem-based approach to learning.'

Titchen (1985, 1987a, 1987b, 1992) has proposed a greater role for problem-based learning in the development of continuing education activities for physiotherapists, and in the multidisciplinary training of health professionals in the UK. Some aspects of problem-based, self-directed learning have been incorporated into the training of health care professionals in the UK, mainly in connection with clinical practice and skills' development modules. The use of learning contracts in the training of nurses and other health professionals in the UK is another way that the principles of constructivist and adult learning are being used in health care education and training.

The Master's Programme in Evidence-Based Health Care at the University of Oxford is built around students bringing clinical problems to the course for which they are supported in self-directed learning to find and appraise the best available evidence. Where there is no such evidence, or the evidence that exists is of questionable validity, reliability or quality, students learn the principles and practices of research design, biostatistics and research protocol development in order that they can establish such evidence. Teaching and learning on the Oxford Master's Programme includes some didactic lectures and plenary sessions, in which students are encouraged to question, interact and participate. Small group learning for private and personal tutorials is encouraged.

There is some evidence that medical students graduating from problem-based, self-directed undergraduate education achieve better professional competence than students from more traditional, discipline-based education and training (Neufeld 1985, Friedman et al 1990, Woodward et al 1990, Patel et al 1991, Shin et al 1993).

Shin et al (1993) undertook a retrospective comparative analysis of family practitioners trained between 1974 and 1985 at McMaster University (using the principles and methods of problem-based learning (PBL) and at the University of Toronto (using more didactic, discipline-based and subject-based methods of learning). The study examined these family practitioners' knowledge of hypertension and its management, especially their familiarity with, and use of, up-to-date evidence-based best practice for the management of high blood pressure. The authors found that doctors trained at McMaster University had significantly greater overall clinical knowledge of hypertension and of the most effective treatments for the condition. They also had significantly greater knowledge of the evidence concerning successful approaches to patient compliance with treatment. A multivariate analysis of possible factors that might have accounted for these differences suggested that the medical school attended by these doctors was the only statistically significant variable. Shin and colleagues concluded that medical training based on self-directed learning and problem-based learning was superior than more traditional approaches in the development of these skills and tasks (though not necessarily others).

This last caveat is important because there is little, if any, evidence that self-directed and problem-based methods of learning are invariably better than other methods, or for all types of learning. Norman and Schmidt (1992), in reviewing the evidence on problem-based learning, conclude that:

1. there is no evidence that PBL curricula result in any improvement in general, content-free problem-solving skills
2. learning in a PBL format may initially reduce levels of learning but may foster, over periods of up to several years, increased retention of knowledge
3. some preliminary evidence suggests that PBL curricula may enhance both transfer of concepts to new problems and integration of basic science concepts into clinical problems
4. PBL enhances intrinsic interest in the subject matter and appears to enhance self-directed learning skills, and this enhancement may be maintained.

Two systematic reviews of problem-based learning in health care (Albanese & Mitchell 1993, Vernon & Blake 1993) provide further evidence that its effectiveness is mixed. Both reviews suggest that PBL is superior to traditional methods of teaching and learning in terms of clinical performance, clinical knowledge, student satisfaction, faculty satisfaction, academic process and study behaviour. On the other hand, traditional methods are superior to PBL in terms of: achievement on NBME Examinations (Part I), other tests of factual knowledge, and knowledge of basic science.

EFFECTIVE TEACHING STRATEGIES

Collaboration, participation and democracy

The principles of adult learning reviewed above have clear implications for effective teaching methods. The effective teaching of adults (and of children) requires the teacher to be a facilitator of learning rather than simply a provider of information, knowledge and skills. Knowles (1990) has identified 16 principles of teaching, none of which mentions directly instructing the student, imparting knowledge or any other oracular activities. Rather, Knowles sees the effective teacher of adults as 'exposing students to new possibilities of self-fulfillment', 'helping each student clarify his/her own aspirations', 'helping each student diagnose the gap between his/her aspiration and his/her present level of performance' and so on (Knowles 1990:85–87). The active role of the teacher, for Knowles, is also seen as democratic and participatory. For instance, 'the teacher shares his thinking about options available in the designing of learning experiences and the selection of materials and methods, and involves the student in deciding among the options jointly'. Similarly, 'the teacher gears the presentation of his own resources to the levels of experience of his particular students' and 'the teacher helps the students to apply new learning to their experience, and thus make the learnings more meaningful and integrated' (ibid).

This underlines the point made earlier that adult and constructivist learning does not mean a disorganised, unstructured, *laissez-faire* approach to teaching. The unprepared teacher is a poor teacher and violates the central principle of democratic, non-hierarchical learning, i.e. that it involves a two-way, contractual commitment to the learning experience. Also, as we have seen, a constructivist approach to learning does not deny a role for didactic teaching. To repeat Knowles' observation, didactic instruction may be appropriate where 'learners are indeed dependent, when they have had no experience with a content area, when they do not understand the relevance of a content area to their life tasks or problems, when they need to accumulate a given body of subject matter in order to accomplish a required performance, and when they feel no internal need to learn that content' (Knowles 1990:64). Moreover, didactic teaching and learning may be appropriate where class sizes are large, or learning situations are not conducive to small group, face-to-face interaction.

Lecturing

Good lecturing involves gaining familiarity with the lecture room, its acoustics, its audio-visual equipment and other teaching aids, such as a white-board/blackboard and flip-chart. Small details, such as the temperature of the room and its opportunities for fresh air and air-conditioning can have a major influence on the success or failure of a lecture (or small group teaching session, or tutorial). If the lecture is part of a sequence of such talks or presentations it is important to ensure that sufficient breaks are organised for exercise and refreshments. The good lecturer will endeavour to present the lecture in such a way that questioning and clarification from students are encouraged, without disrupting the flow of the lecture or having the presentation digress into less relevant areas.

A good lecture will have a presentational structure which has a beginning, middle and end. The first should state the aims and objectives of the lecture and should elicit from students whether these concur with, or differ from, their needs and interests. The second part should include the content of the lecture: ideas, theories, arguments, counter-arguments, data, critically appraised literature, etc. The third part should draw the evidence of the content of the lecture together and draw a conclusion or set of conclusions, with due attention also being drawn to gaps in the current state of knowledge, uncertainty about particular aspects of data, and the direction that learners might take for their own reading and inquiry.

Powerpoint provides a useful aid to presentation and dissemination of a lecture, seminar or workshop, and is now universally available to anyone working in the Microsoft Office environment. Powerpoint presentations, however, have their own rules for effectiveness, including using an adequate font size (minimum 18 point for most presentations), avoiding too much information on any one slide, not having too many slides, and avoiding excessive use of animation. Also, Powerpoint is an aid to effective presentation and not a presentation in its own right. Simply showing Powerpoint slides and reading out what is on them is both redundant and a dereliction of duty to explain, elucidate and illustrate the issues behind the bullet points.

Group work

Small-group work is clearly an important element of adult and constructivist learning, and includes activities, such as seminars, workshops and teamwork. A small group has been defined as consisting of 'not more than twelve people interacting with each other so as to achieve a common goal' (Kendrick and Freeling 1993). Small groups allow its members to learn by sharing their experiences, knowledge and skills, using the group as an experience from which to learn, becoming aware of their own attitudes, and coming to tap their own unknown potential (Schofield 1998). Successful learning in small groups depends on the size of the group, the environment in which the group is working, the duration and frequency of its meetings, the clarity of the tasks it sets itself, the leadership and dynamics of the group and the ground rules that are established by the group at the outset (ibid). Schofield, like Kendrick and Freeling (1993), suggests that the leader of a group acts as a resource to ensure that the perceptions of the group experience are shared and allow a 'safe house' atmosphere to develop. Another role of leadership of small groups is to promote open, critical thinking. Small groups, then, are the embodiment of the constructivist principles of democratic, non-hierarchical, self-directed and problem-based learning.

Teaching and learning opportunities

Opportunities for teaching and learning about evidence-based practice in health care settings will be variable, but tend to divide into 'opportunistic' and 'strategic' possibilities. The former refer to naturally occurring, often routine, activities, such as weekly meetings, grand rounds, research group meetings, staff meetings, etc. These often allow the evidence-based practitioner an opportunity to present some of the principles and practices of evidence-based health care as part of the routine activities and rhythms of their workplaces. Strategic teaching opportunities refer to those that are set up by the evidence-based practitioner specifically to teach the principles, procedures and pay-offs of evidence-based research and practice. They may take the form of seminars, workshops, lectures, searching and critical appraisal sessions, and e-learning opportunities (web boards, chat lines, email conferencing, electronic journals). The goal of opportunistic and strategic teaching in health care settings is to capture and maximise the 'teachable moment' and the 'learning moment' of colleagues.

OVERCOMING RESISTANCE TO TEACHING AND LEARNING

The Evidence-Based Medicine Working Group (1992) has identified four barriers to teaching evidence-based medicine:

1. the rudimentary skills of health professionals in critical appraisal
2. the time factor involved in critical appraisal
3. the lack of high-quality evidence leading to a sense of futility in attempting evidence-based practice
4. the skepticism of colleagues towards evidence-based practice.

The EBM Working Group suggests that these problems can be ameliorated by the use of teaching and learning strategies along the lines of the constructivist and andragogical approaches reviewed above.

There are problems in the social organisation of health care, however, that work against the resolution of uncertainty, doubt and skepticism by teaching strategies alone. Dowd (1994) has suggested that for education to work as a change strategy in health professions it must involve collaborative learning that is non-threatening and democratic, in which the teacher acts as a facilitator, and the learner contributes to solving problems and taking part in discussion. Dowd maintains that the crucial factors are the acquisition of problem-solving skills and a belief in the values of holistic education. Martin (1997) has suggested that the conditions that facilitate successful restructuring in schools include the support from all stakeholder groups, the cooperation and trust between all personnel, the ability to deal with those who resist change, a mutual determination of what will be acceptable, adequate time and technical support, work time to participate in shared decision-making and sufficient local resources to implement change.

Many of these factors are absent in health care settings. Health care is a largely hierarchical form of social organisation with some professions assuming dominant and super ordinate positions in terms of their knowledge base, status and claims to power. Learning in many health care settings has traditionally been top-down, instructional and expository. When combined with the claims to superiority mentioned above, the result is often a form of authoritarianism and professional imperialism that is highly resistant to change or democratic innovation. Under these circumstances, the mutual determination of achievable goals, and ways of reaching them, are uncommon.

Despite the frequent claims to multiprofessionalism and multidisciplinary teamwork in health care settings, this is often largely rhetorical. The social organisation of health care often resembles that of the farmyard in Orwell's Animal Farm: all men are equal but some are more equal than others. Even where interprofessional relationships are more democratic and egalitarian, the pressures of clinical and administrative work, as well as research, often leave little time for educational development or innovation. A further hindrance to teaching and learning in health care settings is the often poor physical environment of hospitals and health centres, many of which lack basic resources, such as vacant rooms, a white-board, projection facilities or even a flip chart.

These structural, environmental and interactional conditions indicate the areas in which action may be necessary if effective teaching and learning are to be achieved. That is to say, the development of non-hierarchical arrangements for learning about, and implementing, evidence-based best practice would seem to be a priority for people working in the health care sector. This might begin by identifying who the stakeholders are in a health care setting and widening the net to include individuals and professions that have hitherto been excluded. Effective teaching and learning can be enhanced by having individuals from all levels of seniority, as well as different professions, responsible for organising workshops, seminars and journal clubs. The more that these can be based on the principles of constructivist learning outlined above, e.g.. problem-solving, needs-based, democratic, experiential as well as experimental learning, and so on, the more effective they are likely to be. The use of consultative techniques, such as the Delphi method, the nominal group method and critical incidence analysis (Ellis, 1988) can help identify common goals and consensus in how to achieve them. Finally, it is important that feedback mechanisms are developed so that teachers and learners can learn from each other about effective and ineffective ways of learning about and implementing evidence-based practice. The need to monitor and evaluate teaching and learning initiatives remains a priority in the development of effective ways of teaching evidence-based health care.

SUMMARY

This chapter has reviewed the nature of evidence in educational and social science research and suggested that this needs to be integrated with that from epidemiological and clinical research. This involves taking a broad approach to knowledge and evidence, and using the full range of research and teaching methods.

The evidence on how individuals learn, especially how adults learn, has also been reviewed and a constructivist approach to learning has been outlined. This has been incorporated by Knowles (1990) and others into an andragogical model of learning, the central elements of which are that adults learn best from solving problems to meet their needs and interests, by drawing upon their existing knowledge and prior experience, and in democratic, non-hierarchic and non-authoritarian environments. The problems that these principles encounter in health care settings have also been reviewed and possible solutions have been considered.

References

Adair J, Dushenko T, Lindsay R 1985 Ethical regulations and their impact on research practices. American Psychologist 40:59-72

Albanese M, Mitchell S 1993 Problem-based learning: A review of literature on its outcomes and implementation issues. Academic Medicine 68:52-81

Anderson G 1998 Fundamentals of Educational Research. The Falmer Press, London

Antman E, Lau J, Kupelnick B et al 1992 A comparison of results of meta-analysis of randomised control trials and recommendations of clinical experts' treatments for myocardial infarction. Journal of the American Medical Association 269:240-248

Barrows H, Mitchell D 1975 An innovative course in undergraduate neuroscience: experiment in problem-based learning with 'problem boxes'. British Journal of Medical Education 9:223-230

Barrows H, Tamblyn R 1976 An evaluation of problem-based learning in small groups utilising a simulated patient. Journal of Medical Education 51:52-54

Barrows H, Tamblyn R 1977 The portable patient problem pack (P4): a problem-based learning unit. Journal of Medical Education 52:1002-1004

Brazier M 1987 Medicine, patients and the law. Penguin, Harmondsworth

Brown A, Campione J 1990 Communities of learning and thinking, or a context by any other name. In: Kuhn D (ed) Developmental perspectives on teaching and learning thinking skills. Karger, Basle

Bruhn J 1992 Problem-based learning: an approach toward reforming allied health education. Journal of Allied Health 21(3):161-173

Bruner J 1961 The act of discovery. Harvard Educational Review 31:21-32

Bruner J 1966 Toward a theory of instruction. Harvard University Press, Cambridge, Mass

Bruner J 1969 The process of education. Harvard University Press, Mass.Cazden C 1988 Classroom discourse. Heinemann, New York

Chalmers I, Hetherington J, Elbourne D et al 1989 Materials and methods used in synthesising evidence to evaluate the effects of care during pregnancy. In: Chalmers I, Enkin M, Keirse M (eds) Effective Care in Pregnancy and Childbirth. Oxford University Press, Oxford

Collins A, Brown J, Newman S 1989 Cognitive apprenticeship: teaching the crafts of reading, writing and mathematics. In: Resnick L (ed) Knowing, Learning and Instruction: Essays in Honour of Robert Glaser, Erlbaum, Hillsdale, New Jersey

Cook T, Cooper H, Cordray D et al 1992 Meta-analysis for explanation. Russell Sage Foundation, New York

Cooper H, Hedges L (eds) 1994 The handbook of research synthesis. Russell Sage Foundation, New York

Davies P 2000a The contribution of qualitative methods to evidence-based policy and practice. In: Davies H, Nutley S, Smith P (eds) Evidence and Public Policy. Policy Press, Bristol

Davies P 2000b The relevance of systematic reviews to educational policy and practice. Oxford Review of Education 26(3 & 4):365-378

Davies P, Boruch R 2001 The Campbell collaboration. British Medical Journal 323:294-295

Davies P 2003a Systematic reviews: how are they different from what we already do? In: Anderson L, Bennett N (eds) Evidence-informed policy and practice in educational leadership and management: applications and controversies. Paul Chapman Publishing, London

Davies P 2003b The contribution of the Campbell collaboration to evidence-based policy and practice. In: Thomas G, Pring R Evidence-based practice in education. Oxford University Press, Oxford

Dewey J 1938 Experience and education. MacMillan, New York

Dowd S 1994 Education as a strategy for allied health, Technical Report. lincoln Land Community College, Chicago, Illinois

Egger M, Davey Smith G, Altman D 2001 Systematic reviews in health care: Meta-analysis in context. British Medical Journal Publishing, London

Ellis R (ed) 1988 Professional competence and quality assurance in the caring professions. Croom Helm, London

Evidence-Based Medicine Working Group 1992 Evidence-based medicine: A new approach to the practice of medicine. Journal of the American Medical Association 268 (17):2420-2525

Fetterman D 1984 Ethnography in educational evaluation. Sage Publications, Beverly Hills

Frankel M (eds) 1987 Values and ethics in organisation and human systems development: an annotated bibliography. American Association for the Advancement of Science, Washington DC

Friedman C, de Bliek R, Norman G et al 1990 Charting the winds of change: evaluating innovative medical curricula. Academic Medicine 65:8-14

Fulford K 1990 Moral theory and medical practice. Cambridge University Press, Cambridge

Gillon R 1985 Philosophical medical ethics. Wiley, Cambridge

Glaser B, Strauss A 1967 The discovery of grounded theory: Strategies for qualitative research. Sage Publications, Chicago

Glass G 1976 Primary, secondary and meta-analysis of research. Educational Researcher 5:3-8

Glass G, McGaw B, Lee Smith M 1980 Meta-analysis in social research. Sage Publications, Beverly Hills

Glass G, Smith M 1979 Meta-analysis of research on class size and achievement. Educational Evaluation and Policy Analysis 1:2-16

Glass G, Cahen L, Smith M et al 1982 School class size: Research and policy. Sage Publications, Beverley Hills

Hammersley M 1990 Classroom ethnography: Empirical and methodological essays. Open University Press, Milton Keynes

Hammersley M 1999 Researching school experience: Ethnographic studies of teaching and learning. Falmer Press, London

Hammersley M, Atkinson P 1995 Ethnography: principles in practice. Routledge, London

Hedges L 1992 Meta-analysis. Journal of Educational Statistics 17(4):279-296

Hobsbaum A, Peters, S, Sylva K 1996 Scaffolding in reading recovery. Oxford Review of Education 22(1):17-36

Hollis V 1991 Self-directed learning as a post-basic educational continuum. British Journal of Occupational Therapy 54(2):45-48

Illsley R 1980 Professional or public health? Sociology in health and medicine. The Nuffield Provincial Hospitals Trust, London

Jacobs T, Lyons S 1992 Give me a fish and I eat today: teach me to fish and I eat for a lifetime. Australian Occupational Therapy Journal 39(1):29-32

Kendrick T, Freeling P 1993 A communication skills course for pre-clinical students: Evaluation of general practice-based teaching and group methods. Medical Education 27(3):211-217

Kimmel A 1988 Ethics and values in applied social research. Sage Publications, Beverley Hills

Knowles M 1990 The adult learner: A neglected species. Gulf Publishing Company, Houston

Kulik J, Kulik C 1989 Meta-analysis in education. International Journal of Educational Research 13(3):220

Lindeman E 1926 The meaning of adult education. New Republic, New York

Martin E 1997 Conditions that facilitate the school restructuring process. Paper presented at the Southern Educational Research Association Meetings, Austin, Texas, January 1997

Mehan H 1977 Learning Lessons. Harvard University Press, Cambridge Mass

Mehan H, Villanueva I, Hubbard L et al 1996 Constructing school success. Cambridge University Press, Cambridge

Morton S 1999 Systematic reviews and meta-analysis, workshop materials on evidence-based health care, extended studies and public programs, University of California, San Diego, La Jolla, California

Neufeld V, Norman G, Feightner J et al 1981 Clinical problem-solving by medical students: a cross-sectional and longitudinal analysis. Medical Education 15:26-32

Neufeld V, Chong J 1984 Problem-based professional education in medicine. In: Goodlad S (ed) Education for the Professions. The Society for Research into Higher Education.

Neufeld V 1985 Education for capability: an example of curriculum change from medical education. Journal for Education and Training Technology 21(4):262-267

Newman D, Griffin P, Cole M 1989 The construction zone-working for cognitive change in school. Cambridge University Press, Cambridge

Norman G, Tugwell P, Feightner W et al 1985 Knowledge and clinical problem-solving. Medical Education 19(5):344-356

Norman G, Schmidt H, Patel V 1990 Clinical inquiry and scientific inquiry. Medical Education 24:396-399

Norman G, Schmidt H 1992 The psychological basis of problem-based learning; a review of the evidence. Academic Medicine 67(9):557-565

Patel V, Groen J, Norman G 1991 Effects of conventional and problem-based medical curricula on problem solving. Academic Medicine 66(7):38-389

Piaget J 1926 The language and thought of the child. London

Piaget J 1952 The origin of intelligence in the child. London

Piaget J 1964 The early growth of logic in the child. London

Piaget J 1970 Science of education and the psychology of the child. Viking, New York

Piaget J 1977 The development of thought: equilibration of cognitive structures. Oxford University Press, Oxford

Polgar S, Thomas S 2000 Introduction to Research in the Health Sciences. Edinburgh, Churchill Livingstone

Premi J 1988 Problem-based, self-directed continuing medical education in a group of practising family physicians. Journal of Medical Education 63:484-486

Rogoff B 1990 Apprenticeship in thinking – cognitive developments in social context. Oxford University Press, Oxford and New York

Rosenshine N, Meister C 1991 Reciprocal teaching: A review of nineteen empirical studies. Paper presented at the Annual Meeting of the American Educational Research Association, Chicago, April 7, 1991

Rosenthal R 1995 Interpreting and evaluating meta-analysis. Evaluation and the Health Professions 18(4):393-407

Schofield T 1998 Teaching and small groups. Lecture notes, module C2, certificate in evidence-based health care, Department for Continuing Education, University of Oxford

Schmidt H 1983 Problem-based learning: rationale and description. Medical Education 17:11-16

Schmidt H 1993 Foundations of problem-based learning: some explanatory notes. Medical Education 27:422-432

Shin J, Haynes R, Johnston M 1993 Effect of problem-based, self-directed undergraduate education on lifelong learning. Canadian Medical Association Journal 148(6):969-976

Smith M, Glass G and Miller 1980 Meta-analysis of research on class size and its relationship to attitudes and instruction. American Educational Research Journal 17:419-433

Spindler D (ed) 1982 Doing the ethnography of schooling. Rinehart and Winston, New York

Tharp R, Gallimore R 1988 Rousing minds to life. Cambridge University Press, Cambridge

Tharp R, Gallimore R 1991 A theory of teaching in assisted performance. In: Light P, Sheldon S, Woodhead M (eds) Learning to think. Routledge/Open University, London and New York

Titchen A 1985 Innovative continuing education: an in-service model. Physiotherapy 71(11):464-467

Titchen A 1987a Design and implementation of a problem-based continuing education programme: a guide for clinical physiotherapists. Physiotherapy, 73(7):318-323

Titchen A 1987b Problem-based learning: the rationale for a new approach to physiotherapy continuing education. Physiotherapy 73(7):324-327

Titchen A 1992 Problem-based distance learning for health professionals. Physiotherapy (78)4:257-262

Vernon D, Blake R, 1993 Does problem-based learning work? A meta-analysis of evaluative research. Academic Medicine 68(7):550-563

Veatch R 1989 Medical Ethics. Jones and Bartlett, London

Verma D, Shannon H, Muir D et al 1988 Multidisciplinary, problem-based, self-directed training in occupational health. Journal of Social and Occupational Health 38:101-104

Vygotsky L 1978 Mind in society: The development of higher psychological process. edited by Cole M, John-Steiner V, Scribner S, Souberman E. Harvard University Press, Cambridge, Mass

Vygotsky L 1986 Thought and language. Mass. MIT Press, London and Cambridge

Walford G (ed) 2001 Ethnography and education policy. JAI, Amsterdam, London

Weiss B 1982 Confidentiality expectations of patients, physicians, and medical students. Journal of the American Medical Association 247(19):2695-2697

Wood D 1991 Aspects of teaching and learning. In: Light P, Sheldon S, Woodhead M (eds) Learning to Think. Routledge/Open University, London and New York

Wood D, Wood H 1996 Vygotsky, tutoring and learning. Oxford Review of Education 22(1):5-16

Woodward C, Fernier B, Cohen M, Goldsmith C 1990 Comparisons of the practice patterns of general practitioners and family physicians graduating from McMaster and Ontario Medical Schools. Teaching and Learning 2:79-88

Chapter 20

Life, the universe and everything
Martin Dawes

This book was written to accompany the Master's course in Evidence-Based Health Care (EBHC) run at the University of Oxford. The tutors were continually trying to find texts that would not only illustrate the concepts of EBHC, but also provide working examples of real-life situations found in all areas of the health service. Students on the course were predominantly from the UK, although we are now getting many more from abroad. This has meant that we have been studying UK-health care delivery situations that are very different from some other countries. However, we believe the concepts remain the same.

The book was never meant to be a stand alone 'how-to-do it' text. In fact it is almost impossible to learn how to search effectively and appraise efficiently without the help of others. Therefore, I would recommend that, as well as having read through the book, you attend one of the many courses now available on searching and appraisal.

The fun of evidence-based practice is the discovery of knowledge. The hard part is the implementation of that knowledge. Both are more enjoyable if the task is shared with others. Working in groups (problem based-learning) is the method we use to teach on the Master's programme. The students come from all backgrounds of the health service, including management and pharmaceutical companies. They have repeatedly told us how much benefit they gain from listening to the views of other students who have differing perspectives on the delivery of care. The implementation of an evidence-based approach to health care requires an acceptance of the worth of the other health professionals working within your team. Their view(s) of the outcome measures you may propose may not be the same as yours. Listening to them will help both in the design of the question as well as the implementation of that evidence.

Share the task of searching and appraising with others. Once you start questioning your practice you will soon find yourself with too many questions to answer and no time to answer them. Use the secondary publications like ACP Journal Club, Evidence-Based Medicine and Bandolier. Strangely enough, the number of secondary appraised sources has increased very little since the 1st edition of this book was written. What I wrote then was: 'I have a section of my computer with references that I have found that are relevant to my practice. These contain information about local conditions as well as generalisable information about clinical conditions. These include likelihood ratios, and NNTs. However, this system is likely to be superseded very soon by commercially available text and computer-based systems that allow you to have a store of for example NNTs. These systems are likely to become available through clinical management systems. What then becomes evident to a few can become widely available.' That prediction has largely come true for therapy but not for diagnosis. Two major additional sources are: Clinical Evidence (is a very useful source if one is looking for therapy), and Inforetriever (a source for handheld computers). What is disappointing is the lack of diagnostic resources. Having illustrated the need for sensitivity, specificity and likelihood ratios for every test we do to be available, there is no one source that has put these together.

Once you have spent time searching, appraising and implementing, it is difficult seeing that information and knowledge disappear under the mountain of new information that arrives on your desk everyday. The advent of computers heralded a new opportunity for information management. Initially their small memory made us structure the information very carefully making it easy to find again. Paradoxically, the rapid increase in the virtual size of computers with the associated wide availability has made them now, in many cases, act like rubbish sacks. It is so easy to think of all medical knowledge to be at your fingertips on a computer but now there are other barriers in your way. To make it easy there are pieces of software that can help. Some of these are available from the Web (http://www.gpfaqs.com).

The concepts of evidence-based health care will still have to be delivered. There will be little point in having all the likelihood ratios for clinical signs and symptoms if the clinicians are not able to understand them. That is putting the horse before the cart. There is no point in having a system with all the information on it if we are not going to ask questions about our practice. This remains the crux of all evidence-based practice.

We must continually seek knowledge. We must seek to confirm that what we are doing is backed up by evidence. That means a commitment to continual questioning of what we do. Evidence-based practice is not a current fashion. It is the means to enable you to be an efficient and competent health professional for the rest of your clinical career.

Index

D

Q

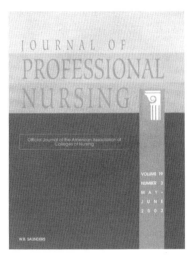